Praise for *Herbal Allies*

"Robert Rogers's herbal journey is inspired by a lifetime of working with and listening to wild plants. In *Herbal Allies*, Rogers shares his deep knowledge and experience. His body of knowledge is expansive and thoughtful in all aspects of plant medicine. A must-have for anyone interested in the medicinal and traditional indigenous use of wild boreal plants! I love how the book is organized by the Cree moon calendar with many stories and legends shared with Rogers by Cree elders."

—BEVERLEY GRAY, herbalist and author of *The Boreal Herbal: Wild Food and Medicine Plants of the North*, and *A Field Guide to Medicinal Plants of Canada*

"Part memoir, part herbal, *Herbal Allies* will entertain you with stories while divulging interesting herbal information you won't see anywhere else. Brew up a cup of tea and sink into this delightful book written by a distinguished herbal elder."

—ROSALEE DE LA FORÊT, RH (AHG), author of *Alchemy of Herbs*

"In *Herbal Allies*, Robert Rogers shares with us knowledge that only many years of patience, observation, and right of honor can bring. His extensive plant knowledge mirrors his deeply spiritual connection to the medicines and natural cycles of this land. *Herbal Allies* is a perfect balance between the spiritual, energetic, and technical aspects of plant medicine."

—TIFFANY FREEMAN, RH (AHG), registered acupuncturist, and Traditional Chinese Medicine doctor

"*Herbal Allies* is truly a unique offering. It provides a rare and personal orientation to the living tradition of herbal-nature wisdom, along with a precious compendium for practicing herbalists. The essence that also comes through these pages is the great importance of relationship, not only our relationship to plants but to each other and to our diverse global traditions of healing. This book will serve many generations of budding herbalists to come."

—CHAD CORNELL, master herbalist, Hollow Reed Holistic

TITLES BY ROBERT ROGERS

available from North Atlantic Books

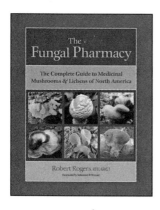

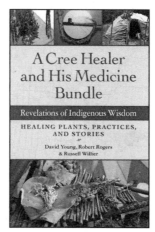

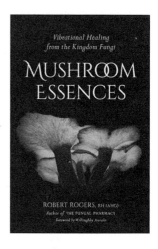

The Fungal Pharmacy
978-1-55643-953-7

Cree Healer and His Medicine Bundle
978-1-58394-903-0

Mushroom Essences
978-1-62317-045-5

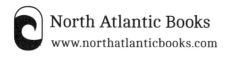

North Atlantic Books
www.northatlanticbooks.com

North Atlantic Books is an independent, nonprofit publisher committed to a bold exploration of the relationships between mind, body, spirit, and nature.

HERBAL ALLIES

My Journey with Plant Medicine

ROBERT ROGERS, RH (AHG)

Foreword by *Matthew Wood, RH (AHG)*

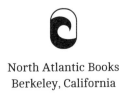

North Atlantic Books
Berkeley, California

Published by   Cover art © iStock: Photo_Hunt
North Atlantic Books   Cover design by Howie Severson
Berkeley, California   Interior design by Happenstance Type-O-Rama

Printed in the United States of America

Herbal Allies: My Journey with Plant Medicine is sponsored and published by the Society for the Study of Native Arts and Sciences (dba North Atlantic Books), an educational nonprofit based in Berkeley, California, that collaborates with partners to develop cross-cultural perspectives, nurture holistic views of art, science, the humanities, and healing, and seed personal and global transformation by publishing work on the relationship of body, spirit, and nature.

North Atlantic Books' publications are available through most bookstores. For further information, visit our website at www.northatlanticbooks.com or call 800-733-3000.

MEDICAL DISCLAIMER: The following information is intended for general information purposes only. Individuals should always see their health care provider before administering any suggestions made in this book. Any application of the material set forth in the following pages is at the reader's discretion and is his or her sole responsibility.

Library of Congress Cataloging-in-Publication Data

Names: Rogers, Robert Dale, 1950– author.
Title: Herbal allies : my journey with plant medicine / Robert Dale Rogers, RH (AHG).
Description: Berkeley, California : North Atlantic Books, 2017.
Identifiers: LCCN 2016043560 (print) | LCCN 2016046262 (ebook) | ISBN 9781623171391 (print) | ISBN 9781623171407 (ebook)
Subjects: LCSH: Rogers, Robert Dale, 1950– | Indian healers—Alberta—Biography. | Herbalists—Alberta—Biography. | Cree Indians—Alberta—Biography. | Herbs—Therapeutic use—Alberta. | Medicinal plants—Alberta. | Cree Indians—Medicine. | Indians of North America—Medicine—Alberta.
Classification: LCC E99.C88 R64 2017 (print) | LCC E99.C88 (ebook) | DDC 971.2004/97323092 [B]—dc23
LC record available at https://lccn.loc.gov/2016043560

1 2 3 4 5 6 7 8 9 SHERIDAN 22 21 20 19 18 17

Printed on recycled paper

North Atlantic Books is committed to the protection of our environment. We partner with FSC-certified printers using soy-based inks and print on recycled paper whenever possible.

Acknowledgments

THIS VOLUME IS DEDICATED TO LAURIE, the beloved soul mate in my life. You have helped make our ongoing journey joyful, precious, and fulfilling.

I would also like to dedicate this book to First Nations healers and their ongoing commitment to the health and well-being of their people.

I dedicate this book to my herbal teachers, past and present. Special mention goes to Norma Meyers, Bernard Jensen, John Christopher, Rose Auger, Michael Moore, William A. Mitchell, Robert Pearman, Mors Kochanski, Russell Willier, James Green, Kahlee Keane (Root Woman), and other early mentors.

I would also like to thank my contemporary herbal companions, including Matthew Wood, Stephen Buhner, David Winston, Terry Willard, David Hoffmann, Rosemary Gladstar, Jim McDonald, Sean Donahue, Guido Massé, 7Song, Margi Flint, Mindy Green, Thomas Easley, James Christian, Chad Cornell, Todd Caldecott, Abrah Arneson, Christopher Hobbs, Anna Rósa Róbertsdóttir, Bev Gray, Tieraona Low Dog, Donald Yance, Francis Brinker, Claudia Keel, Rosalee de la Foret, Chanchal Cabrera, Mark Blumenthal, Kris Hill, Darcy Williamson, Frans Vermeulen, David LaLuzerne, and professional members of the American Herbalist Guild. You have been my supportive community for the past many years and I am very thankful.

Special thanks to my students, past and present, from Prairie Deva College, Grant MacEwan University, and the Northern Star College of Mystical Studies.

You have enriched my life in so many ways. I am truly grateful.

Special thanks to Doug Reil, for believing in this project.

Contents

Foreword

WOW! AN EXCITING BOOK: an amazing autobiographical experience, lived on the northern frontier of the settled world, mixed together with a lifetime of herbal lore learned directly from the woods, backwoods neighbors, medicine men and women, scientific papers, and direct clinical experience. Although herbal lore may be thought too technical for the nonherbalist, in places, the adventure of discovering and putting these plants into use, related by the author, gifts us with an exciting onrushing narrative that instead is hard to put down. Into this are inserted the life lessons of the herbalist himself.

If you have never met an herbalist, you are in for a treat. In order to follow this calling a person has to be unique, unconventional, daring, willing to learn all the time, and quite bright, if not brilliant. If ever there was a group in the midst of our modern world that was not composed of muggles and house elves, it would be herbalists. For most of them this is a spiritual calling, not just a way to make money. Actually, it is not a very good way to make money at all. As one Appalachian herbalist said to me, "I didn't want to be an herbalist, because all the ones I knew lived in shacks." And indeed, Robert begins his journey in a shack.

Not only is there no money in the matter, at least for the beginner, in the 1970s, when our autobiographer began his journey, herbalism was quasi-illegal. All of us, back then, looked behind our backs, as well as forward, to practice. I feared the Federal Drug Administration would arrest me every day for the first five years of my practice—not understanding that it was actually a matter for the state Board of Medical Practice until one of my friends received her cease-and-desist order. But by that time, whoever they were, they'd left the barn doors open, and there was stuff all over the fields. We fought back and we won. Then there were a few people that actually hated us. One herb store was burned to the ground in the 1970s. I worked at an inner city herb store; we were robbed at gunpoint. But I wouldn't trade it for anything, and neither would Robert Rogers.

Money, law, safety, and practicality aside, the calling won't let a person alone. The herbalist is driven for a lifetime. Not an easy life, but an entertaining one for sure. Not just for oneself, but for anyone lucky enough to hear an herbalist tell his or her stories. And now, Robert takes us on that trip with him, not only sharing his life adventures but his plant discoveries and allies.

I grew up in what Robert calls the "north," in comparison to his bio-region, which he rightly calls the "far north." So many of his plant allies are my friends and companions.

I remember them from hikes in the woods, plant-picking excursions on beautiful days in the crisp northern sun, afternoons in the herb shop, or clinical hours in my old office, farm house, or on the road. And so often, there I am again, out in the woods, walking a path of beauty and wonder, and getting paid for it. Robert shares that beauty and wonder as well as the knowledge of how to use those "far northern" herbs and how they were used by indigenous peoples—and understood by white-coated scientists as well. This is not just an autobiography, but a working herbal.

But the herbalist is not always or necessarily an outsider, and Robert tells many stories about his work with academia, agriculture, and the medical profession in the far north. This is not a story about integrative medicine, but about cooperation between wildly different disciplines that meet with respect in the middle. I say "not integrative" because my experience of that movement in conventional (muggle) medicine is that it is just an attempt to commandeer products and knowledge from unconventional healers without incorporating them into the integrated system. And guess what? The herbs even started to make money for ordinary people. Robert helped launch a new crop worth millions of dollars for farmers in the far, far north—the famous *Rhodiola rosea* only grows in the cold north.

Herbalism is not just a bunch of medicinal substances that are poorly understood by modern biomedicine and need to be studied, sanitized of their origins, and moved into the sleek shining offices of modern health professionals—no shacks here. Herbalism is a whole system with its own understanding of how herbs work. This understanding is often empirical (experiential), historical and traditional (stories, stories, stories), and sensory (what does it taste like, smell like?). The herb is a slurry of medicinal substances that work together in a whole array, each one too weak to act on its own, but together in a natural plant vessel a powerful presentation of survival chemicals suited to environmental stresses—phytochemicals that have carried those plants through billions of years of "clinical trials" in the seething evolutionary iron kettle of Mother Nature. Can modern medicine boast of anything like that? The slurry of compounds work together to nudge the body in a certain direction—I like to call this nudge-opathy.

How do we learn about those hidden properties? It will not be through isolation of constituents, or clinical trials too simple to capture the nuances of whole plant medicines. It is through wood-lore—knowledge of the wilderness—such as Robert and his friends, indigenous and otherwise, learned through careful observation. It is through experience in the clinic, of which Robert has almost two decades. It took me fifteen years to learn how little I knew and how much I knew. After that, I finally felt like I knew what I was doing. The neat thing about medicinal plants is that there is always something more to learn. It is not like conventional medicine, which pretends to know it all as it leaves behind old information and gathers new every year, so that one decade in medicine barely resembles its predecessor.

The herbal constituent is not necessarily suited to a specific bonding site but to broad tissue functions and imbalances where tannins, demulcents, aromatic volatile oils, bitters, and relaxants work gently, mostly across the organism. But it takes skill to understand how herbs work, just as it takes skill to work with drugs. It is not a matter of forcing herbs into the conceptual universe of the modern medical world, but of learning to think as they think, in natural patterns of hot and cold, damp and dry, tense and relaxed, excess and deficiency, fast and slow, yin and yang. The medicinal substances of herbs are their own alphabet, independent of the biomedical ABCs.

The best way to learn about herbs is through stories, and that makes this book one of the best available for learning about these herbs, because it is full of stories, though not neglecting modern science. When we read a story, we remember it, and that is how the best teachers instruct. It is close to effortless. So, my friends, learn from one of the best teachers in the field and enjoy your read, as I have.

Matthew Wood
Martell, Wisconsin

Introduction

Where is the wisdom we have lost in knowledge?
Where is the knowledge we have lost in information?
—T. S. ELIOT

I HAVE LONG CONSIDERED completing this project. Over the years I collected an overflowing library of hundreds of herbal books for my home office and assembled another complete herbal library at our college. Some are truly excellent, and I really cherish the works of Stephen Buhner, Matthew Wood, Michael Moore, Peter Holmes, David Winston, Nancy Turner, Darcy Williamson, and numerous other great herbal allies and professional members of the American Herbalist Guild. These books are very special to me.

Most of the herb books written by various PhDs, pharmacists, and biochemists were disappointing and disappeared from my shelves long ago. The reason is simple: many herbal books on the market repeat the same findings and mistakes over and over. The writings are seldom based on actual field or clinical experience with medicinal plants.

In fact, during my early explorations into plants of the boreal forest in the early 1970s, there were very few books on medicinal plants. Most books were authored in England, and irrelevant to northern Canada, or totally useless, without mention of the plant part, preparation, dosage, or even the correct Latin binomial. The first book that spoke to me was the *School of Natural Healing* by John Christopher, published in 1976. It still sits in my library.

I admit to having a bit of a split personality, with one foot in the wilds of the boreal forest and another as assistant clinical professor in family medicine at the university. My wife did me the great honor many years ago of writing a fictional story for children about ecology, the environment, and listening to your inner self. She made two of the main characters Mr. Fun Guy, a guitar playing, fun-loving hippie living in a log cabin in the forest, and Dr. Bo Tanic, a professor doing research at the university. They were best of friends and had numerous herbal adventures. The book is called *The Path of the Devas* (Szott-Rogers, 2004).

This bias will show in my writing. But this is how I learned and connected with my herbal allies. I took in, over the past forty years, various teachings on regional plants by traditional First Nation healers in my part of the world and then investigated their plant constituents. I would look into the world of organic chemistry and surmise other potential uses for my new herbal allies. I marveled at the potential synergy between different plants and how an herbalist can increase efficacy by putting several plants together in a formula.

Today I am increasingly occupied with the potential of herbal medicine to treat drug-resistant bacterial, viral, and fungal infections. By increasing the efficacy of some older class of antibiotics with herbal medicine, the ability to inhibit MRSA (methicillin-resistant *Staphylococcus aureus*) and other newly developed pathogens is increased twofold, tenfold, and sometimes six-hundredfold. I am also intrigued by the ability of plant and mushroom medicines to increase natural killer cells or induce apoptosis (programmed cell death) in various cancer cell lines.

I was given the opportunity and privilege of working with tens of thousands of clients over an eighteen-year period in clinical practice. I was able to assist many individuals with severe and chronic health conditions, which were very difficult, or impossible, to treat with drugs or surgery.

Many years ago, I picked up a love of photography. I don't believe my skills with a camera have gotten much better, but the quality of modern digital photography has enhanced my own personal enjoyment. Plant pictures are an important element of this book, as so often herbal books have no photos or are of a size that makes identification very difficult.

I hope this small contribution will present to both the budding and experienced herbalist an opportunity to relook at our boreal plant allies with renewed possibilities.

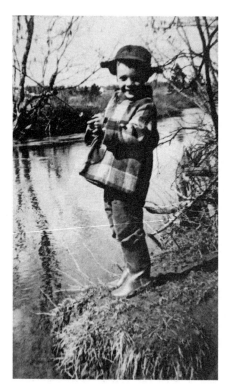

Robert fishing at age 6

1

Discovering My Herbal Allies

I WAS BORN IN CHARLOTTETOWN, Prince Edward Island, a small maritime province in eastern Canada. I nearly did not make it, as I was birthed with the umbilical cord wrapped around my neck. Astrologically, I am Aquarian with my moon in Cancer.

My early years were spent in Truro and Halifax, Nova Scotia. In the mid-1950s, my uncle came back to Canada after serving in the Korean War. He arrived and stayed at our home, suffering from tuberculosis. Being susceptible to respiratory conditions, I was quickly infected and aggressively treated with massive doses of antibiotics. I remember vividly awaking one night with my entire body covered in large red hives that burned like fire. I was six years old at the time.

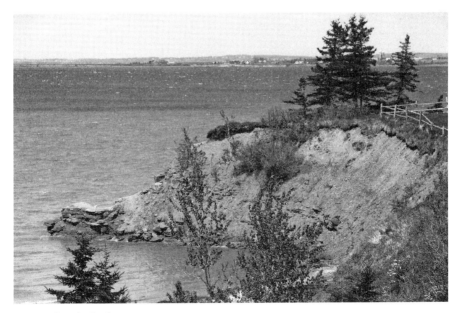

Prince Edward Island

That summer I began to collect glass canning jars from my mother's kitchen and scrounging others from neighbors. I carefully filled these with water from our rain barrel and then filled each jar with different-colored flowers from our yard and surrounding areas. I carefully placed these on top of large amethyst stones in full sun. At night I would cover and place them under the porch, and the next day they would go back into the sun. I began to drink the waters, choosing orange-colored water one day, or yellow or blue water the next. These were my first herbal allies. Only much later in life, in the early 1970s, when I was introduced to the flower essences developed by Edward Bach, did I understand how my inner guides were assisting my healing process.

I have always loved plants and nature. At age nine, I found, under our balsam fir Christmas tree, a microscope. This was so exciting! Everything I could find went under the scope and helped me enter this previously hidden world. Today, my digital microscope takes high-resolution pictures with great detail and preserves them on my computer.

I was never a great student, as it was all too easy. I always had top marks in the class, as this was the expectation of my parents. But my respiratory health was not good. When I was ten years old, I was walking through the aisles of our local library when a small pamphlet-sized book fell on the floor in front of me. Curious, I picked it up. It was titled *Arnold Ehret's Mucusless Diet*. I took it home.

Arnold claimed mucus-forming foods, especially anything white like sugar, dairy, and flour, were disease-producing. He was a great exponent of fasting and did several fasts of twenty-one days, twenty-four days, thirty-six days, and finally forty-nine days. Both his father and brother died of tuberculosis, which held great meaning for me. It is rumored he traveled to the Mediterranean island of Capri with Paul Bragg, of health product fame. Arnold believed a fruitarian diet was ideal. Having long suffered allergies, hay fever, and asthma, I asked my mother if I could eat differently than the rest of family for a while. In two weeks my health was greatly improved, and in six weeks I no longer had need for medications or an inhaler.

My mother was of German Protestant background, from the south shore of Nova Scotia. When I was young, only ten years after the end of World War II, I was told everyone in the region was of Dutch ancestry. Her grandfather, Delbert Webber, was the local blacksmith. Today, in Chester Basin, Nova Scotia, there is a small memorial in the central square honoring Del Webber. He suffered asthma as well, probably due to the coal smoke associated with his profession.

I joined Cubs when young, and then Scouts, and received my Queen's Scout badge, equivalent to an Eagle Scout in the United States, at fourteen years of age. We had moved from Saint John, New Brunswick, to Calgary, Alberta, during my last months of grade nine. My father used to take me for walks, collecting spring fiddleheads and dandelion greens. I learned from him how to appreciate these wild herbal allies in my diet. Years later, in the 1970s, I discovered fiddleheads in northern Alberta and created a company called Fiddlehead Farms. The first year, my partner and I harvested six hundred pounds for a city food chain.

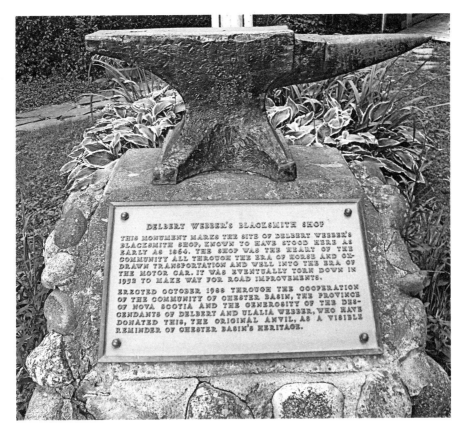

Memorial to Delbert Webber

I loved camping, even winter camping, and all living things in the forest. Grant Mac-Ewan presented to me the award of Queen's Scout during a ceremony at the Southern Alberta Jubilee Auditorium. Forty years later, I taught herbal medicine at the university named in his honor.

Cubs and Scouts were good for me. The family move to Calgary was good in many ways. The clear skies and sunny weather were a welcome relief from the damp and foggy coast of New Brunswick. Away from the fog, pulp and paper mill, and oil refinery, my respiratory system gained much relief. And then came high school and girls. My favorite teacher taught biology, and I loved the subject.

I entered the University of Alberta in 1968 with the intention of gaining a Bachelor of Science degree, leading to medicine. After two years I began to realize I would be a very poor biomedical doctor, as I was somewhat faint at the sight of blood and not a big fan of pharmaceuticals. I worked at the University newspaper, *The Gateway*, during my years on campus. I struggled to find my journalistic style, a trait that has followed me all these years. I finished my science degree in botany, and during those last two summers, volunteered in the Alberta Service Corps, somewhat similar to the Peace Corps. The last summer, living in the city, I took the opportunity to visit the downtown library and scour the herb section. It consisted mainly of English herbal books, but I set up my own card filing system, listing conditions.

The Alberta Service Corps led to friendships, resulting in seven of us buying 160 acres of land and a house near Joussard, on the south shore of Lesser Slave Lake, Alberta, in early 1973. It was quickly named Hippie Hill by the local residents. Having been raised in cities all my life, this was an exciting new venture. Building a log cabin, growing a garden, wild-crafting herbs, milking a goat, making cheese from the milk, raising rabbits and bees, owning and riding my first horse was all new and exciting. I experimented with wind power and solar ovens, built a root cellar, and generally learned valuable survival skills.

My first painful introduction to devil's club, an important member of the ginseng family, happened in the hills south of my cabin. An herbal ally indeed, but a painful reminder of the power of plants. I barely grazed a stem and a few spines touched the pad of my left hand under my small finger. Forty years later, that same area has thickened scar tissue.

The town of Joussard was a small fishing village, largely of francophone heritage, and full of interesting and amazing people. One day I met Jean Chancelet, who was in his late eighties at the time. He traveled from France at an early age to Montreal, then took a train to Edmonton, a wagon train to Athabasca, and a steam barge on Lesser Slave Lake. He built a log home on the lakeshore and lived there most of his life. He took kindly to this young naive hippie, shared his twelve-year-old black currant wine, and told me "You know nothing," which was true.

He lived right on the lake and had an amazing garden. He introduced me to the use of Dr. Schuessler cell salts, which I use to this day and have suggested their benefits to many clients and students over the years. This was in the days before the Internet. A book company, Health Research, out of Mokelumne, California, took out-of-print books and made photocopies, or Gestetner copies. I still retain in my library a copy containing *Biochemic Pathology of Disease* and *The Twelve Cell Salts of the Zodiac* by George Carey. The modern practitioner may find a newer book, with great color photos by David R. Card (2005), a good investment on the topic.

Jean grew half an acre of white, red, and black currant bushes. He taught me how to clip the top leaves of first-year raspberry canes to double fruit production the next year. Each winter I would watch him grow weaker, and in the spring he would eat his own fresh asparagus and dandelion buds with home-produced apple cider vinegar, and a spring came back to his step. Two more herbal allies I value to this day.

One summer I decided to go on a four-week water fast. I had no idea what I was doing but had read about fasting, trusted Arnold Ehret's opinions, and thought it was a good idea.

The first four days were pretty rough, but soon after, things smoothed out, and I found I could do some basic gardening, haul water, and such. It was day twenty and a hot, sunny afternoon. I was wearing a white T-shirt and as I went to my outdoor shower (a bucket painted black and hung on the south side of the house with a hose), I took off my shirt. As it pulled over my face I had a flash of memory. I was eight years old and sitting alone on a wooden bench in a long dark-green hallway. It was the doctor's office where I got my allergy shots. I remember thinking, how strange, and then I turned the shirt around and saw two yellow-orange spots on the back, right where the kidneys sit. I smelled the spots, which were phenolic and acrid. I stopped my fast the next day.

I opened a health food store in Joussard in 1977, called the Bodhi Shop. It was mainly whole foods sold in bulk. It did not last long, mainly due to personal distractions like marriage, divorce, and my house burning down. Sort of what would be expected during a Saturn Return phase of life when you are not paying close attention.

To the east of Hippie Hill was Driftpile Reserve, where resided the Cree healer Rose Auger. I relate some of my adventures with her in the chapter on wild sarsaparilla. Barbara Tedlock (2005, 269) wrote, "Recently women's prophecies have taken on a new ecumenism with feminist overtones. Brooke Medicine Eagle, an intertribal healer who trained with a Cheyenne woman shaman, insists that a return to women's traditions is necessary for balance, growth, and healing."

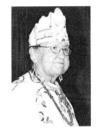

Rose Auger

Rose Auger, a Woodland Cree prophet, agrees. At a 1995 international meeting of elders, she demonstrated the power of feminine spirituality. During the council, one of her spider guardians, who always accompanies her to listen and help, hopped onto the lap of a young holy man, who began to tremble. As he reached out to swat the spider—an unthinkably brutal act—an elder sitting next to him gently picked the creature up and handed it back to Rose. She smiled and prophesied that during the final days of the earth's forthcoming purification, Spider will return to correct what has gone wrong with the younger generation.

Rose made herself available to anyone needing help. "We have to get back to our traditional life, because then you become whole, you're happy, you're at peace. You can put in a garden, you can pick your own medicines, your own natural foods. There is so much you can do for yourself which keeps you healthy" (Meili 1991).

To the west of my little log cabin was Sucker Creek Reserve, the home of noted indigenous activist and author Harold Cardinal. I soon ran into Russell Willier, who had recently begun healing work with herbal medicine on the reserve and elsewhere. He struggled with this burden, like many, as he received support from some people in his community but was demeaned by those who were either jealous or did not understand. There were many residents on the reserve who believed medicine-making is inherited (in his case, it was), as Russell had had passed down to him a tenth-generation medicine bundle. We would see each other here and there, but I really never sought out the opportunity to study with him.

Some of my early herbal allies in the mid-1970s were Norma Myers, Bernard Jensen, John Christopher, and local indigenous healers such as Rose Auger. Norma was a wonderful person and a great herbalist who started Green Vale Herbal College. One summer in the mid-1970s I hitchhiked from northern Alberta to Vancouver Island on my way to

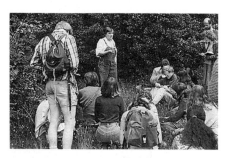

her summer herb gathering at Alert Bay. I met James Green, author of *The Herbal Medicine-Maker's Handbook*, for the first time at this gathering, and he introduced me to the Bach flower remedies.

I was standing by the road just north of Nanaimo with my thumb out when a newer-model Volvo stopped and picked me up. It was Nancy Turner, the famous ethnobotanist, and her husband Robert who drove me to the north end of the

Norma Myers (courtesy of Don Ollsin)

island to catch the next ferry. Only years later did I realize who she was and her life's work with west coast First Nations healers. Forty years later, she generously wrote some kind words for the back cover of *A Cree Healer and His Medicine Bundle*, cowritten with Russell Willier and David Young.

Many years later I was a guest lecturer for a medical anthropology course taught by David at the University of Alberta. I introduced a film and shared my adventures with Eduardo Calderón, a shaman who lived near Trujillo, Peru, where I studied herbal allies from 1982 to 1984. Eduardo was an amazing healer. I would visit his small concrete home where he lived with his wife and eight children. It was important to buy some cold *cerveza*

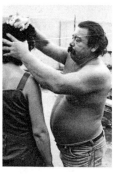

to share, which I did as often as possible. We laughed together a lot, even though my Spanish was terrible.

He diagnosed patients using *cuye*, or guinea pig. The small animal would be rubbed all over the body, making sure all the organ systems and meridians were energetically activated. Eduardo, also known as the Wizard of the Four Winds, would then kill the rodent and examine the internal organs to determine the source of the illness. That part was removed. The animal was then dressed up, and later eaten for dinner.

One of his favorite herbal allies for séance and spiritual journeys was the mescaline-rich San Pedro cactus (*Echinopsis*

Eduardo Calderón
(courtesy of Jeff Salz)

pachanoi*) of the northern coastal region of Peru. The cactus has been used for at least three millennia by healers of Peru,

Ecuador, and Bolivia. It is easily purchased at local markets and is legal to grow in North America. This cactus contains up to 4.7 percent mescaline by dry weight. This was sometimes combined with other plant allies to create an entheogenic brew, known in Quechua as *achuma*. Eduardo paid particular attention to the phases of the moon. Tuesday and Friday were his favored evenings for healing ceremonies.

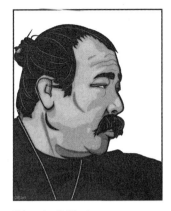

Eduardo Calderón

"Eduardo opened his séances by picking up his deer hoof, which symbolized curiosity, swiftness, and elusiveness, and held it out to detect and exorcise attacking spirits. As he put it, 'the altar is nothing more than a control panel by which one is able to calibrate the infinity of accesses into each person'" (Tedlock 2005, 166).

There are several books and films on his life. *The Seer and the Blind Man* is one such film. A manuscript of the film, *Eduardo the Healer* (1978), was translated into English, and published by North Atlantic Books in 1982, the same period of time I spent with him.

One of my favorite memories of my time in Peru was traveling to Machu Picchu. It was the spring equinox and I snuck in and camped out on the site in my sleeping bag. I awoke in the morning to the sight of a giant condor drifting high above me. It was revelatory.

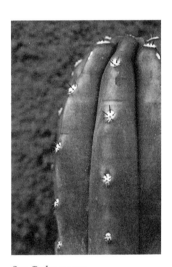

San Pedro cactus

In the fall of 1984, I moved back to Edmonton. My father had suddenly passed away, and my mother was living by herself. I found a small second-floor office near the High Level Food Co-op in Old Strathcona in Edmonton. I had previously worked at this cooperative from 1978 to 1980 as the store herbalist. I thought the city was ready for a full-time herbalist, but by December I had only a handful of clients and my meager funds were running low. I actually thought briefly about moving back to Joussard and my cabin in the woods. One day, a reporter from the *Edmonton Journal* newspaper phoned and asked if she could interview me for a story on iridology. I had studied the art and science of iris diagnosis with Bernard Jensen in the early 1970s and found it a valuable addition to my herbal practice. It was a day or two after Christmas when the full-color story came out, including interviews with some of my few, yet satisfied, initial clients.

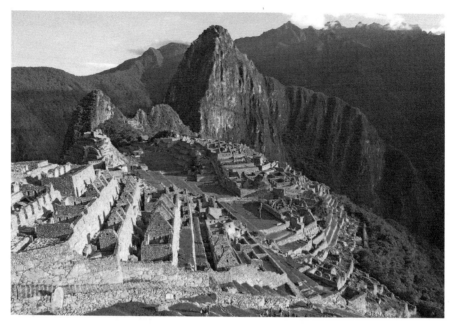

Machu Picchu

Operating at a barebones level, I checked my telephone message machine the next morning, and there were seventy-two calls. The next day, a further thirty-five messages were waiting, and I was booked solid for the next three months. Things began to look up. My herbal allies had intervened on my behalf.

From 1984 to 2002 I helped educate tens of thousands of people on the benefits of herbal medicine and learned an enormous amount myself. I began to intensively study and work with the plants and mushrooms of the boreal forest. This special part of the world became my spiritual temple and helped me reconnect, through my plant allies, with my inner place of balance. For the next forty years, I compiled and recorded information from journals, books, and most importantly, from First Nations healers and other herbal allies. I read books by the Eclectic physicians and their insights and indications for indigenous herbs growing in my region.

I began to look at the chemistry of our local plants, and by studying some major constituents, began to think about their medicinal use in a different manner. If this defines me as an untraditional herbalist, then so be it. I believe it is true that writing down the names of several hundred constituents of a medicinal herb does not mean you know that plant, any more than the chemical constituents of a human allow you to understand their soul and personality. However, inquiry into these components led to the creation of some highly effective synergistic herbal combinations. Two or more herbs, together as allies, will increase their efficacy and medicinal benefit by several factors.

In the late 1980s, I traveled to Newfoundland to visit a friend. Her father was a seventy-five-year-old Irish Orangeman and medical doctor. He was unimpressed with this young hippie herbalist, but after sharing a few rounds of Irish Whisky and some banter and laughter, we developed a certain level of comfort. At one point he looked at me, and with his index finger summoned me closer. He asked if I would like to know the secret of helping people with health issues. I nodded affirmatively, and he said, "If you let people talk long enough, they will tell you what is wrong with them." I never forgot his advice, and it made all the difference to my clinical practice.

The herbal allies I met and spent time with and learned from over the decades are too numerous to name, but you know who you are. I thank you from the bottom of my heart. I am especially grateful to my clients, who over the years taught me more about plant medicine than I could ever learn from a book.

In 1990 I met the amazing Laurie Szott. She was a student in my medical anthropology class, talking about Eduardo. We instantly fell in love. She has made all the difference in my life, and has been a huge support for the past twenty-seven years. I love her immensely and my life would not be the same without her.

Now back to my connection with Cree healer, Russell Willier. His medicine name, Mehkwasskwan, translates as "Red Cloud." David Young and colleagues, including Stephen Aung, conducted a psoriasis project involving some of Russell's plant allies. It was filmed and led to a book, authored by David and others, called *Cry of the Eagle: Encounters with a Cree Healer* (Young, Grant, and Swartz 1989). The project treated ten people with psoriasis using local plants, prepared in the form of an ointment applied externally, combined with medicine-lodge sweats and prayer. The project was very successful, in my opinion, considering the poor outcomes for this condition using the biomedical model.

Willier taught me about herbal combinations. "You have to know your herbs in order to put the combination together. Once you get the combination, you pretty well have it for the rest of your life until you pass it over to somebody else. And the ones that have been lost, if the medicine man didn't pass them over to someone before he died, they can sometimes be given back by the spiritual world. For example, the spirits might give back a combination to someone by telling them about it in a dream" (Young, Grant, and Swartz 1989, 62). Nearly thirty years later, David, Russell, and I collaborated to write *A Cree Healer and His Medicine Bundle*. It reveals for the first time, of which I am aware, the contents of a tenth-generation medicine bundle.

One day in the mid-1980s I got a phone call from Robert, a psychologist and friend. He informed me that an herbalist in Red Deer, Alberta, had recently passed away, and his widow had a garage full of herbal tinctures. I immediately drove my powder-blue Volvo 122 down the highway and filled it to the brim with hundreds of quarts of tinctures. Some were quite rare, such as mother tincture of Nux Vomica and Rauwolfia. I asked her how much she would like as payment, and she said, "How about fifty dollars?" I reached in my pocket and gave her a hundred-dollar bill.

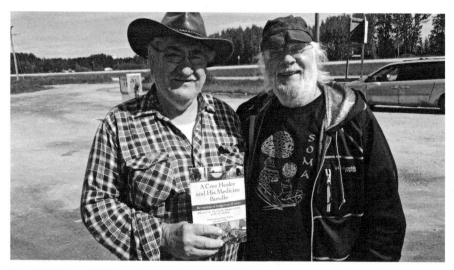

Russell Willier and Robert

I now had several hundred herbal allies and the beginnings of an apothecary. I could put together herbal formulas specifically for my clients and their conditions at the time. My practice at this point consisted of offering nutritional advice, herbal medicine, iridology, and flower essences. In the mid-1970s, while living in the north, I sent to Mount Vernon in England for a set of Bach Flower remedies. I remember the cost, twelve pounds for the entire set, and all forty came in small two-milliliter bottles with tiny curved glass droppers. Years later, my wife and I developed the Prairie Deva flower essences, mainly from herbal allies of the northern prairie and boreal forest. Today, at Northern Star College, we co-teach flower essences to a new generation of students.

In the fall of 1987 I traveled down to the Napa Valley for the first conference of the American Aromatherapy Association. All the big names were in attendance, including Robert Tisserand, Daniel Pénoël, Victoria Edwards, Kurt Schnaubelt, Julia Lawless, and if I remember correctly, Len and Shirley Price. It was a grand aromatic event, and nothing to sniff at, for sure.

Rae Dunphy, from Calgary, and I were the two lone Canucks. I shared a room with Robert Seidel from The Essential Oil Company. One evening, he asked me if I had ever smelled true Bulgarian Rose Otto. I replied that I probably had not, so he took out a small carrying case with hundreds of small vials. He took one, put a toothpick into it, and handed it to me. "Place this in your mouth, close your eyes, and wait." The sensation was like a rose explosion in my mouth and olfactory nerves. And to this day I have not been fooled by diluted nor adulterated rose oil.

I returned to Edmonton and decided to carry a small line of essential oils. One night, after a sip or two of single-malt scotch on the rocks, the name Scents of Wonder came to me. I met Laurie soon after, and this became the name of our small line of essential oils. We traveled to the south of France on our honeymoon and visited several farms growing plants and distilling various essential oils.

In the mid-1990s I was invited by the provincial government's Alberta Agriculture to a roundtable discussion on diversity. I suggested building a small portable steam distillation unit to explore native plants and their essential oils. In the first year after construction, volunteer members of the Alberta New Crops Network steam-distilled some seventy plants in the province, from spruce to yarrow, and several unusual choices like *Caragana* and calamus root. Later, I became chair of the newly named Alberta Natural Health Agricultural Network and pioneered, with the help of members, the introduction of *Rhodiola rosea* into the province.

I retired from clinical practice in 2002 after eighteen years. Almost immediately I began to teach an introductory herbal program at Grant MacEwan College, now MacEwan University, and did so for the next decade. Laurie and I taught a flower essence program to students enrolled in the successful Holistic Health Practitioner Program. We also taught at our Prairie Deva College, which morphed into the Northern Star College in 2005. When MacEwan College became a university, they only wanted to fund bachelor's degrees, and the program was, unfortunately, disbanded. This period of time helped me conduct further research and write about over six hundred medicinal herbal allies and medicinal mushrooms of the boreal forest. I have chosen, for this book, twenty herbal allies.

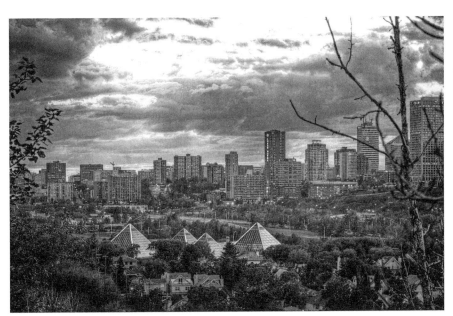

Edmonton

Today, in the river valleys of Edmonton, I continue to pick plant medicine for my own use. One of my favorite spots, just outside the city, is known in Cree as *maskêkosihk* trail, meaning "Land of the Medicines." I am most fortunate to live in a city with the largest urban parkland in North America.

These herbal allies represent the sequence of their collection for medicine, from spring to fall. In the far north we have but twenty weeks of plant growth, if that, and so I present them according to the lunar cycles of the northern Cree.

2

How to Use This Book

DUE TO THE FLOWING NATURE of content, this book will make more sense to the reader if enjoyed from the following perspective. As a student, clinician, and now herbal educator, I have been exposed to and have used a variety of learning and teaching methods over the years. The twenty individual plants examined in this book are presented according to Cree lunar cycles, following the seasons in the north from April through September. That is, from the last snowfall in spring to the first frost of fall. The journey with herbal allies involves plants and people as well as various stages of life. From the early emergence of plants in early spring to the formation of flowers and then seeds—this is the natural cycle of birth and death and rebirth.

Having lived nearly fifty years in northern Canada, I have seen snow fly in every month. It may not stay long on the ground from June to August, but I have been witness to snowfall under every lunar month. The plant sections follow a more-or-less similar pattern. I first share some of my personal experience with my herbal allies, either right at the outset or somewhere near the beginning. Briefly, in most cases, I explain the origin of common and binomial names of the plants. I then give a background into traditional use of the plant by various First Nations and indigenous peoples of Turtle Island (North America). These include common names, collection, and usage for food, clothing, survival skills, toolmaking, and health benefits.

I then wander into the medicinal use of these herbs by various peoples around the globe, with special attention on the nineteenth-century Eclectic physicians and Physio-Medicalists. These dedicated individuals contributed insights into an array of medical plants native to North America that were truly remarkable. Born a century earlier, I suspect my herbal path would have led me to the birthplace of this remarkable group in Cincinnati. In this city, you will find the famous Lloyd Library, which preserves hundreds of thousands of publications dedicated to plant medicine written by these remarkable medical practitioners.

At some point I wander into my own observations on plant use in herbal medicine, offering insights into various plant combinations I have found useful in clinical practice and for treating various health conditions. And then, my untraditional herbalist colors really begin to show, and I venture into the world of phytochemistry.

I don't believe you can understand plant medicine by looking at a list of organic chemicals, but I sometimes see picture patterns that excite me.

Some of my observations are speculative, and others are on a tangent and direction that may help lead other practitioners into newer insights, and possibly new patterns of synergy and potentially useful combinations. You will note lilac and bear root are little discussed in most herb books. I like to use plants bioregional in nature, whether indigenous or introduced. I include, when available, other insights into plants from the perspective of the homeopaths. When given at mother tincture dosage, the differences between herbal and homeopathic preparations and use begin to blur and blend. In one chapter I write about bees and the products they gather from plants for our health benefits. Many people call it bee pollen, but really, it is various flower pollens, gathered by bees.

I used a variety of gemmotherapy preparations when in clinical practice, mainly as drainage remedies. These extracts are prepared from fresh buds or plant shoot tissues, chopped and left to macerate in a blend of water, glycerin, and alcohol. After three weeks, this mixture is pressed and filtered. The remedies take advantage of the fresh embryonic plant tissue. I have been experimenting with ginkgo, linden, and sea buckthorn with some success. If various parts of the plants yield themselves to preparation as carrier oils, I include this information as well.

I am a true fan of fresh plant preparations, but for many plant parts containing up to 80 percent water, a twenty-four-hour wilt of the plant part will give a superior product, with less danger of contamination by mold. This is especially true of plant oils.

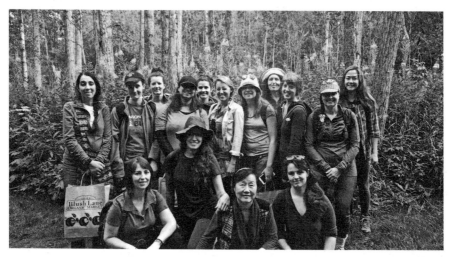

Field trip with students from Northern Star College

14

In the north, the sun method rarely works well for oil preparations from buds, flowers, or leaves. I have found the low-temperature setting on a crock pot ideal for this type of medicine-making. I enjoy steam distilling our native plants and include information on the health benefits of the essential oils and hydrosols in most sections.

I used essential oils and hydrosols in clinical practice with great success, using techniques learned from Daniel Pénoël and other aromatherapy-oriented medical doctors from France. I am extremely enthusiastic about the use of medical aromatherapy and teach its benefits to our students at our small college. The use of aromatograms to culture unknown pathogens and their reaction to essential oils was very helpful in a number of difficult-to-treat conditions.

Those alchemists interested in producing hydrosols from plants in their own region will find a microwave distiller (www.oilextech.com) a wonderful additional tool. After gathering the plant material, the hydrosol is produced in just six minutes. I have made wonderful hydrosols with this method, including wild mint, linden, and mock orange flowers.

About ten years ago I discovered the beautiful poetry of Sylvia Seroussi Chatroux, and where possible I have included her delightful take on the plants in this book. Thank you, Sylvia.

Plants are more than an assemblage of constituents, as mentioned above. I have therefore included observations on the personality traits and spiritual properties of the plants. Many of these insights may help us understand plants as living beings that speak to us in a language we can learn. Yes, I hug trees. I also listen to what they offer and feel comforted by what they communicate in their own unique manner. All plants have spirit. Not all people are attuned to communication with plants, but many healers have shared this special gift with all of us. Learning about plant spirit and personality can take a lifetime and is not easily shared in a single book. I have included, when possible, some insights into herbal allies from amazing people like Pam Montgomery, Laura Aversano, Dorothy Hall, and others. Thank you so much for your deep insights and for sharing them.

Healing with plants may involve plant and animal totems, the sharing of sweat lodges, ceremony, fasting, and various techniques of connection. All of these techniques have helped shape my plant view of the world. My wife, Laurie, and colleague Catherine Potter at Northern Star College have a deep interest in the world of astrology. I have therefore endeavored to include astrological insights when they have come my way. I am not well trained in medical astrology but appreciate the connection. Hippocrates, Greek father of medicine, wrote, "A physician without a knowledge of astrology has no right to call himself a physician."

And finally, there are recipes of preparation. I admit a bias toward fresh plant tinctures but include both fresh and dried plant preparation. This may include cold or hot infusions and decoctions as well as maceration tinctures. The ratios are based on my own observations, and the alcohol content is based on the fact that I am of one-quarter Scottish heritage and very frugal. For many years I relied on corn-based Everclear, which is 95 percent alcohol or 190 proof. About ten years ago I tried to contact the producers and ask if they used GMO corn. I asked several times, and with no response, I made up my own mind. I now suggest using a beautiful Polish vodka made from potato that is 96 percent alcohol or 192 proof. It is so pleasant compared to Everclear that my wife uses it in her aromatic perfumes. It is called Spirytus Rektyfikowany. In the United States there are several great companies that offer organic alcohols from grapes, wheat, corn, and sugarcane at good prices.

The taxonomic names are up to date as of the last edit. That can change quickly, so I have made sure to include older, alternate Latin binomials that may be more familiar to botanists, herbalists, and homeopaths.

I hope you enjoy the journeys with my various boreal herbal allies.

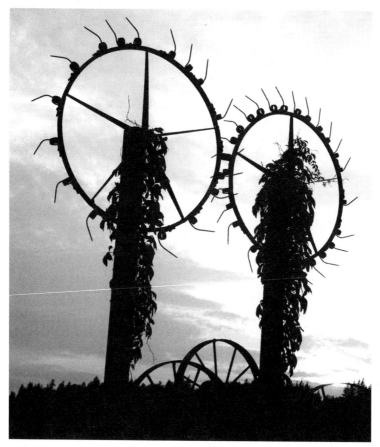

Plant totem

3

Herbal Allies and the
Cree Moon Calendar

*The moon is the mediator, intercessory and gateway between
the realms of celestial influences and the earthly realm.*
—HYEMEYOHSTS STORM (1972)

THE GATHERING AND PREPARING of wild-crafted plant medicines is dependent upon awareness of the seasons. In my part of northern Canada, spring can start in early April up until the end of May. It is not unusual for the seasons to be six weeks early or late, and one has to adjust to the pace of nature. Global warming is definitely influencing these cycles, contributing to changes in plant hardiness zones. The area in which I harvest herbs was considered zone 2 about forty years ago and is now zone 3b.

The life cycle of plants, known as phenology, indicates environmental and seasonal changes, related to gathering for food and medicine. Traditional phenological knowledge is relatively stable in temperate regions, and the plant life cycle rather predictable. Often, the flowering of a shrub or the ripening of fruit is associated with the appearance of a mammal, bird, or fish.

The picking of plant medicines requires a deep connection with the seasonal cycles. The timing can vary, but depending on which part of the plant is required, an optimal time will be noted.

The boreal forest crosses the top of North America from Newfoundland to Alaska, and then down the top of the Rocky Mountains to New Mexico. Many of the herbal allies in this book are widely available for medicine. For every thousand feet of elevation, the appearance of the plant after winter is delayed by two weeks. This is important to remember when looking for these plants in your region of the continent.

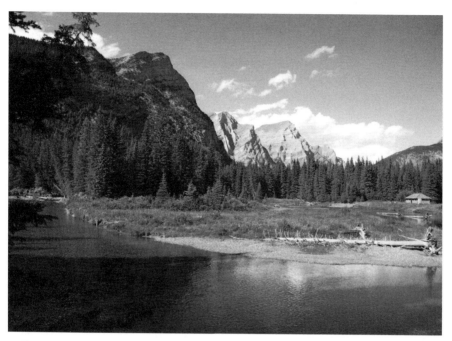

Rocky Mountains of Alberta

Leaves are often collected in optimal condition before the flowers appear. Sweet colts-foot is an exception, as the flowers appear on a separate stem almost a month before any leaves. Bark is most easily collected in the spring, and roots in the fall, after a frost.

The Cree moon calendar was traditionally based on thirteen lunar cycles. This only makes sense. Today, however, the Cree lunar calendar has been adapted to fit into the twelve months representing our Western view of an annual transit around the sun. In this book I am following one of the commonly used models. It should be noted that the Cree people are widely spread across the aspen parkland and boreal forests of northern Canada. Therefore, there are different words and pronunciations representing the lunar calendar. The word *month* is derived, of course, from the same root word as *moon*.

It will be observed that spring and summer seasons come earlier to regions of Ontario and Quebec, in some years, so a variation is noted.

When you look at the moon phases for each year, you will see that there are thirteen moons in the calendar year. These differ from year to year. In 2016, for example, there were two new moons in September, one at the beginning and another twenty-eight days later. It will vary throughout the years based on when the new moon first appears. The moon cycles run from new moon to new moon and thus do not fit neatly into our twelve months. The thirteenth moon moves each year and is difficult to place in any one season.

The Greeks viewed the new moon as a time of fertility and rebirth, as the moon and sun joined together in the same part of the sky. This is a time when the forces of plants are concentrated downward into the roots. The Greeks thought the curved sliver of a new moon looked like a newly sprouted seed.

The thirteen moons relate to the thirteen phases of life in humans. The first phase begins from birth to age seven, then to fourteen, twenty-one, and so on. Lessons learned help transform each period of time and influence the following trials and initiations required to become whole.

Another aspect of healing relates to the Medicine Wheel. The four colors and directions relate to how how individuals see themselves and the world. It can vary with the regions of North America, but for the northern Alberta Cree, west is black, north is white, south is yellow, and east is red.

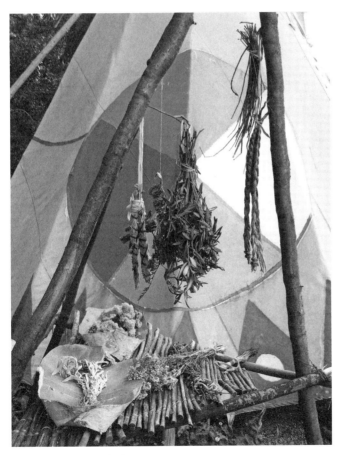

Medicine Wheel and herbs

The knowledge of the west is emotion and reason, or figuring-it-out knowledge. It is about connecting head and heart. The west or Nepawanuk takes away the sun each night. In Cree, Nepawanuk means "the place where the sun goes down." The west is the destination for people when they die. It is a wind that dries the land.

The north is about movement, mental activity, or doing-it wisdom, and our relationship to culture. The Cree call this Kewatin, a cold north wind that brings winter. Kewatin was the brother who wished to rule the earth, and when denied, he turned against the planet.

The south is represented by Kewatin's brother Sawin, the healing wind, and is about time, physical health, relating, and understanding, including ecological respect for the land. Sawin allows the birds to return north and raise their young. Egg-laying, egg-hatching, and molting months are three Cree lunar signposts related to geese and other migrating birds.

The east is about vision and the ability or awareness to see. This direction is concerned with local knowledge but a worldwide vision, and it involves stories, teachings, and ceremony. The east wind is Wapun, which, in Cree, means "the dawn of a new day." With sunrise you can see red in the clouds.

Hyemeyohsts Storm (1972) writes:

> At birth, each of us is given a particular Beginning Place within these Four Great Directions on the Medicine Wheel. This Starting Place gives us our first way of perceiving things, which will then be our easiest and most natural way throughout our lives. But any person who perceives from only one of these Four Great Directions will remain just a partial man. For example, a man who possesses only the Gift of the North will be wise. But he will be a cold man, a man without feeling. And the man who lives only in the East will have the clear, far sighted vision of the Eagle, but he will never be close to things. This man will feel separated, high above life, and will never understand or believe that he can be touched by anything. A man or woman who perceives only from the West will go over the same thought again and again in their mind, and will always be undecided. And if a person has only the Gift of the South, he will see everything with the eyes of a Mouse. He will be too close to the ground and too nearsighted to see anything except whatever is right in front of him, touching his whiskers.

In the same manner, an herbalist will look at his or her client from the perspective of the Hippocratic, Traditional Chinese Medicine, or Ayurvedic system of constitution and the inherent strengths and weaknesses of the individual. In all cases, the goal is to help bring balance to the individual, to steer him or her onto the pathway of health and well-being, or *niitsitapiipaitapiiyssin*.

The herbalist learns and grows through the experience of working with plant allies and healers. The various phases of growth, like the lunar cycles, test and reveal deeper levels of maturity and wisdom. In my own experience over years of clinical practice, I observed that less heroic interventions produced better results in the long run.

The following is a list of the twelve moons of the Cree, according to the *Alberta Elders' Cree Dictionary* (LeClaire and Cardinal 1998).

Pisim means moon. The moon is also known as "night sun" or *tipiskaw pisim.*

January: the cold moon, Kisepîsim

February: the eagle or bald eagle moon, Mikisopîsim

March: the goose moon, Niskipîsim

April: the frog moon, Ayîkiwipîsim

May: the egg-laying moon, Opiniyâwewipîsim

June: the egg-hatching moon, Opâskahopîsim

July: molting moon, Opaskowipîsim

August: the flying moon, Ohpahopîsim

September: the mating or rutting moon, Onôcihitowipîsim

October: the freeze-up moon, Kaskatinowipîsim

November: the frosty moon, Iyikopiwipîsim

December: the tree-cleaning moon, Pawahcakinasîs

Turtle Island

"There are always thirteen on Old Turtle's back, and there are always thirteen moons in each year. Many people do not know this. They do not know, as we Abenaki know, that each moon has its own name, and every moon has its own stories. I learned those stories from my grandfather" (Bruchac and London 1992).

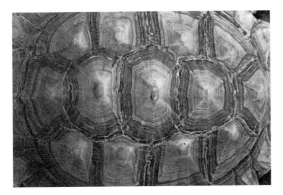

Turtle shell

Turtles have a special meaning to indigenous people. The pattern of scutes on a turtle's shell defines the lunar calendar cycle. Around the edge are twenty-eight individual scales that represent the days of the lunar cycle. And in the center of the shell are thirteen larger scales, representing the year's lunar calendar. It is traditional to use thirteen poles when setting up a tipi.

Turtle Island is the name given to North America by various native peoples. The "original" legend was passed on from the Lenape (Delaware) people, but it has been embraced, with slight variation, throughout the continent. Sky Woman fell to earth and was carrying child. The whole planet was water with nowhere to stand or sit. A giant turtle was swimming in the great abyss and was a refuge for various animals. In order to create a land base, various creatures dove deep into the water, attempting to retrieve some soil. After many tried and failed, muskrat made the journey. He was gone a long time, and when he floated to the surface, he was dead. But between his paws was a small piece of mud. Sky Woman was so grateful she breathed life back into the little hero. The soil was spread over turtle's back and became Turtle Island, now called the continent of North America.

The turtle represents perseverance, longevity, and steadfastness, all traits to be admired. Gary Snyder authored *Turtle Island* in 1974 and won the prestigious Pulitzer Prize for Poetry the following year.

Frog Moon—Ayîkiwipîsim or Ayikîpîsim

Generally speaking, frog moon is associated with the month of April. This can vary, of course, depending upon the harshness of winter and how prolonged the melt of spring is. This is the lunar cycle of frogs croaking in the swamps and their ritualistic sounds of mating.

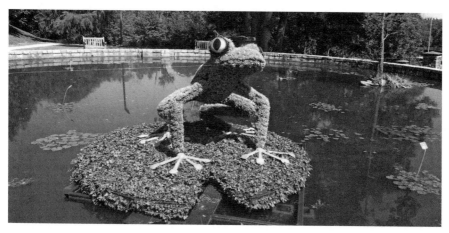

Frog at Atlanta Botanical Gardens

To the Anishinaabe people, frogs represent transformation and growth. In the Pacific Northwest, the amphibians represent renewal and springtime. Frog is sometimes carved onto totem poles on the west coast of Canada. The Frog clan is found in various tribes, including the Chippewa, Zuni, and Tlingit. Frog Dance is a celebrated ceremony of the Creek tribe. In the mythology of the Innu (Montagnais-Naskapi) of Quebec, Anikaeu is the master of frogs and toads.

A Cree legend records the origin of the frog moon:

When the world was young, Wis-a-ked-jak, the Trickster, met with all the animals to decide how many moons would be winter. Moose answered, "There should be as many moons of winter as hairs on my body." Amik, the beaver, said, "There should be as many moons as scales on my tail." Then O-ma-ka-ki, the little frog, said, "There should only be as many moons of snow as toes on my foot." Wis-a-ked-jak decided that this was right. So it is that winter lasts only five moons, and when it ends, the small frogs sing their victory song in this moon with their name. (Bruchac and London 1992)

Sweet coltsfoot flowers make their appearance during frog moon. Their bright white flowers shine like diamonds under a full moon, sparkling at night for all to see. The flowers and stems are collected, cooked, and eaten. The Cree have several names for the plant, including moose ear, frog leaves, owl's blanket, and wolverine's foot. It is a favorite springtime food of bears. Much later the leaves appear.

The warm days and cool evenings are the right time to tap birch trees for their delicious and nourishing sap. Birch bark is easily collected during this moon, as the inner bark is well lubricated and easy to remove. Birch bark scrolls, known as *wiigwaasabak*, were used as writing material. These were marked with bone, or charcoal, sometimes colored with red or blue pigments. Various songs and healing recipes were recorded dating back at least four hundred years. The pages were stitched with split spruce roots, and then rolled and placed in the birch bark containers, naturally formed from dead trees. Birch bark biting, known as Mazinibaganjigan, is a beautiful artwork of the Cree, exhibiting geometric and mandala-like representations.

This is the time to collect the inner bark of poplar, with its rich carbohydrate strips of nourishment. Because the sap is rising, the bark strips off the tree like butter, making for easy collection. The strips of inner bark were eaten fresh, or dried and then added to pots of hot water and cooked in a manner like pasta. Birch bark containers were filled with water, and hot rocks from the fire were added to create the boiling needed for the poplar strips.

According to some native tribes, burning the bark of black cottonwood (*Populus balsamifera* ssp. *trichocarpa*) will cause a strong wind. Thirteen balsam poplar poles are sometimes used to build the symbolic arch for the Thirst Dance, sometimes called the Sun Dance.

Egg-Laying Moon or Leaf-Budding Moon—
Opiniyâwewipîsim or Sâkipakâwipîsim

One variation in the north is Apiniyâwepîsim. We are now in the month of May, with long days and short nights. In parts of the north, the sun barely sinks below the horizon, and everyone is energized by the long days of warmth and light. Birds are building nests and setting on eggs to keep them warm. Fish are laying their eggs in the shallow of lakes, and the leaves of trees and herbaceous plants are beginning to open.

The Budding Moon is recorded as a Huron legend:

One year Old Man Winter refused to leave our land, and so our people asked for help from our great friend, Ju-ske-ha, known to some as the Sun. He knocked on the door of Winter's lodge then entered and sat by Winter's cold fire. "Leave here or you will freeze," Winter said, but Ju-ske-ha breathed and Winter grew smaller. Ju-ske-ha waved his hand, and a white owl flew down to carry Winter back to the deep snow of the north. The lodge melted away and the trees turned green with new buds as the birds began to sing. And where the cold fire of winter had been was a circle of white May flowers. So it happens each spring when the Budding Moon comes. All the animals wake and we follow them across our wide, beautiful land. (Bruchac and London 1992)

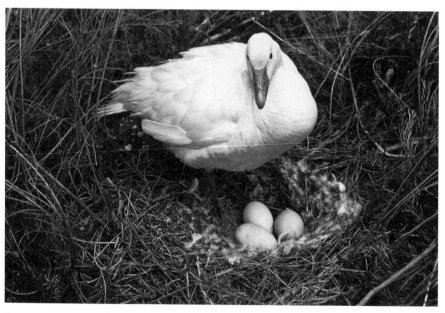

Snow Goose with new eggs

Bees are well established in their hives and working overtime to collect the propolis, nectar, and pollen that is so abundant. At this time the days are long and warm. Pollens are flying about and bees are actively feeding brood and collecting poplar resins to produce propolis. This powerful antibiotic substance helps maintain health in the hives.

This is a good time to collect the fresh spruce needles, which taste more like citrus than at any other time of the year. The fresh, soft needles are lighter in color and found on the very tips, making them easy to collect. These are the needles I gather to make spruce beer, giving a still robust but lemon or orange flavor to the brew.

The inner bark and needles of tamarack are collected at this time, and preserved for later use as food and medicine. The needles are soft and easy to collect. When the needles turn yellow in fall, this is the time female black bears are entering their dens. The sugary sap is collected and stored for later use.

Egg-Hatching Moon—Opâskahopîsim or Opâskâwewowipîsim

This lunar cycle is based around June, when nature is in full growth. The days are twenty or more hours in length, with a vitality and vigor not seen the rest of the year. It is a time of annual gathering at meeting places, where neighboring tribes sit together in friendship and share stories and meals. Ceremonies such as the once banned Thirst Dance (Sun Dance) are conducted, stretching a young man's endurance in the presence of his peers. The full ceremony has been legal in Canada since 1951.

Drumming, dancing, and song, along with fasting and ceremonial pipe and prayer, are practiced at these cultural events. In some cases, young men are fastened to a central pole with rawhide thongs through their pectorals. Filming today is strictly forbidden, but in 1960 the National Film Board of Canada released the documentary *Circle of the Sun* after filming a Kainai Nation ceremony the year before.

June 21, the longest day of the year, also known as the summer solstice, was declared National Aboriginal Day in Canada in 1996. The Onöndowága (Seneca) call the sixth moon Strawberry Moon.

In late spring a small boy whose parents had died went hunting game down by the river where the Jo-ge-oh, the Little People who care for the plants, live. He shared what he caught with those Little People. In return they took him in a magic canoe up into the cliffs, taught him many things, and gave him strawberries. He was gone just four days, but when he returned, years had passed and he was a tall man. He shared with his people what he was taught and gave them the sweetness of the red strawberries. So, each year, the Senecas sing songs of praise to the Little People, thanking them again for this moon's gift. (Bruchac and London 1992)

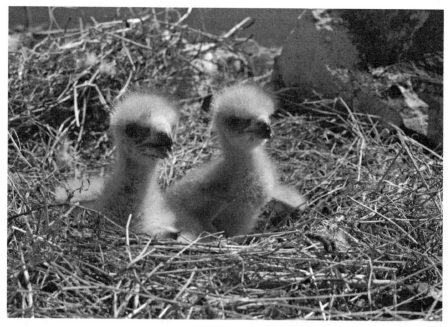

Bald Eagles just hatched

In June 2016 we had a true Strawberry Full Moon, the first since 1967. This means that the full moon falls on the summer solstice in June, and it will not happen again until 2062.

This is the time of collecting leaves and flowers of many medicinal plants. The white berries of red osier dogwood are beginning to ripen, and the inner bark is harvested for smoking mixtures. Native traditions suggest the bush be talked to and presented with tobacco before bark or branches are removed. The berries will appear from new flowers over a two-month period, extending well into the mating moon.

Fireweed is blazing a beautiful magenta over vast areas of countryside and is prime for collection of its valuable leaves and flowers for medicine. When fireweed is blooming indicates the time to hunt mule deer. In some areas the flowers are a phonological indicator that the moose are fat enough to hunt. Later, the mature seed fluff will be gathered to make waterproof clothing and insulate bedding.

The cultivated lilac is beginning to bloom and leaves, bark, and flowers can be gathered and prepared for medicine. The Cree enjoy the beautifully scented flowers and named the introduced plant *nîpisîsa ka wâpikwanekiy*.

Labrador Tea is blooming with its heady fragrance and it is time to pick both flowers and leaves for tea, medicine, and perfume.

Molting Moon—Opaskowipîsim

The young birds and ducks are shedding their soft young feathers and bringing forth their adult plumage. It is July, and nature is in its full splendor. The Pomo of California related the seventh moon with the appearance of acorns, a staple food:

> *When the world was new it was covered with water until Earth Elder, the Creator, reached down to the mud below and placed it onto Turtle's back. Earth Elder shaped the sun and the stars, then sat for a moment, thinking of what was most needed, what would help the humans still to come. That was when Earth Elder made the first tree, a great oak with twelve branches arching over the lands. Then, sitting down beneath it, the sun shining bright, Earth Elder thought of food for the people, and acorns began to form. So it is, each year, when the sun shines brightest, these first acorns come and our Pomo people gather this moon's coming harvest.* (Bruchac and London 1992)

The unusual eerily white ghost pipe is popping out of the ground and is ready to harvest and prepare for medicine. I love to watch the translucent white "flowers" and stem turn a beautiful turquoise and then quickly a deep violet color when exposed to alcohol. It is almost alchemical in its transformation. It is known as wolf's urine, and said to grow where the animals void their bladder.

In the swamp, the marsh scullcap is found in full bloom, growing along with wild mint and bugleweed. It is a far more effective medicine when prepared and preserved fresh, so time is of the essence.

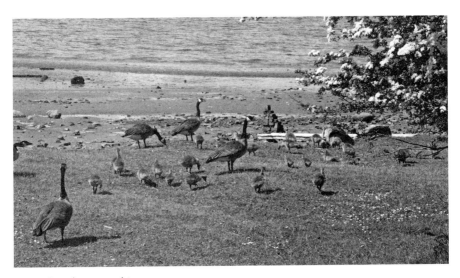

Young Canada geese molting

The green mature seeds of cow parsnip are ready for picking. They are easily gathered by the handful but do come with small insects that need to be removed, one way or the other. They can be dried on nylon screens for later use in food or medicine or freshly crushed and prepared as a tincture. On Haida Gwaii, the blooming of cow parsnip is a sign the seagull eggs are no longer good to eat. At this time of year you can practically watch and hear the giant cow parsnip grow.

Flying Moon—Ohpahopîsim or Ohpahowipîsim

The lunar cycle is now in August, and there is a sense of coolness in the air. The lake plants are beginning to ripen with seeds, including the important wild rice. The Mamaceqtaw (Menominee), of northern Wisconsin and Michigan, harvest wild rice, a staple food. Their name, Omaeqnomenew, given to them by neighboring Huron and Ojibwe, comes from the word for wild rice. In legend, the eighth lunar cycle of the year was the Moon of Wild Rice.

In the old days, they say, Bear came out of the ground and became a man, but found he was lonely. He called to the sky: "Thunder Eagle, come down to earth and be my brother." Then the giant Eagle, who made thunder and lightning by flapping his wings and flashing his eyes, flew down and he, too, became human. Then the Creator, the Good Mystery, made

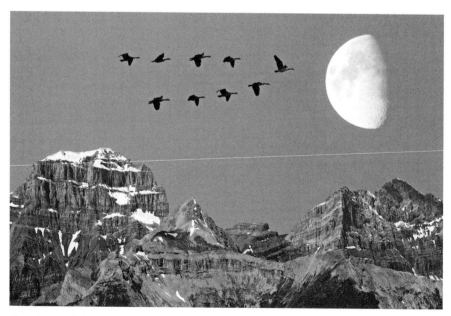

Canada geese flying

the Thunder People the water-bearers, gave them the gifts of corn and fire. To the People of the Bear, the Good Mystery gave another gift—wild rice. When the Thunder People came to visit the Bear village near the mouth of the Me-nom-i-nee River, they brought with them water and fire and corn. The Bear People gave them wild rice in exchange. And so it came to be that those two families live together and harvest this special food in the Wild Rice Moon. (Bruchac and London 1992)

The bears are seeking buffalo berry and beginning to fatten up for winter. For the Secwepemc of British Columbia, the ripening of berries indicates the beginning of the sockeye salmon migration to fresh water. It is the time to harvest the inner bark and ripe berries of high bush cranberry.

The muskrat root (calamus) is prime and awaiting harvest at the edge of shallow lakes. It is a busy time for wild-crafters. The cold water and long summer days help develop a hot, pungent taste in the root not found in other parts of North America. Many herbalists say that the farther north the plant grows, the stronger its taste, and I believe this is so. I once was offered a piece of root growing in New Mexico, and it hardly tickled my tonsils.

The introduced mullein is now in full flower and ready to pick for preparation into oil for lymphatic and ear problems. Some of the flowers are allowed to go to seed, and harvested during the mating moon for other purposes.

Mating or Rutting Moon—Onôcihitowipîsim

It is September and time to harvest roots. The energy of the plants after the first frost has moved downward and is now stored in the underground roots. The bull moose and male elk are scraping velvet from their antlers and getting ready for mating season. I enjoy a visit to the mountain parks at this time of year, with a touch of frost in the air and the bellowing of male elk echoing through the valley. This is moose-calling time. Those hunters with special skill will bring out their birch-bark moose callers.

The days are warm, but the evenings bring a touch of freezing, and the aerial parts of plants are dying. The leaves are turning yellow and storage of food for the long winter begins. Winter is coming.

The Mi'kmaq (Micmac) of eastern Canada call the ninth lunar appearance Moose-Calling moon.

In this season when leaves begin to turn color, we go down to the lakes and with birch-bark horns make that sound that echoes through the spruce trees, the call of a moose looking for a mate: Mooo-ahhh-ahhh, Mooo-ahhh-ahhh. *If we wait there, patient in our canoes, the moose will come. His great horns are flat because, long ago, before people came, Glooskap asked the Moose what he would do when he saw human beings. "I will throw them up high on my sharp horns," Moose said. So Gloos-kap pushed his horns flatter and made him smaller. "Now, Moose," he said, "you will not want to harm my people." So the moose comes and stands, strong as the northeast wind. He looks at us, then we watch him disappear back into the willows again.* (Bruchac and London 1992)

The wild sarsaparilla rhizome is easily gathered at this time, especially in areas of sandy soil. Also known as rabbit root, the fall rhizome is preferred, but care must be taken not to wait too long, as finding them after the bright yellow leaves have fallen can be quite difficult.

Wapos is the Cree name for the rabbit in the moon. It can be clearly seen this time of year when the moon is bright orange and full.

The cultivated *Rhodiola* roots, the size of turnips, are harvested and sliced thinly for medicine. Their common name, roseroot, is obvious as the scent arising is reminiscent of rose petals. Although cultivated in northern Canada, roseroot grows wild all over Iceland. Many households plant the hardy sedum in their front or back yards, and even with their loved ones in local cemeteries.

Bear root *(Hedysarum alpinum)* is harvested at this time. The pea- to thumb-sized corms are easily pulled from the ground. You will sometimes find crisp white tender roots of a good size, up to an inch in diameter and a foot long. Care is needed as black and grizzly bears are also seeking out this nutritious food source, and sharing is not in their nature. Often you will find large holes in the side of hills where bears have taken the largest roots

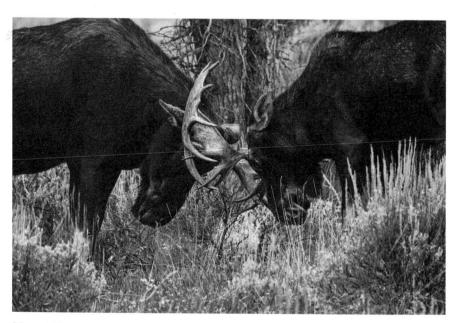

Moose rutting

and left others. This is not a good place to camp for the night! Bear root or osha (*Ligusticum porteri*) is a well-known and prized medicinal herb, found in the southern Rocky Mountains.

Herbalists of northern Canada do not have direct access to this species but utilize the related Canby lovage (*L. canbyi*). Its furry, oily rhizomes can be used for a similar purpose. Native people would smoke the powder with tobacco, or smudge the root as a good luck charm. The root was used to prevent babies catching cold, revive unconscious people or those who have gone into a trance, or when possessed by spirits, such as the blue jay spirit. The highly prized root was rubbed on clothing and the face before a dance. The root works nearly as well as yarrow root for toothache.

4

Nine Tips for Budding Herbalists

HERE ARE MY NINE TIPS for new herbal students. I hope they may help you, in some small way, with the process of becoming a more complete clinician. None of this information was given to me as a young man, but over time as a clinical herbalist, these tips helped me shape a connection with my herbal allies.

One. I will attempt to paraphrase Carl Jung: *Only the wounded healers heal, and only they can heal to the extent they have healed themselves.* I put this saying on a parchment and hung it above my desk during my eighteen years of clinical practice.

It means, do your own work! Accept your own vulnerability and remember the times in your own life when you overcame health issues. As an herbalist, you would never consider suggesting to your client an herbal tincture that you had not ingested and experienced yourself. You cannot ask a client to go on a journey you have not traveled. Be a living example of health and well-being, but do not be so dogmatic that you stop enjoying your own journey.

One day I was sitting in a blues bar, listening to music and sipping a beer. One of my clients walked over to me, and said she was shocked to find me there. I reminded her this was something I enjoyed. So be authentic. You will attract to you, and your practice, like-minded individuals who feel a connection.

Two. Become more culturally aware. You will be working with a wide range of ethnicities, religious beliefs, and social mores. The belief system of your client is paramount to his or her healing process, and imposing your own may well short-circuit this important aspect. Because all healing is from the head down, the mental, emotional, and spiritual needs of the client come first. Statistically speaking, the average human has one breast and one testis. Be aware of your own limitations when dealing with the other sex. You may believe that you fully understand the female reproductive system if you are male, but you probably don't. Vice versa is also true.

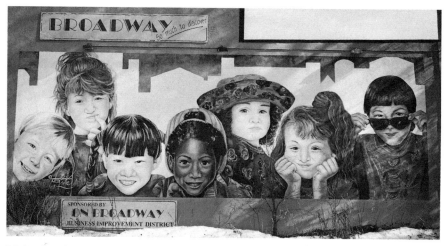

Multicultural mural, Saskatoon, Saskatchewan

Three. Many clients, particularly those dealing with chronic conditions, have been to a number of other health care practitioners. If they had been helped, they would not be seeing you. Be respectful but do not indulge in criticizing other health modalities, be it biomedicine, naturopathy, body work, homeopathy, or whatever route the client has previously traveled. Avoid any indulgence in negative opinion, no matter how tempting.

Criticizing other health modalities does not make you a superior clinician. I gave and received many referrals from other health practitioners. Help create a community of holistic health providers in your part of the world.

Four. Set healthy boundaries. Some clients who are desperate for help will express their needs via personal confrontation. The best mode of action is none. I once had an older woman who came into my office, quickly sat down and before even introducing herself, said, "Fix me!" I asked her what she meant, and she replied that she had seen everyone, and that she had been told I was a good herbalist, and I should fix her.

I carefully responded that I did not sit in the chair for her, but for my own good, and that a relationship or partnership was necessary to achieve any success. I said that I was sitting here for me so that we both could learn and grow together. She stood up and said, "That is quite the statement," at which point I suggested this was not going to work, and there would be no charge for the appointment.

Two weeks later, my receptionist let me know this particular client was on the line. I answered, and she told me that no one had ever spoken to her as I had. I said nothing. She asked if she could come for another appointment, and I agreed. In the next six months, her health condition improved by over 80 percent, and she became not only an improved client but referred me to her family and friends.

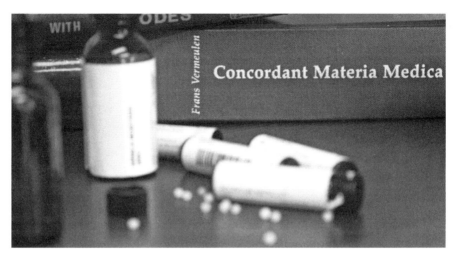

Homeopathy

Five. Take the time to create a good apothecary of herbal tinctures. There are no better herbal medicines than those you produce, especially from wild-crafted plants. Focus on becoming a bioregional herbalist and study the plants that thrive where you live.

It may seem that Australia or Africa or South America offer unusual plant medicines, and they do, but can you access them in their prime state? And don't get me started on the contaminated and adulterated condition of some herbs exported from China and India.

There are many reasons to be leery of herbs prone to contamination with heavy metals and other pollutants. This is not to say that organic medicinal plants are not available from North American suppliers. If you know your local herbs, you will always have a ready supply and can harvest them at the peak of their perfection. I do not believe exclusively in fresh plant tinctures, as some herbs require drying, but it is hard to do fresh extractions when you don't live near the plants.

Under the present law in Canada, a registered herbalist can produce their own herbal medicines and dispense them to their clients. Study your local herbs and rely on them!

Six. In the beginning of an herbal practice, you may find it useful to share office space with other practitioners of natural medicine. I shared space and a receptionist for eight years with Robert Pearman, a great naturopath and homeopath. I learned so much from his respectful, thoughtful approach to clients and clinical intake. It is very important to continue studies in the field of herbal medicine, and sharing case studies in confidence as well as ideas with colleagues are great advantages.

Seven. Join a professional organization such as the American Herbalist Guild. Subscribe to magazines such as *Herbalgram* and other online and paper publications that help you keep up to date with the latest findings and studies. *Plant Healer Magazine* has great articles by many knowledgeable herbalists. View Internet herb sites with a jaundiced eye.

Build a library, and weed it over time, condensing down to the books you find most useful time and again. Attend the occasional herb gathering or conference, and in time, when the occasion arises, give a presentation yourself. Connect with herbalists in your area and support their work by buying their authored books or attending their plant walks and events.

American Herbalist Guild

Alberta had no herbal gatherings until 2011 when Abrah Arneson and I helped facilitate the first event after being inspired on the long drive home from the Montana Herb Gathering.

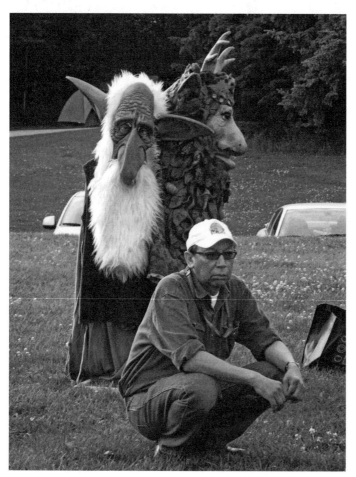

Clifford Cardinal and friends at the Alberta Herb Gathering

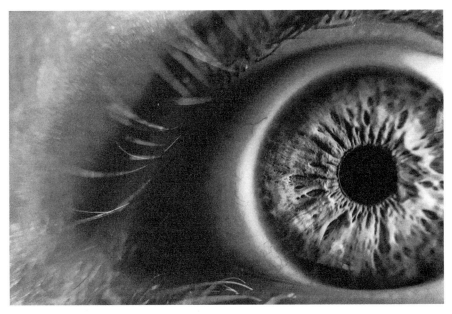

Iridology

Eight. Study various diagnoses and healing techniques. Iridology; facial, skin, ear, teeth, tongue, and pulse diagnosis; reflexology; reiki; touch for health; urinalysis; hair analysis; enzyme therapy; body language; neurolinguistic programming (NLP); and other modalities will help make you a better clinician.

The Practicing Herbalist book by Margi Flint is highly recommended, due to its vast compilation of body signs, helping guide the novice herbalist to read their client's constitution and predispositions. It is continually being updated, so purchase the latest edition.

Nine. Instill hope in your client. Everyone needs hope. In cases where the client has given up, try Gorse, one of Bach's great flower remedies. Or Wild Rose where there is resignation. Without hope there can be no healing.

5

Frog Moon Herbal Allies

Coltsfoot

Arrow-Leaved Coltsfoot ◆ Owl's Blanket ◆ Wolverine's Foot ◆ Moose Ear Leaf ◆ Frog Leaf—*Petasites sagittatus* (Banks ex Pursh) A. Gray ◆ *P. frigidus* (L.) var. *sagittatus* (Banks ex Pursh) Cherniawsky ◆ *P. dentatus* Blankinship

Arctic Coltsfoot ◆ Snowleaf Coltsfoot—*Petasites nivalis* Greene ◆ *P. hyperboreus* Rydb. ◆ *P. frigidus* (L.) Fries var. *nivalis* (Greene) Cronq. ◆ *P. warrenii* H. St. John

Palmate Leaved Coltsfoot—*Petasites palmatus* (Ait.) Gray ◆ *P. frigidus* var. *palmatus* (Ait.) Cronq.

Grape Leaved Coltsfoot—*Petasites frigidus* var. *x vitifolius* ◆ *P. hookerianus* (Nutt.) Rydb. ◆ *P. speciosus* (Nutt.) Piper. ◆ *Nardosmia arctica* (A.E. Porsild) A. Love & D. Love

Vine Leaved Coltsfoot—*Petasites x vitifolius* Greene ◆ *P. frigidus* var. *x vitifolius* (Greene) Chern. ◆ *Nardosmia vitifolia* Greene

Sweet Coltsfoot ◆ Butterbur ◆ Butterfly Dock—*Petasites hybridus* (L.) P. Gaertn., B. Mey. & Scherb. ◆ *P. officinalis* Moench ◆ *Tussilago petasites* L.

> *I love coltsfoot that they*
> *Make their appearance into life among dead grass:*
> *Larches, that they*
> *Die colorfully among somber immortals.*
>
> —David Constantine

Petasos is from the Greek meaning a large-brimmed hat worn by shepherds, in reference to the size of the leaves. The plant is common to the northern prairie but is often mistaken in texts for the English Coltsfoot, *Tussilago farfara*. In fact, it is much closer in nature to Butterbur, *Petasites hybridus*, a native of Europe, in its medicinal makeup. The genus, at least in North America, is a taxonomic mess. I have included both newer and older binomials so the average reader can search on the plant in older texts and plant-identification books.

Tussilago aerial parts are cool, bitter, salty, somewhat astringent, and decongesting and useful in dry or wet coughs. In France, the coltsfoot leaf was painted on pharmacy doors, advertising herbal medicines were available at that location.

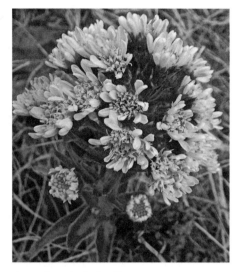

Petasites root is more warming, pungent, bitter, and both stimulating and relaxing in nature. It was known as plague flower or pestilence plant for its use during the great epidemic in Europe and is called bog rhubarb for its preferred moist location and appearance. The white to pink flowers and stems arrive in spring long before the leaves and make an acceptable asparagus-like potherb. In a large patch, the sweet floral fragrance is strong enough to make one dizzy.

Arrow-leaved coltsfoot flower

The flowers, as mentioned, pop up at least one month before the leaves. This is very unusual in plants and suggests a powerful reserve of energy in the roots to sustain a stem and flower for a month before leaves appear to photosynthesize and recharge. It is a very important herbal ally.

Traditional Uses

The Saskatchewan Cree call the flower *wapathaman* and the leaves *mosotawakayipak*, "moose ear leaf," or *yuwskiyhtiypuk*, "soft leaves." Alberta Cree call arrow-leaved coltsfoot *piskehtepask*, meaning "separate leaf," in reference to the leaf and flower coming at separate times. Another name is *miyokatayinipiya*, meaning "frog leaves." In northern Alberta, the Cree know it as *puskwa* and commonly refer to the herb as "wolverine's foot" or "owl's blanket" due to its insulating value. The furry undersides of the leaf are gathered by birds to line their nests. The Dené Tha (Slavey) call the plant *ya yenoshetia*, meaning "bear eats it." In British Columbia, the Ditidaht word for *P. frigidus* means "elk's food."

In Alaska, the Dena'ina call arctic and palmate-leaved coltsfoot "owl's blanket," *k'ijeghi ch'da*. The roots are soaked in hot water and the tea is taken internally for tuberculosis, sore throat, stomach ulcers, and similar health issues. It appears to stop the internal bleeding associated with these conditions. Various indigenous northern people used coltsfoot for coughs, colds, and other bronchial complaints.

Women healers of the past used root decoctions to bring on menstruation that stopped due to shock or cold, or simply to relieve painful periods. This is interesting, because the women of various British Columbia tribes would dry and work the leaves with their hands to produce a cottony material to use as a sanitary napkin. Ukrainian settlers in Alberta used *pidlibuk* leaves in the form of poultices, often combined with fresh milk for wounds.

The fuzzy side was placed against the skin to reduce skin rashes. "When someone had a skin condition that would not heal, it was treated with large greenish-white, rhubarb-like leaves [coltsfoot?], which were collected from slough edges" (Mucz 2012, 209). Decoctions of fireweed were also used as a wash. The leaves were dried and later soaked in warm water and applied to open sores and ulcers. The dried roots were grated and applied to boils or running sores. For eczema, the root of palmate coltsfoot is boiled and when cool, applied as a wash. The flower heads can be decocted and taken for treating coughs.

The Karok use the root for ulcerated sores that do not heal in the form of a crushed poultice. A salve was prepared from the root, combined with self-heal, Johnny jump-up, and dried wormwood blossoms, according to Josephine Peters (2010) in her delightful book on herbal medicine. For psoriasis, scabies, and ringworm, combine the root with plantain, wormwood, and violet.

The leaves were rolled into balls, dried and burned, and used as a salt substitute rich in sodium, calcium, and potassium. This works best if done in a container that restricts oxygen flow, producing a powder that is less smoky. The large succulent stems of arrow-leaved coltsfoot can be eaten raw or steamed. They contain small amounts of pyrrolizidine alkaloids, so I would limit the intake. They taste somewhat like celery, perhaps a little sweeter.

The plant is governed by the planet Venus and the water element and represents maternal care. Leaves were smoked to create visions, and the tiny seeds were used in love divinations, sown by hopeful maidens. Arrow-leaved and arctic coltsfoot possess triangular leaves, while palmate-leaved coltsfoot is just that, with several fingerlike (palmate) segments. All are used identically. Grape-leaved coltsfoot is considered a hybrid between arrow-leaved and palmate-leaved varieties. Sweet coltsfoot (*P. hybridus*) is a red-pink flowered European import that is now growing wild all over the northeastern United States. It is fully hardy to the prairies, but since we have several effective species growing wild, there is little need to plant it. Several sources suggest the female plant root is best dug up in spring, and the androdynamic plant roots in fall; I'm not sure why.

Medicinal Uses

Constituents: *P. palmatus*: S-petasin, iso-S-petasin and related esters, saponins, petalsipaline, triterpene saponins, pyrocatechol tannins, bakkenolide, resins, potassium, helianthinin, inulin, various alkaloids, including small amounts of pyrrolizidine alkaloids in the young leaves, but not the root, and essential oils (0.65%). The first two active ingredients are found in both leaf and root.

P. hybridus root: esters of the eremonphilane-type sesquiterpene alcohols petasol, neopetasol, and isopetasol, with S-petasin (0.36%) iso-S-petasin (0.15%), neopetasitine and aneglicoyl-neopetasol as principal components; fukinone, bakkenolide A, dodecanal; benzofuran derivatives, the alkaloids sececionine, integerrimine, senkirkine, as well as petasitenine, neopetasitenine, and the nontoxic alkaloids neoplatyphylline, isotussilagine, and tussilagine in total amounts of 1–100 mg/kg; flavonoids isoquercitrin and astragaline, inulin, mucilage, tannins, 0.1% essential oil, including dodecanal. Petasin content ranges 7.4–15.3 mg/g dry weight from rhizomes and 3.3–11.4 mg/g dry weight from leaves.

The leaf contains less than one-tenth this amount in similar composition, as well as flavonoids such as isoquercetin and astragaline. Some chemotypes contain furanopetasin and 9-hydroxyfuranoere-mophilone as the major alkaloids of both root and leaf.

Various pyrrolizidine alkaloids (PAs) such as senecionine and integerrimine are found in the immature leaf and flower stalk, but less in the mature leaf and root. One study in Switzerland found PA content in rhizome from 5 to 90 ppm and leaves between 0.02 and 1.5 ppm (Wildi et al. 1998). The PAs are usually highest in thickenings on roots just below leaves. Medicinal plants free of these alkaloids are now cultivated in the eastern United States. Some authors recommend collecting leaves at hand size, but this contradicts the science.

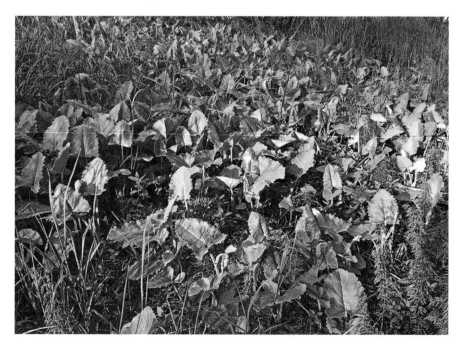

Coltsfoot leaf or root preparations will assist the body by inducing perspiration and relieving chest pain. It stimulates the lungs to expel phlegm and eases asthmatic wheezing with its antispasmodic action. Combined with sundew, it is useful in whooping cough, bronchitis, asthma, and other difficulties. It combines well with freeze-dried nettle leaf for relieving hay fever and allergic rhinitis.

It stimulates the immune system and fights infections of the bladder, on the skin, and, of course, in the lungs. Like its traditional use, coltsfoot root decoctions are helpful as a wash for external ulcers and chronically weeping wounds.

I personally prefer the fresh root tincture, but as mentioned, the flowers come well before the leaves. The best time to harvest is in fall when the leaves have turned dark, even after a bit of frost. The root is more pungent and bitter, but like the leaf, it is warm and drying.

The fresh leaves are applied to sprains and strains of the joints and ligaments. For dressing wounds and stopping bleeding, press the white underside of the leaf as a compress bandage to the affected area.

Petasin, a sesquiterpene of petasol and angelic acid, is the most active antispasmodic component. It suppresses a protein in the blood that plays a role in triggering bronchial spasms, according to Kahlee Keane (2012), also known as Root Woman, an accomplished Saskatchewan herbalist.

Research in Italy found *Petasites (officinalis)* active on stomach and biliary systems. Extracts show benefit for acute and chronic gastritis and biliary tract spasms, especially when there is cardiac involvement.

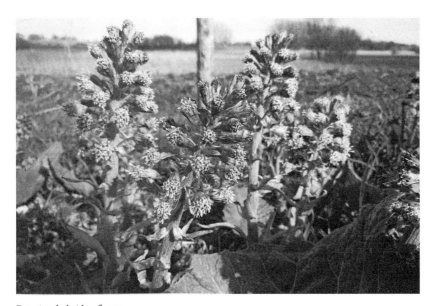

Petasites hybridus *flower*

Studies by Bickel et al. (1994) found isopetasin helps inhibit vasoconstrictive peptido-leukotrienes, validating traditional *Petasites* use for gastric and antispasmodic activity. Petasin is the most active spasmolytic agent in the plant and is fourteen times more effective than papaverine, an antispasmodic derived from opium.

The leaves can be smoked or combined with mullein leaves for respiratory problems. In fact, you can take a large leaf and extract the large thick stem and then roll it up like a cigar. In a dry climate this will dry through for a ready smoke in three or four months. Vaporizers work best for leaf powder.

Migraine-type headaches and lower back pain due to slipped discs have been treated successfully using fresh root extracts.

Studies on cancer patients show marked antitumor and analgesic effect.

Vogel (1986, 179) states that *Petasites hybridus* affects tumors strongly and yet is quite harmless: "Petasites is particularly beneficial in the fight against metastases, because it can prevent them."

One drop may give rise to a strong reaction in sensitive patients, especially those whose respiratory systems are affected. It is not widely known, due to U.S. Food and Drug Administration (FDA) and Health Canada regulations, but petasin is used in Germany for diabetes, prostate cancer, and menopause. The root will bring on delayed menses and relieve painful spasmodic dysmenorrhea. I have used it successfully in irritable bowel syndrome. I once treated a young woman for migraines associated with a long menstrual cycle and used it in a formula along with feverfew and crampbark. She was pleased on her next visit with her more normal cycle and relief of headaches and then revealed to me her long-standing issue with irritable bowel. After that, I began to see the pattern in other clients and found it useful not only in menstrual issues but lung issues such as asthma associated with skin eruptions appearing premenstrually. Chin-line acne was often resolved with simple supplementation of vitamin B_6 in many cases.

Taken as s warm decoction or root tincture dropped into hot water, it will promote sweating and expectoration, helping remove excess mucus from lungs. It combines well with mullein leaf and crampbark for asthma.

It may be useful in resolving eruptive fevers, according to Peter Holmes (1997, 162):

In many ways Butterbur root could substitute for the Chinese Hairy angelica root (Angelica Du Huo). Both share pungent, bitter, warm effective qualities and are used in lung wind cold conditions with headache, along the lines of acupuncture points LI 4, LU 7, GV 14 and 16, and Gb 21. Wind damp type neuralgias and myalgias will similarly benefit from Butterbur.

Zhi-Hong Wang et al. (2015) appear to validate Vogel's use in prostate cancer. Both S-petasin and iso-S-petasin induce apoptosis via the activation of mitochondria-related pathways in prostate cancer cells. A study by Adachi et al. (2014) appears to validate petasin as a compound that modulates glucose metabolism, suggesting use in type 2 diabetes.

In one randomized study utilizing 8 mg of petasin per tablet, a CO_2 extract of the root was found as effective for seasonal rhinitis as the antihistamine cetirizine, but without the sedative side effects (Schapowal 2002). A larger study of 330 patients at several participating clinics found butterbur and fexofenadine worked equally well for those suffering intermittent allergic rhinitis (Schapowal 2005). An extract with 25% petasins was given for eight weeks in doses from 50 to 150 mg in children and adults with asthma. Just 28% were being treated with corticosteroids, 53% with beta-agonists, and 19% with other medications.

In another study, the extract decreased the number, duration, and severity of asthma attacks. More than 40% reduced their asthma medication (D. K. Lee et al. 2004).

One interesting study of fifty-eight young children by Oelkers-Ax et al. (2008) looked at pediatric migraines and treatment with *Petasites*, music, and placebo. After an eight-week baseline, children received one of three methods, and follow-ups were conducted at eight weeks and then six months later. Post-treatment, only the music therapy was superior to placebo, whereas both music and *Petasites* were superior in the follow-up period. The style of music offered was not mentioned. It was probably not Led Zeppelin or AC/DC.

Weber & Weber, a German company, recently introduced a high-potency *Petasites* product to the North American market. It is specific for migraines, helping maintain proper muscle tone in cerebral blood vessels. A CO_2 extract was found superior to placebo in a clinical trial (Grossmann and Schmidramsl 2000).

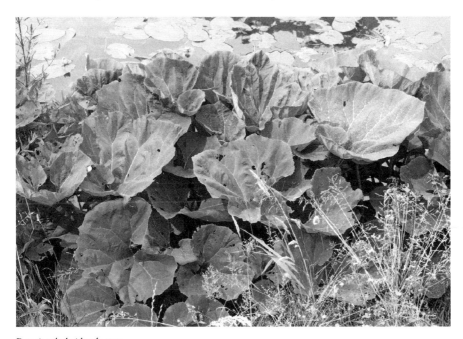

Petasites hybridus *leaves*

45

A large placebo-controlled randomized controlled trial (RCT) was conducted by Lipton et al. (2004) on 233 adults with episodic migraines. The group taking 75 mg twice daily had a reduction of migraine frequency of 45%. *Petasites* may be helpful for pediatric migraines, considering the significant side effects and questionable therapeutic value of other medications (Utterback et al. 2014).

According to the BGA (Federation of German Wholesale, Foreign Trade, and Services), the rootstock may be applied to acute convulsive pain in the abdomen. The daily administered dose must not contain more than one microgram of the PA alkaloids or alkaloid N-oxides and can only be taken for a duration of four to six weeks per year.

Petasin and isopetasin constituents are anti-inflammatory, antispasmodic, antihistaminic, and antidopaminergic in activity. Isopetasin inhibits synthesis of prostaglandins, which are important mediators of inflammatory response. Petasin appears to relax smooth muscles by inhibiting the intracellular release of calcium and is anti-inflammatory. It appears to have an affinity for blood vessels in the brain. Three clinical trials recorded a decrease in the number of migraine attacks per month, reduced symptoms, and diminished duration and intensity of pain. Petasin helps lower hypertension via vasorelaxation (Wang et al. 2010). The herb appears to affect peptido-leukotrienes, but not prostaglandins, with some gastrointestinal protection (Bickel et al. 1994). Extracts from *P. hybridus* inhibit airway hypersensitivity and production of Th2 cytokines IL-4 and IL-5 (Brattström et al. 2010). Benzofuran derivatives from the root modulate the immune system and show significant toxicity and induce apoptosis against MCF-7 breast cancer cell lines (Khaleghi et al. 2014; Soleimani et al. 2015).

The rhizome is approved in Germany for acute spasmodic pain associated with kidney stones and for an irritated urinary tract and as a muscle relaxant for the bladder. Weiss (1988, 91) was a pioneer in German herbal medicine. "The butterbur thus has completely new indications, primarily neurovegetative disorders affecting the stomach and biliary system, producing an 'irritable stomach' and biliary dyskinesia. It appears that this plant has particularly useful compensating, neurosedative, and at the same time, spasmolytic properties." He considered wormwood and butterbur a good combination for nerve and colic conditions. I agree.

Homeopathy

In my early days of clinical practice, I had access to the homeopathic product Petadolor from Europe. *Petasites (hybridus)* is a remedy that produces severe aggravation in those with cancerous growths and tumors. In homeopathy, this is a favorable sign, indicating its need. The mother tincture is not well tolerated, so higher potencies should be given. If the mother tincture is used, start with one drop in a glass of water and sip throughout the day. Increase as the body becomes accustomed. The mother tincture may be used in severe or obstinate neuralgia in the small of the back or down the loins. It may be used for pain in the frontal sinuses, and irritation of the urethra. It should be remembered in cases of spasmodic coughs, prostate inflammation, as well as orchitis and spermatic cord pain.

Renal and biliary colic may be present. The patient may have a disinclination to be spoken to, and in the evening when tired, voices seem unpleasantly loud. There may be a slight feeling of faintness. Profuse perspiration is suffered at night, and the supraorbital muscles feel as if drawn upward, especially with headaches located above the right eye.

Dizziness may be present in morning, with headache starting on the left side of head and then settling over the right eye. Soreness of the tip of tongue in morning may be present, and toothache is aggravated by cold water. There may be pain around pyloric valve, made worse from pressure, and the joints are stiff at night. Lumbar pain is worse upon rising from a seat.

Dose: 1st to 3rd potency. The mother tincture is prepared from the fresh root. Start with one drop in water. If the aggravation is too strong, dilute to 2X or even 3X. It will still work, but with less intense effects.

The first proving of *P. hybridus* was on six people with the tincture by Küchenmeister in 1847. Berridge self-experimented in 1865 with the tincture and added some additional indications.

Essential Oil

Constituents: root of *P. hybridus:* 0.1–0.4% essential oil composed of 1-nonene, eremophilone, and furanoeremophilone; petasyle and isopetasyle acetates and angelates; two lactone sesquiterpenes, eremophilanolide and furanophilanolide; and two sesquiterpenes, petasitene and pethybrene.

Eremophilone exhibits cytotoxicity against P388D1 mouse lymphoblast cells in vitro (Beattie et al. 2011). This compound is in a rare class of biologically active, bicyclic sesquiterpenoids.

The properties of the steam-distilled oil mirror those of the tincture. In France, *Petasites* oil is used for asthmatic crises and for asthmatic bronchitis. It combines antispasmodic and anticatarrhal properties, making the mucus more solvent. It is an ideal lung medicine.

Dose: Two to three drops in honey water, as needed. It may be diluted in carrier oil to a 5% dilution and rubbed into chest region, or in the case of menstrual cramps or neuralgia, applied to affected area.

Flower Essence

Coltsfoot is one of the first flower essences I ever produced. It is part of the Prairie Deva Flower Essence line. I believe its early spring appearance, up to one month before the leaves, gave me a strong inclination to study this amazing plant.

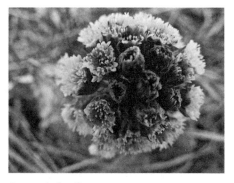

Sweet coltsfoot flower

Coltsfoot (*P. frigidus* ssp. *sagittatus*) flower essence may help us breathe deeply, ground our bodies, and subsequently gain perspective. Deep breathing helps us merge back into our own skins, release grief, and open to the present moment. Coltsfoot is an essence of orientation.

It is a good essence to take while meditating or planning, especially when making important decisions and learning to create priorities. The essence helps to heal old love wounds and clear traumatic emotions. When we are back on track to our true soul purpose, energy and optimism reemerge to guide the way.

Astrology

Ernst Michael Kranich (1984) looked at coltsfoot's astrological influence. The moon's influence remains very strong on the earliest of our composite plants, like the coltsfoot.... The shoots grow in the moist, often somewhat loamy soil as rhizomes.

RECIPES

Extract: Take 1 cup of fresh leaves to 2 cups water. Simmer slowly down to half. Add 2 teaspoons each of honey and vegetable glycerin. Stir well and store.

Dose: 1 teaspoon as needed.

Petasites extract: Standardized to 7.5 mg of petasin and isopetasin. 50–75 mg twice daily with meals. Use a lower dose for allergic rhinitis.

Tincture: *Petasites* rhizomes can spread up to forty feet or more. Wash carefully and use fresh for best medicine. Make a fresh leaf or fresh root tincture at 1:3 and 40% alcohol. The precipitate is largely inulin.

Dose: 1 teaspoon as needed, up to three or four times daily.

Mother tincture: Make 1:1 with fresh root and 60% alcohol. Use one drop in water and test reaction. Dilute more if necessary.

Fresh juice: *P. hybridus* plant juice is available commercially but can also be made from the fresh root and leaves.

Dose: 1 tablespoon every hour diluted 6 times in hot water.

Syrup: Slow simmer the fresh root in honey at 1:5 ratio at 80–90°F for 6 hours. Strain and use for respiratory conditions. Take 1 tablespoon as needed.

Caution: Due to the plant energetics, do not combine sweet coltsfoot with Goldthread. Avoid use in individuals with phase 2 liver detoxification problems. One study found hepatic toxicity when taken at 200 times the normal daily dose. Do not take during pregnancy or while nursing. Do not combine with anticholinergic drugs or herbs with similar action. May lower blood sugar and *may* interfere with anticoagulants. The aerial leaves from boreal forest contain pyrrolizidine alkaloids, similar to those found in comfrey. Long-term use is contraindicated. The root may contain PAs. Short-term use is suggested.

Birch

Paper Birch—*Betula papyrifera* Marsh.

Water Birch—*Betula occidentalis* Hook.

Bog or Dwarf Birch • Scrub Birch—*Betula glandulosa* Michx.

Swamp Birch—*Betula pumila* L.

> *Meanwhile the old men went on drinking mead and passed the Birch Bark snuff box to and fro.*
>
> —Pan Tadeusz

> *I was sitting on the lake and I took some bark off a birch tree. If I light it, the beaver smells it. It is going to swim to me. Even when we trap them, we put a piece of birch on the trap. I nail it there and if the beaver smells that, it has to come to that trap. So the best beaver food that I know of is birch.*
>
> —Victor Stewart

Birch is likely derived from the Anglo-Saxon *birk* or *bircha*, meaning "white" or "shining white." A more remote possibility is from the Sanskrit *bharg*, meaning "shining," or *bhurga*, meaning "a tree whose bark is used for writing upon." The whiteness is due to tiny grains of betulin, described below, found in the vacuoles of bark cells. In the Himalayas, the birch is worshipped as a radiant white goddess whose vehicle is a white swan. Saraswati, the Indian goddess of healers, singers, and scholars, corresponds, in some ways, with the Celtic goddess Brigit.

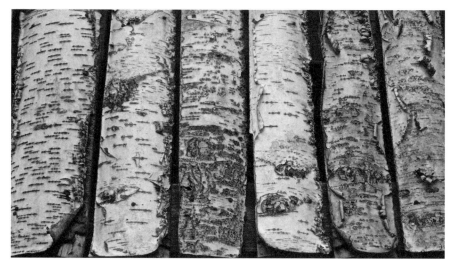

Birch logs

Another possibility of its origin is the Latin, *batuere*, "to strike," referring to the use of birch rods for punishment, or birching. This is based on driving out evil spirits and returning sanity to those who turned mad. Birch twigs were traditionally used to "beat the bounds" of a piece of land. In medieval times, birch rods were carried in front of the magistrate on his way into court as a symbol of authority and means of correction. Vermeulen and Johnston (2011) write:

> *Roman warriors used equal length white birch rods tied together with leather straps to form bundles called fasces. Since the end of the Roman Empire, numerous governments and other authorities have used the image of the fasces as a symbol of power. The most notable example was the Italian fascist movement, which derives its name from the fasces.*
>
> *Despite its recent unsavory associations, there are a surprising number of place having fasces symbols today. It can be seen in the President of the United States' Oval Office above the door leading to the exterior walkway and above the corresponding door on the opposite wall that leads to the President's private office. The fasces depicted have no axes. One of the most powerful embodiments of freedom, Abraham Lincoln sits in a chair comprising fasces in his monument in Washington, D.C. The official seal of the United States Senate has a pair of crossed fasces.*
>
> *This emblem remains on the front cover of French passports and as part of the French coat of arms. Both the Norwegian and Swedish police have double fasces in their logos. The coat of arms of Ecuador and Cameroon, the flag of Columbia, as well as the crests of several fraternities and political parties all contain fasces as symbols.*

Betula is derived from the Celtic *betu*, and may be related to the Anglo-Saxon *beorgan*, meaning "to protect or shelter." *Beith* is the first letter of the Druidic tree alphabet, and the sacred Beth of Cerridwen represents beginnings and births. *Beth*, in Hebrew, denotes two in kabbalah numerology. It stands for the power that "opens creation's process of taking form." *Beth*, *beith*, and *bith* correspond to meanings such as "world," "existence," and "enduring." The association with birth is obvious.

The whiteness of the bark suggested its connection with the White Goddess, who was both birth-giver and death-bringer, in her crone form as the carrion-eating white sow. The white bark denotes connection with the fairy realms. Brigid, the Irish goddess of returning light, is derived from the Sanskrit *bhereg*, meaning "wrapped in brilliance."

I first became familiar with paper birch during my first winter in a log cabin. They say firewood heats you up twice, once while cutting it and then again when it is burned. Up to this point I had used spruce for quick kindling for the woodstove, and burned well-seasoned alder and poplar for the larger overnight unit. That summer I cut down and split some larger birch from my quarter-section and let it dry. I was so impressed with the quiet, constant heat units of birch, I never considered another overnight fuel for my woodstove. I was fortunate to live on the south shore of Lesser Slave Lake, in northern Alberta, where paper birch towers over one hundred feet tall and two people can barely touch hands around the diameter at base.

Later, I learned that during World War II, these magnificent trees were cut into lumber to build Mosquito fighter planes. One day, a neighbor told me about making birch syrup. I sent away to a company in Quebec and bought some metal spiles. I already had lots of five-gallon white pails from the local fish plant, so I was ready that spring. It was early April, with snow still on the ground, but above freezing temperatures during the day. I tapped into the south side of five large birch trees within walking distance of my cabin.

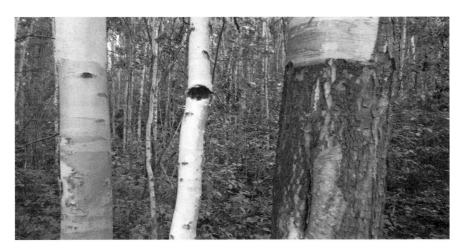

Birch of different ages

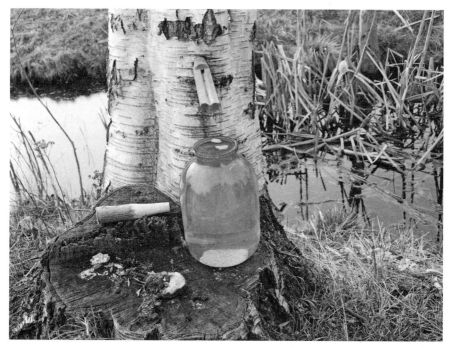

Birch sap collection

The next morning I was surprised to find them all half full of birch sap. I took a sip and enjoyed the flavor, slightly sweet with tinge of mineral aftertaste. The production was amazing. One morning I went out and the overnight flow of sap from one tree was nearly five gallons. But I was determined to make birch syrup, said to be comparable to maple syrup produced in Quebec and Vermont. Over the next ten days I would drag my cache of sap to the cabin and pour it into a large enamel pot on the woodstove. I moved it from direct heat to the far right of the stove to ensure a gentle boil. As I found out, it takes one hundred gallons of sap to produce less than two gallons of syrup. It was a lot of work, but well worth the effort.

Traditional Uses

I later learned that Russia produces over 3.7 million gallons of birch syrup a year that is sold in glass bottles for general consumption. Birch wine, *berëza*, is also popular in Russia. In China, birch juice is widely enjoyed, with birch syrup, birch cola, and birch honey peach products produced in Inner Mongolia. Products such as Birch Haw Drink and Senhua Champagne are exported to South Korea and Hong Kong.

On its own, birch sap is a rejuvenating springtime tonic, rich in vitamins and minerals. The Cree call the sap *waskwayiska*, using it to cleanse the body after a winter diet of meat and fat. To preserve it for later use, the sap was put into containers made from birch bark and the surface was covered with a layer of oil. The Cree of Alberta call it *waskwiyî* and used the bark traditionally for baskets, canoes, bowls, and moose callers.

The spring bark is easiest to work. It is cut to the proper shape and then bent and laced with the split root of black spruce. Birch bark has several layers that contain resin and will harden rather quickly. Charcoal and spruce sap is applied to the outside to complete the waterproof seal. If it will be used as a cooking pot for an open flame, the orange inner bark is on the outside, and the white outer bark is on the inside of the cooking vessel. If it will be used for cooking with hot rocks, this is less relevant.

The fall wood is used for making snowshoes and is good for dry snow. When the snow is wet, the shoes absorb too much moisture and become too heavy. Small-diameter trees with bark left on are ideal for files and other handles, as they do not split. Twigs are used for brooms.

Birch wood is used to make toboggans, drum frames, canoe paddles, and hide stretching racks. Moose calls from rolled birch have been found in Mesolithic North American caves. Mors Kochanski, my good friend, wears a birch bark hat that suits him well.

Some canoes could be made from a single piece of birch bark by folding and sewing it onto a frame of willow. Some canoes of the Athabaskans were so well constructed they could be dismantled and folded for portage around waterfalls.

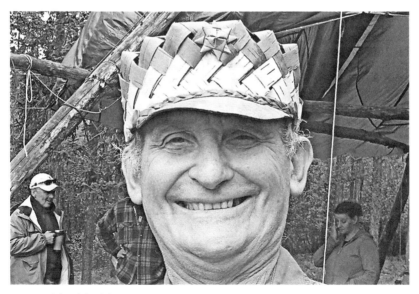

Mors with birch bark hat

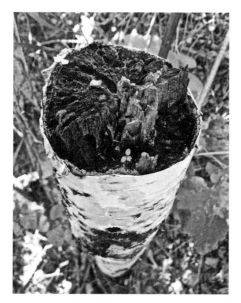

Rotten wood of birch

A beautiful art form I like to collect is birch bark biting, created by biting very thin, folded layers. These are truly mandalas of the woods, but making them is quickly becoming a lost art. Birch bark can also be used as an emergency eye protection from snow glare in winter, the natural slits or lenticels in the bark allow in enough visibility but cut out the most extreme brightness.

Another beautiful form of art is birch bark baskets embroidered with dyed porcupine quills. These are made while the bark is still wet so that the woven quills will be firmly set when everything dries. Birch bark can be tightly wrapped and tied with dogbane twine as a wilderness torch. It burns intensely and brightly, but be careful of any dropping ash.

The white and rotten wood was boiled with leaves of Labrador Tea by the Cree. This extract was dried and powdered and used as a dusting powder on chapped skin. The dry powdered rotten wood was used as baby powder. Rotten wood of birch, or white spruce, was valued for tanning hides, especially brain-prepared moose hide.

For gonorrhea, the buds were used, while for lung trouble, the bark infusions were combined with hemlock (spruce). The Secwepemc (Shuswap) of British Columbia steeped birch leaves in water as a shampoo and combined them with children's urine and alkali clay from certain lakes to make soap for washing the skin. The white papery bark makes a pleasant tea with a faint caramel flavor.

The Blackfoot call it *si ko ki ni* and used the paper birch for making bowls (rogans), utensils, and moose and elk calling cones. The Stl'atl'imx of British Columbia used birch bark funnels on food cache poles so that rodents could not pass. The Dene (Chipewyan) call birch trees *k'i*. They made ceremonial rattles by bending a strip of birch wood into a figure 9 and covering it with caribou hide and pebbles. This was called *deldhere*.

The leaves can be chewed and plastered on wasp stings. The buds can be mixed with lard or goose fat for skin sores and infections. The Cree of northern Manitoba collected birch bark from the east side of the tree and boiled it with another plant to help women who could not get pregnant. The Anishinaabe know paper birch as *nimishoomis-wiigwaas*.

Several herbalists have noted that placing birch posts at the perimeter of compost heaps seems to encourage a faster fermentation and breakdown of organic materials.

Scandinavians use wet birch twigs to gently whip the body in saunas. Some indigenous peoples place birch bark on hot rocks in sweats. The twigs make excellent chewing sticks for those attempting to quit smoking.

Medicinal Uses

Constituents: *B. papyrifera* leaf: polyphenols (9%), saponins, hyperosides, tannins, campesterol, beta-sitosterol, alpha- and beta-amyrin, salicylic acid, methyl esters, gallic acid, betulin ($C_{30}H_5O_2$), luteolin, quercetin, a whole range of bi- and tri-flavonoid procyanidins, xylitol, betulinic acid ($C_{30}H_{48}O_3$—up to 0.3%), sakuranetin, dammarane triterpenoid esters, essential oils, ascorbic acid, and minerals. Dry leaf contains up to 23% protein.

Bark: betulin (10–30%), betulinic acid, lupeol, allobetulin, betulinic aldehyde, oleanolic acid, erythrodiol, ursolic acid; various acyclic diarylheptanoids, including papyriferoside A, 5-O-beta-D-apiofuranosyl-(1>2)-beta-D-glucopyranosyl-1,7-bis-(4-hydroxyphenyl)-heptan-3-one, platyphylloside, aceroside VII, and 1,7-bis-(4-hydroxyphenyl)-4-hepten-3-one; phenolics including chavicol-4-O-alpha-L-arabinofuranosyl (and apiofuranosid)-(1>6)-beta-D-glucoside; (+)catechin 7-O-beta-D-xylopyranoside and nudiposide.

Inner bark oil: trans alpha-bergamotene (18%), ar-curcumene (12%), E-beta-farnesene (12%), Z-beta-farnesene (10%), and cis-alpha-bergamotene (8%).

Twig bark: (+)-catechin-7-beta-D-xylopyranoside.

Total flavonoids average about 3% in young leaves. The seeds contain about 12% protein and 19% fat. The sap contains 49% fructose, 35% glucose, xylitol, and 15% sucrose. It contains 0.5–2% glycosides and trace minerals, particularly potassium 124.8 ppm, manganese 21.7 ppm, zinc 2.05 ppm, and magnesium 120 ppm, as well as small amounts of copper and iron. Spring sap contains myo-inositol, a sweetener used by animals and microorganisms as a growth factor. It contains 17 amino acids, including glutamic acid.

B. pumila: paperyferic acid, deacetoxy-paperyferic acid, dammar-24-ene-12b-O-acetyl-20(S)-ol-3-one.

Bud exudate: acacetin.

Birch sap strengthens the immune system and encourages the body's ability to heal. It is a safe, general tonic for the body that can also be applied as a wash for eczema or even to the scalp to remove dandruff.

Birch leaves and buds can be used as a hot infusion in the treatment of headaches and rheumatic pain. This is in part due to the anti-inflammatory effect of the methyl salicylate common as well to poplar and willow. A tincture of birch buds was found to provide good results in 108 patients with purulent wounds (Zakharov et al. 1980).

Birch bud tincture, taken cold, helps reduce the size and congestion of swollen lymph glands. Combine with cleavers and/or *pipsissewa* for neck, breast, and underarm congestion and with ocotillo for pelvic lymphatic swellings. Combine with nettle leaf for more chronic conditions.

For lipomas, combine birch leaf and chickweed, along with lipase enzymes taken on an empty stomach between meals. The birch juice, derived from fresh birch leaves, is an efficient blood cleanser, with a stimulating effect on the kidneys. It offers relief in the treatment of rheumatic and other swollen, inflamed conditions.

Birch sap is used in cosmetics for astringent action on the skin and could be added to soaps, shampoos, and balms for sore lips by creative manufacturers. Various shampoos for thinning hair use birch extracts, including the commercial product Prograine.

Birch leaf juice reduces the protein content of urine and promotes elimination of uric acid, a contributing factor in gout and kidney stone formation. Work by Havlik et al. (2010) identified birch as having high xanthine oxidase activity, a scientific measure of gout inhibition. Paper birch showed activity against a number of bacteria and fungi in recent work by Vandal et al. (2015).

Early herbalists attributed the diuretic effect to betulin, a terpenic alcohol. Weiss noted that although not a true diuretic, birch seems to have the ability to remove purines from the body. This would certainly explain its excellent results in gout, water retention, and other rheumatic conditions. Taken as a hot tea, the leaf will induce diaphoresis, so the tea is taken best cool.

Hyperoside, a flavonoid, is today recognized as an important active principle. A higher level of total flavonoids, however, is found in younger leaves. Studies by Keinänen and Julkunen-Titto (1996) indicate flavonoid glycosides of birch are highest in the fresh leaves, indicating a preference for fresh plant juices or tinctures. The leaves are gathered when young and in the morning while retaining their essential oils. Dry on shaded, well-ventilated screenings.

Michael Moore (2003, 53) writes, "A cup of tea a day will help wheezy and irritated bronchial mucosa during the winter, the kind of chronically impaired breathing you get from too much wood smoke, too much dry forced air … and general lung grunge."

The wet, internal side of fresh birch bark gives quick external relief to rheumatic pain.

When decocted, the fresh birch bark turns a beautiful rose color. The water is strained and used as a fomentation for skin rash, dermatitis, cradle cap, and on the elderly suffering paper-thin skin. Birch bark extracts exhibit significant wound healing efficacy (Ebeling et al. 2014).

Early Ukrainian settlers in Alberta decocted birch bark and then added a small amount of vinegar as a liniment for aching muscles. Birch leaves and branches were decocted and added to bathwater for painful cramping and twisting in different parts of the body. Decoctions of birch and aspen poplar bark, together, were used for hypertension. Internally, when cooled, the inner bark decoction will help resolve boils. Taken cold, before bedtime, it will help relieve night sweats.

The bark is more active on the liver, and the leaves on the kidneys, but they work well together. Biliary congestion is relieved, especially when combined in equal parts with black currant leaf and Oregon grape root. When bark and leaves are combined, the tea is a mild sedative and diuretic, very good for treating anxiety related to PMS and to calm sciatic pain.

The Tsilhqot'in and other Athabaskans used the flexible stems of water birch (*B. occidentalis*) to manufacture baby-carrying frames. Water birch roots were decocted by the Niimíipu (Nez Perce) as a general tonic as well as steam for fevers. The tea was taken internally for sore throats, stomachache, and such.

Swamp birch branches were placed among spruce boughs by the Gwichin of the Mackenzie Delta to keep the flooring in tents fresh smelling. The Dena'ina and others used leafy branches of swamp birch for padding on their backs when carrying meat or an underlay for cutting meat and fish.

Swamp birch female cones were dried and burned on coals by Makandwewininiwag (Pillager band of Chippewa people). This incense helped relieve catarrh and pulmonary complaints. A tisane from the same cones was used as an after-birth tonic, or to relieve painful menses. Acacetin, from the cones, was found to improve asthma symptoms in a mouse model (Huang and Liou 2012). The compound shows activity against lung cancer in several additional animal studies.

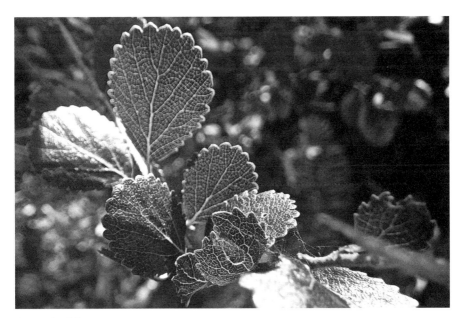

Swamp birch leaves

Acacetin inhibits amyloid precursor protein associated with Alzheimer's disease (Xue Wang et al. 2015). Acacetin induces apoptosis of oral squamous carcinoma cell lines, suggestive of cancer inhibition (C. D. Kim et al. 2015). Acacetin is found in safflower seeds and other plants and flowers. The compound was rediscovered in the herb damiana by J. Zhao et al. (2008) when studying anti-aromatase activity. Acacetin showed potent aromatase inhibition in the manner of chrysin, derived from poplar catkins. Aromatase inhibitors are used to treat hormone-sensitive cancers.

Swamp birch (*B. pumila*) cones, fresh or dried, can be set on low coals and the smoke inhaled for severe and chronic sinus inflammations. It is sometimes difficult, at first glance, to distinguish between bog and swamp birch. Generally, swamp birch is taller, up to 2–3 meters, while scrub birch may reach 150 cm. They both contain resin glands, but swamp birch leaves have a very distinct reddish tinge on the underside. Bog or scrub birch produce cones in the fall that were combined with Labrador Tea by the Cree of Alberta for treating pneumonia. The tree is known as *apstewaskwei*, according to Cree healer Russell Willier.

The twig tips can be decocted to stop both internal and external bleeding. The Dene (Chipewyan) call the shrub *intanbandhaze*, "little round leaf," and the Dene Tha (Slavey) *di bili di yoseti*, meaning "spruce grouse eat." The name bog birch is unfortunate, as the shrub is rarely found in bogs, and more often indicative of fen-like situations, black spruce swamps, and alpine slopes.

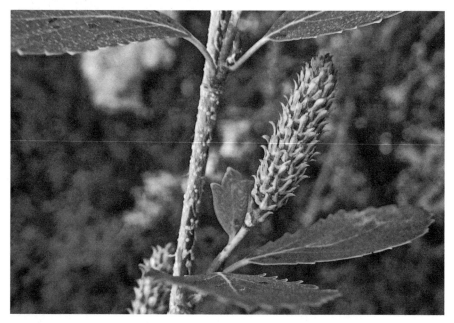

Dwarf birch

Dwarf Birch (*B. glandulosa*) is known to the Inuit of West Greenland as *avaalaqiat*, related to the word *avaaq*, meaning "back of the head." In Nunavik it is used for cooking and bedding and to make fishing spears.

The cones of *B. pumila* were heated over coals by the Ojibwe as a smoke for catarrhal patients. They brewed cone infusions for relief of menstruation, and to give strength during or after childbirth. The Meskwaki (Fox) steeped the tiny cones as a tea for new mothers, or for difficult menstrual periods. *Meskwaki* means "red earth people," probably based on the use of ocher on the skin to prevent insect bites.

Taxonomically, *B. glandulosa* and *B. nana* are both known as dwarf birch, but the latter is very small and has no resinous glands.

Birch contains xylitol, which has been used as a sweetener since 1975, after Finnish research showed it reduced cavities. Xylitol is derived naturally in various fruits and fibrous vegetables, or hardwood like birch, and is produced by the human body during normal metabolism. At one time in Russia xylitol was used as a raw material for the production of ascorbic acid. Unlike six-carbon sugars, xylitol is a five-carbon sugar that is not converted to acids by oral bacteria. It has 40 percent fewer calories and does not affect blood sugar fluctuations. It is sometimes produced from corncobs (GMO?) through catalyzation and hydrogenation, and sometimes through fermentation with *Candida* yeast species. Xylitol is used as a moisture-retaining agent in cosmetics, toothpastes, alkyd resins, surfactants, and plasticizers.

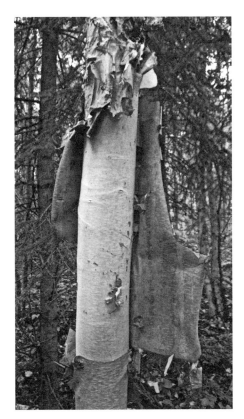

Studies by Matti Uhari (2000) at the University of Oulu in Finland have shown regular doses of xylitol in chewing gum cut chronic ear infections in children by up to 50 percent. Xylitol inhibits plaque and dental caries by 80 percent, relieves dry mouth, protects salivary protein, retards demineralization of tooth enamel, and reduces nasopharynx and mouth infections. Xylitol helps reduce the acid damage to teeth of individuals suffering bulimia. A spray containing xylitol for sneezing allergies has recently hit the market. Xylitol is toxic to dogs.

Birch bark peeling

The bark of the birch contains betulinic acid, an active ingredient showing promise in treating melanoma in vitro and in vivo without toxic effect. Betulinic acid is active against malignant brain tumors and possesses anti-HIV, anti-inflammatory, antitumor, antiviral, and anticarcinoma activity. Betulinic acid is believed to down-regulate the mutant p53 suppressor gene responsible for allowing proliferation of oncogenes (Pisha et al. 1995). In other words, betulinic acid promotes tumor cells to self-destruct or commit self-programmed death, or apoptosis (Fulda et al. 1997). Cancer cells treated with betulinic acid show enhanced mitochondrial membrane damage leading to apoptosis (Fulda et al. 1999). Recent work by the same author suggests use of betulinic acid against a variety of human cancer cell lines (Fulda and Kroemer 2009). Birch bark standardized extracts of 160 mg daily were given to 42 patients with chronic hepatitis C for twelve weeks. Fatigue and abdominal were pain reduced sixfold and asparate aminotransferase by 54% (Shikov et al. 2011). The extract contained 75% betulin and 3.5% betulinic acid. Betulin has been found to activate GABA(A) receptor sites, suggesting use in anxiety or depressive mental states (Muceniece et al. 2008).

C. J. Lee et al. (2004) found betulin stimulates mucin release by directly acting on airway mucin-secreting cells, suggesting the use of birch bark decoction in chronic respiratory disease. Betulin lowers cholesterol by blocking a pathway and may help fight obesity and related metabolic disease. Betulin targets the sterol regulatory element binding proteins, a transcription factor important in the expression of genes involved in the production of cholesterol, fatty acids, and triglycerides. Betulin made mice more sensitive to insulin and reduced atherosclerotic plaques (Tang et al. 2011).

Cyclodextrin-solubilized triterpenoid extracts from birch bark have shown activity against 42 human tumor cell lines at very low doses (Hertrampf et al. 2012). New studies suggest it may attenuate kidney, lung, and liver injury, albeit in rat studies. Betulinic acid kills colon cancer stem cells, at least in vitro. Birch bark, betulin, and betulinic acid show promise against stomach and pancreatic cancer cell lines that are drug-sensitive and drug resistant (Drag et al. 2009).

Let us recap: betulin possesses antitumor, antiviral, antidepressant, hepato-protective, expectorant, anti-inflammatory, cholagogue, and antimalarial properties, while betulinic acid is antitumor, antibacterial, antiprotozoal, antiviral, and anti-inflammatory.

Platyphylloside, isolated from the inner bark of paper birch, is strongly cytotoxic (Mshvidadze et al. 2007). One diarylheptanoid in paper birch, 1,7-bis-(4-hydroxyphenyl)-5-hepten-3-one, shows therapeutic potential against liver fibrosis (Lee et al. 2012). Another compound, nudiposide, shows protection against glutamate-induced neurotoxicity in HT22 cells in vitro (Lee et al. 2015).

Lupeol, a lupine-type triterpene in birch bark, inhibits melanoma cancer cell lines (Hata et al. 2000). It shows potential against prostate cancer and reduces skin cancer cell proliferation. Its great advantage is significant anti-inflammatory potential with no toxicity to normal cells. Lupeol reduces oxalate kidney stone formation, inhibits cold sore (herpes simplex) replication, reduces inflammation, and modulates immune function. Lupeol shows remarkable activity against MRSA in another study (El Sayed et al. 2016).

Birch bark extracts betulin and lupeol influence skin wound healing in diabetic donors. Poor circulation and difficult-to-treat foot and leg sores are a major concern in diabetes, often leading to amputation (Wardecki et al. 2016). Lupeol shows strong inhibition of osteoclast differentiation and bone loss. It may be useful for osteoporosis, Paget's disease, osteolysis associated with periodontal disease, as well as multiple myeloma (Im et al. 2016).

Rheumatoid arthritis patients have lower levels of kynurenic acid in synovial fluid around the joints. A study by Zgrajka et al. (2013) found birch leaves contain high levels of this metabolite of kynurenine, which is antioxidant, analgesic, and anti-inflammatory. Other herbs with high levels of this compound are peppermint, stinging nettle, and horsetail.

Birch inner bark has been traditionally applied to teenage acne, reducing the sebum production of skin pores. The birch doctrine of signatures lies in its skin-like layers of bark, indicating its affinity for human skin conditions. This follows anthroposophic medicine in corresponding the dry, hard, mineralized bark to human skin and sclerosis. Rudolf Steiner discerned a somewhat similar duality of process in the life of the birch:

> *On the one hand, there is the concentration of vegetable proteins in the young leaves of the birch, the enfoldment of which in the spring he saw as a "vegetable reflection" of the processes at work in young human beings; on the other, there is a demineralization process—analogous to that which takes place at the level of the skin in man and woman—which results in the bark of the tree containing comparatively high concentrations of potassium salts.*
>
> *The functional polarity between bark and young leaf manifests itself in all trees, but is most marked in the birch. As a consequence of this it is held remedies derived from birch bark, which so efficiently carries out a vegetable demineralizing process, are often effective against the sclerotic, hardening, processes which, at the level of the skin, manifest as dry dermatoses such as psoriasis.*
>
> *Conversely remedies derived from the young leaves of the tree may be prescribed … for the treatment of wet skin complaints such as weeping eczema.*
>
> *Therefore birch bark extracts are not invariably administered to sufferers from sclerotic, dry skin dermatoses, or leaf extracts to those patients who have wet skin disorders. (Felter and Lloyd 1898)*

Recent work by Martin et al. (2012) looked closely at the potential of oleanolic acid and erythrodiol, two compounds in birch bark. They found both triterpenes restrict the development of autoimmune encephalomyelitis (multiple sclerosis) by switching cytokine production toward a Th2 profile, with lower levels of Th1 and Th17. Earlier work by Freysdottir et al. (2011) found ethanol extracts of birch bark suppress human-dendritic-cell-mediated Th1 response with increased IL-10 and IL-17 increased response. This suggests an immune modulating effect.

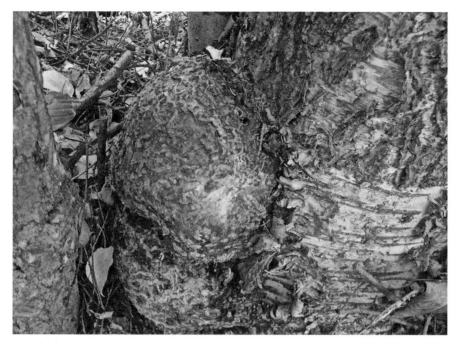

Birch burl

Erythrodiol promotes apoptosis and arrests breast cancer cell growth (Sanchez-Quesada et al. 2015). Earlier work by Manayi et al. (2013) found the compound active against colon carcinoma and 6.4 times more selective than methotrexate (positive control). This compound is also present in purple loosestrife aerial parts and olive leaves.

Birch bark standardized extract ointments are effective in the treatment of actinic keratoses based on a study of 28 patients in a prospective nonrandomized pilot study. Half were treated with birch ointment and other half a combination of cryotherapy and ointment. Clearing of more than 75% of lesions was found in 79% of patients treated with birch bark ointment, and the combined therapy response was 93% (Huyke et al. 2006).

An excellent review of the *Betula* genus use in medicine was recently written by Rastogi et al. (2015).

Personality Traits

Vermeulen and Johnston (2011) contribute:

> *Betulaceae's special aptitude is to perceive the potential of prosperity and vitality in what appears to all others to be perpetually desolate, barren, and discarded. Betulaceae are undeterred by harsh, depleted, and adverse conditions.*

In fact, they even excel when having to work hard with few resources. These new endeavors seeking individuals explore new realms and embrace new beginnings as the world's pioneers, trailblazers, and groundbreakers.... What distinguishes this family most is that they take the depleted and replenish it.... Tough conditions toughen their resolve and resourcefulness. Their groundbreaking labor appears to be generous, caring, and benevolent because it helps the less hearty or entrepreneurial to follow their successes with relative ease.

Sporting the scars of overcoming a harsh life, one experiences an inner transformation. The regeneration, cleansing, and healing casts a lightness, serenity, and grace equally renew as a springtime breeze.

Harry Van Der Zee writes:

There is the idea of rejuvenating power, of cleansing, blessing, comforting, and healing. The idea of a child bringing joy into the life of the old and of a young person who brings life-force and a refreshing light into the life of the sick. Betula seems to represent a young, female energy.... In society, we find the image of the nurse who lightens the burdens of the sick and the old … just like a nurse who will not bother the disabled person with her own complaints. She will hide herself behind her white apron and put on her professional smile. On a physical level we may expect Betula to be indicated in cases of loss of too much fluid, like polyuria or menorrhagia, with symptoms of weariness and depletion. (Vermeulen and Johnston 2011, 946)

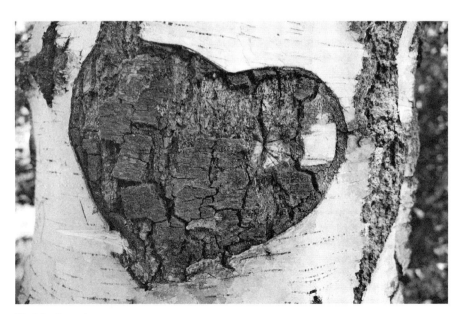

Birch bark carving

Essential Oil

Fifteen years ago I became chairman of the Alberta Natural Health Agricultural Network, a group of entrepreneurs who received government assistance to build a portable distillation unit. In the first year after construction, over seventy plants were harvested, distilled, and sent to Quebec for analysis.

Birch bark essential oil, which is hydro-distilled, was briefly discussed and dismissed as a market opportunity. Nearly all the "birch" oil on the aromatherapy market is cheap, synthetic methyl salicylate, which makes up 98.9% of the natural essential oil. Minor amounts of ethyl salicylate and linalyl acetate are present, but the average person cannot tell the difference. It is toxic and should be used with care, even externally.

Birch tar is produced by destructive distillation of bark and wood. The main constituents are guaiacol and cresol. The latter compound is prohibited in cosmetic products in Canada.

The hydrosol, or water left over from distillation, is anti-inflammatory, astringent, antiseptic, and toning. It may be a useful sunscreen spritzer, like fireweed, used before or after sun exposure. It has a distinct wintergreen scent that is well known. One fun thing I discovered is that crunching on wintergreen Life Saver in a dark closet will sent florescent green sparks flying from the mouth. It is worth doing once.

Bits and Pieces

Birch pollen is second only to grass pollens as a major spring source of rhinitis, asthma, and other sensitivities. Cross-reactions with various fruits and vegetables may cause oral allergy syndrome and exaggerate atopic eczema. Apples, almonds, cherries, pears, peaches, plums,

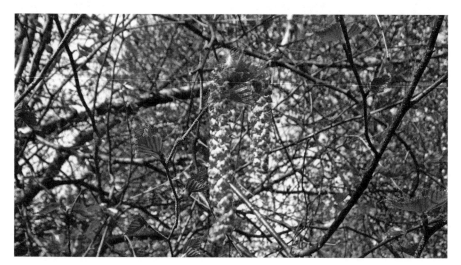

Birch pollen

oranges, kiwis, walnuts, carrots, celery, fennel, parsnip, and hazelnuts are the major cross-reactive allergies. Hazelnut also produces pollen that rivals the irritability of birch. A British study relates childhood bed-wetting with hazelnut and soy food allergies. Work by Sénéchal et al. (1999) found 70% of patients allergic to birch pollen are hypersensitive to fruits, especially apples. Some 16% of Swedes are allergic to birch pollen, posing a significant health risk.

Sancho et al. (2006) found allergies to a variety of fruits, including apples, pears, cherries, and plums, as well as vegetables such as celery, potatoes, and carrots, and nuts such as hazelnuts and walnuts are associated with allergies to birch pollen. Pollen production is highest in late afternoon, but very low between midnight and early morning.

Medicinal Mushrooms

Birch trees host four important medicinal mushrooms, but you will rarely find any two on the same tree. Chaga *(Inonotus obliquus)* is very popular at the present time and has a lot of anecdotal and empirical evidence for its use in chronic health conditions, including cancer. One of my main concerns with chaga is sustainability. The sterile conk is being widely harvested and utilized in an inappropriate manner. Unlike other polypores, the sterile conk does not reproduce. Only at the last stages of life, when the birch is finally succumbing to old age, do microscopic fruiting bodies appear for a day or two. If the spores from these rare mushrooms drift into the crevice of an adjacent birch, there will be an infection and the organism's life continues.

If all the sterile conks are harvested in an area, then the odds of survival are greatly reduced. They can be more plentiful where found on birch, but only one in 20,000 trees

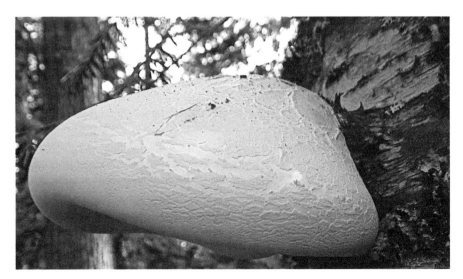

Birch Polypore (Polyporus betulinus)

65

will have a sterile conk. The sterile conk requires decoction and, perhaps, fermentation to become a useful health product. Sprinkling a bit of dried powder on top of a coconut cream whip or an organic mocha latte does nothing but waste a valuable resource.

Two birch polpores were found on the clothing of Ötzi, the Iceman. His six-thousand-year-old intact body was exposed by a retreating Swiss Alpine glacier some twenty-five years ago. He had a piece of the annual birch polypore (*Polyporus betulinus*), which was

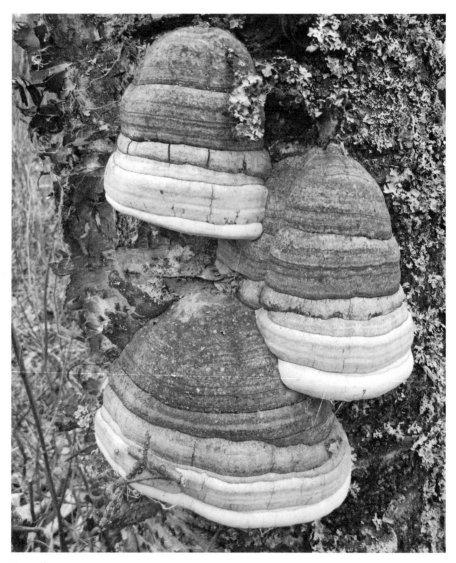

Fomes fomentarius

possibly used as a pad for making fire with a bow drill. Early speculation around its use as parasiticide is doubtful. Recent studies suggest strong angiotensin-converting enzyme (ACE) inhibition in cardiovascular problems and antimicrobial activity against highly resistant *Enterococcus faecalis* (Vunduk et al. 2015).

The third polypore, the false tinder conk *(Fomes fomentarius)*, was present as a dung water prepared context, carved from under the surface. This served as a medium to accept a spark or friction fire heat to begin smoldering. The context was widely used to make vests and hats, or today, to dry fly fishing lures. I have a hat, made in Romania, prepared from this mushroom, given to me by Solomon Wasser, editor in chief of *The International Journal of Medicinal Mushrooms.*

The dried polypore was used by the Cree of Northern Canada to carry smoldering coals so that a campfire could be easily started after a journey. It was also tossed into soups and stews, serving two purposes: it is highly antibacterial and helps prevent salmonella and listeria spoiling food undergoing alternating hot and cold conditions; and during boiling, the mushroom released polysaccharides and oligosaccharides into the food, helping optimize immune function during the cold winter months.

Research has found several hospital-acquired drug-resistant bacteria, *Klebsiella pneumoniae* and *Serratia marcescens*, are strongly inhibited by this medicinal mushroom.

Iqmik *(Phellinus igniarius)* also lives on birch. It is widely harvested in Yukon and Alaska and reduced to ash under anaerobic conditions. This ash is added to tobacco to help deliver nicotine more quickly and efficiently to the brain. It has a number of medicinal uses, including significant activity against various cancer cell lines as well as

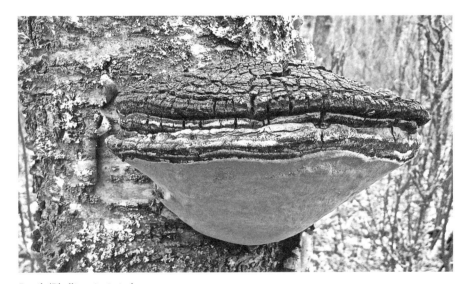

Iqmik (Phellinus igniarius)

influenza A and B, H1N1, H3N2, H9N2, and relief of symptoms associated with multiple sclerosis (MS).

Years ago, I read that Highland Birchwoods in Scotland was growing shiitake mushrooms on birch. I have since trialed it in northern Canada on paper birch, and the much desired edible and medicinal mushroom really enjoys eating birch. It also likes alder and oak, but alas, we have few of the latter tree growing in my part of the world.

Considerably more information on these mushrooms and some two hundred others can be found in my publication *The Fungal Pharmacy: The Complete Guide to Medicinal Mushrooms and Lichens of North America* (2011).

Myths and Legends

Diane Ferguson (2001) recorded this older legend about birch. The Penobscot people tell a story of a young woman who was to marry one man while loving another. In the weeks before the wedding she grew more and more despairing, and people sat and prayed with

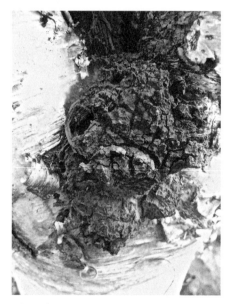 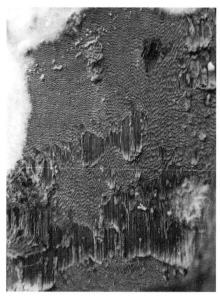

Chaga (Inonotus obliquus)

Chaga fruiting body (courtesy of Lawrence Millman)

her to no avail. Finally, the conjure man was sent, but she had already decided that death would be preferable. When she died it broke the spirit of the man she loved, and he too grew sick and died. The conjure man felt sorry and made a gift to the couple, turning them both into birch trees, standing side by side. This is why, when you walk the woods, you'll find birch trees growing together as a pair, and smaller ones clustered around, the children of the lovers from long ago.

An old legend from Czech Republic goes like this: A shepherdess sat at the edge of a grove of birch trees spinning flax into linen thread. Suddenly a strange women dressed in white appeared before her.

"Do you like to dance?" she asked.

"I'd like to dance the whole day," said the shepherdess, "but my mother has given me all this flax to spin."

"Tomorrow is another day," said the woman, and away they whirled and danced.

This was repeated for several days, with the women waving her hands and spinning the flax into fine linen thread. The days passed, and one day, after dancing, the woman placed some golden birch leaves in the shepherdess's apron and then disappeared. The girl returned home, gave her mother the thread, and told her of the woman.

"It was the wild woman of the birch wood," exclaimed the mother.

"She said my dancing pleased her, and she gave me these birch leaves," said the young woman with a laugh. But when she emptied her pockets, she found the leaves had turned to solid gold.

This Siberian legend was preserved: On a high hill grows a giant birch. The roots spread underground to surround the earth and the branches surround the heavens. At the base of the birch is a spring, roofed over with white sheets of birch bark. On the edge is a birch wood container. In this is a ladle of silvery birch bark. On the bottom of the ladle is a decoration of the sun and the moon. As the sun moves through the heavens, the ladle turns with it. They say that if you fill the container from the spring, and dip into it the ladle and drink deeply, you will live forever, as this is the water of life.

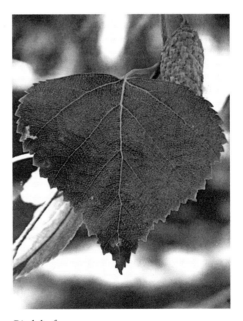

Birch leaf

RECIPES

Birch sap: To collect sap, it is necessary to drill a ½-inch hole 2 inches deep on the south side of the tree. Drill into large trees only, at a slight upward angle. In Alberta, the sap can begin to flow in early April and as late as mid-May. Metal taps can be purchased, or you can use elder stems. Tap them into place and attach five-gallon buckets. In the height of the harvest you may collect up to 5 gallons daily, up to 75 gallons per season, from a large tree. This sap may be drunk fresh or frozen or preserved for medicinal usage. For the latter, combine sap with 96% alcohol at an 8:2 ratio. Standard dose for diuretic and other benefit is 1 cup daily (*French Pharmacopoeia* 1998).

Birch syrup: Filter the sap through cheesecloth. Place it in a large pot on the stove and bring it to a boil. It creates a lot of humidity indoors and probably should be made outside. As soon as it thickens, move it to low heat. Be careful not to burn it at the final stage. At the desired consistency, bottle and store it in the refrigerator. Freeze any extra. It is tedious, taking up to 100 gallons of sap to produce 2 gallons of syrup.

Birch beer: Take 4 gallons of sap and boil for 10 minutes. Remove from the heat and add 1 gallon of honey. Put 4 quarts of birch budding twigs into this and allow it to cool down to 70°F. Strain into a fermenting vessel and add good yeast. Allow to work until fermentation is complete. Then bottle by priming with ½ teaspoon sugar, and cap. It's ready in 10–14 days (Buhner 1998). A simpler recipe involves throwing a handful of corn into a jug of sap and allowing fermentation.

Birch sap wine: Take 12 parts birch sap and 1 part honey. Combine in a double boiler and heat to 105°F. Then add a muslin bag containing brewer's yeast. Allow this to ferment for two weeks at room temperature. Rack off and age for up to two years. An excellent hair lotion for redheads and blonds is made by combining birch leaf and twig infusion with one-tenth part of birch sap wine.

Birch tea: Put a small handful of the fresh young buds and leaves into 2 cups of boiling water and steep for 20 minutes. Drink 1–3 cups daily. Add ½ teaspoon sodium bicarbonate to infusions for a better effect. Dried leaves can be used as well.

Birch bark decoction (for melanoma): Bring 1 quart of water to boil and add 1 heaping cup of birch shavings. Simmer for 4 minutes, remove from the heat, and steep for 40 minutes more. Drink 3 cups daily on an empty stomach. Birch bark is most easily gathered in early spring when the sap is flowing, and close to a full moon.

Tincture (best from buds): 1 teaspoon three times daily. Make 1:5 tincture at 70% alcohol.

Tincture of buds, leaves, and bark: 1 teaspoon three times daily. Make a fresh tincture of 3 parts leaf, 2 parts bud, and 1 part birch bark by weight, combined with 20 parts of 40% alcohol. Let sit for two weeks, then strain. Another option is to take the birch bark decoction above, add leaves and buds after simmering, and combine 1:1 with 60% alcohol. An apple cider vinegar extraction of the fresh leaves is good for bone and immune health; use the same ratios.

Birch bark powder capsules: The bark is ground to a fine powder and placed in 00 size capsules. Take two capsules up to three times daily. In Finland, the birch bark is turned to ash and then capsuled for medicine.

Birch juice: May be made fresh or bought commercially. 1 tablespoon is taken three times daily.

Betulin extraction: A 23% yield of betulin can be achieved with ultrasonic extraction of birch bark. Use 96% alcohol at a ratio of 1 part bark to 42 parts solvent at 122°F for three hours at 5 kHz vibration.

Birch leaf ointment: Cover 12-hour-wilted birch leaves with canola or olive oil in large jar. Let stand in a warm spot for two weeks. Strain and filter. This is excellent when combined with balsam poplar bud oil 2:1 for rheumatic and arthritic pain of joints and muscles. Use a crock pot in cooler climates, using low temperature for 6 hours or more.

Bath: Take 2 pounds of birch leaves and twigs and simmer in water for up to 20 minutes. Strain and add to a hot bath for rheumatic and urinary complaints.

Caution: Potentiation of warfarin was found in eleven patients concurrently using an ointment containing methyl salicylate. Some bleeding events took place in four people. In one case, pro-thrombin time doubled after using the ointment on arthritic joints. Natural or synthetic methyl salicylate may affect vitamin K metabolism or displace warfarin from protein binding sites; this is speculative (Brinker 2010, 58–59).

Birch oil is contraindicated during pregnancy and breastfeeding. Individuals with sensitivity to salicylates should be cautious. According to Robert Tisserand, this often applies to people with ADD/ADHD. It is also contraindicated in gastroesophageal reflux disease (GERD).

The maximum level for methyl salicylate in topical products in Canada is 1%.

Poplar

Black Poplar • Balsam Poplar—*Populus balsamifera* L. • *P. balsamifera* var. *balsamifera*

Balm of Gilead Poplar—*Populus candicans* Aiton • *P. tacamahaca* Mill. • *P. balsamifera* L. var. *candicans* (Ait.) A. Gray

Black Cottonwood—*Populus trichocarpa* Torrey & Gray ex Hook. • *P. balsamifera* L. ssp. *trichocarpa* (Torrey. & Gray) Brayshaw

Trembling Aspen • Aspen Poplar—*Populus tremuloides* Michx.

Cottonwood • Plains Cottonwood—*Populus deltoides* W. Bartram ex Marshall • *P. deltoides* ssp. *monilifera* (Ait.) Eckenwalder

Narrow-Leaved Cottonwood—*Populus angustifolia* E. James

He spake, and, trembling like an aspen-bough,
Began to tear his scroll in pieces small …

—John Keats

The Poplar is a French tree
A tall and laughing wench tree
A slender tree, a tender tree,
That whispers in the rain.

—Christopher Morley

O'er all the giant poplars, which maintain
Equality with clouds halfway up Heaven,
Which whisper with the winds none else can see,
And bow to angels as they wind by them.

—Philip James Bailey

My early exposure to poplar in northern Alberta was colored by local residents' dismissal of it as a wood with little heating value. This is not really true, especially of aspen poplar, when it's well-dried and seasoned. Poplar wood gives a cool Moon heat, as compared to the Mars heat of oak or the hot, dry Saturn heat of pine.

My log cabin was over seventy years old and built of aspen poplar logs. The lumber can be made into suitable furniture and hardwood flooring. Today, aspen is used extensively as a source of pulp and fiberboard, as well as specialty items like chopsticks, tongue depressors, venetian blinds, ice cream sticks, sauna benches, playground equipment, hockey stick handles, and matchsticks, due to its lack of splintering.

The word *balsam* derives from the Hebrew *besem*, meaning "a sweet smell," or perhaps *bot smin*, the "chief of all oils." *Balsamifera* means balsam-bearing. *Tremuloides* is derived from the Latin *tremulus*, for "trembling." *Arbor populi* is a Latin term meaning "tree of the people." *Aspen* may derive from the Anglo-Saxon *aespe*, or German *esp*, later its adjective *aspen*. *Poplar* is derived from the Greek *paipallo*, meaning "I shake"; *papeln*, "to babble"; or *pappalein*, "to move." It then became the Old French *pouplier* or *peuple*, and hence into English. *Deltoides* means "triangular," referring to the shape of the leaves. The Syrian name is *khashafa*, meaning "to be agitated."

Aspen was the letter *E (eadha)* in the Druid's tree alphabet and used for phyllomancy, or divination by leaf-rustlings, because the leaves are tremulous and create soft sounds. The Onondaga of North America call it *nut ki e*, meaning noisy leaf. The Celts called aspen the shield tree, the making of shields for protection. Incense from poplar is often burned for protection during Samhain (Halloween), when the veils between the worlds are at their thinnest and old fears can be cast aside.

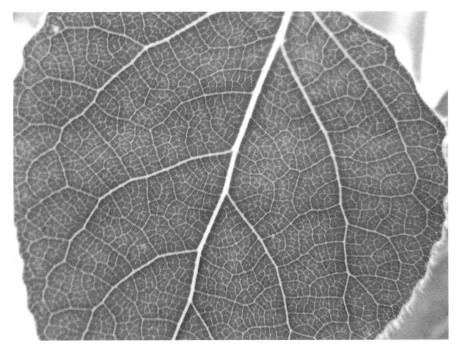

Aspen poplar leaf

The Greeks believed poplar came from the Heliades, the grief stricken sisters of Phaethon, who saw their brother struck by lightning as he drove the sun's chariot. The sisters were turned into poplars by Zeus, their tears falling into a brook as amber. The Greeks dedicated poplar to Heracles, who wore a crown of the tree's leaves when he retrieved the three-headed dog Cerberus from Hades. The leaf tops were scorched by fire, and the undersides turned bright from reflecting the hero's radiance, hence the two-sided leaf colors. Thus, poplars are a sign there is a return from the realm of the dead.

In several languages the local name translates as "woman's tongue." To the superstitious, the connection of death and the underworld gave aspen a reputation as unlucky. An aspen wand, known as a *fe*, was traditionally used to measure bodies and graves. The Christian church theorized that aspen trembled in memory of its wood being used for Christ's cruci-fixion. The shivering or trembling of aspen may be viewed in the doctrine of signatures as representative of its use for the treatment of ague and fever.

Aspen poplar is associated with November 2 and lamentation, while balsam poplar represents relief and September 10. Aspen is associated with the 14th Norse rune, *peorth*. In Russia, the bark was used traditionally to make stoppers for flasks. In China, the poplar tree served the people, while pine was reserved for rulers, *Thuja* cedar for princes, and the pagoda tree *(Sophora)* reserved for high officials. Poplar leaf is a symbol of duality in China, with the dark green on top representing the sun and the white downy underside representing the moon.

Poplar was traditionally embedded between fractured bone ends to act as a bridge for rejoining, regenerating, and reuniting bones. Juniper wood was also popular in the past for this procedure. According to legend, the native tipi design was discovered, by twisting a cottonwood leaf between the fingers to form a conical pattern.

Balsam poplar produces enormous biomass, yielding over nine tons per acre annually. Leaf litter, richer in nitrogen, phosphorus, potash, and calcium than most other hardwoods, may yield over twenty-five tons per acre of nutrient-rich humus. The seed production is enormous, with a single female tree producing up to fifty-four million seeds.

Traditional Uses

Traditionally, the wood was used to make canoe paddles, tipi poles, and snow shovels. Springtime stems can be used to make whistles while the bark is slippery. Even the rotted wood or driftwood is used to smoke hides or fish, as it burns and smolders longer.

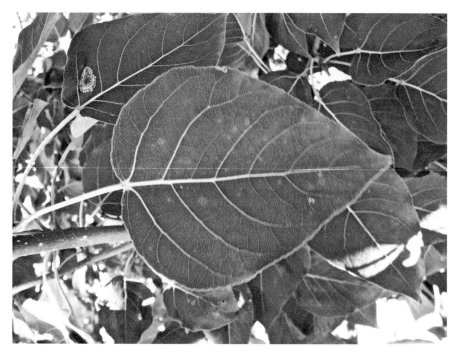

Balsam poplar leaf

Inuit used the thicker balsam poplar bark at the base of the tree as fishing floats that do not get waterlogged and carved sun goggles from the thick curved bark. The inside of the goggles were blackened with charcoal to further reduce glare. The tiny peepholes sharpen the vision. Try this for yourself and you will understand. Close your hand into a fist, and then put it up to your eye. Open your hand slightly and you will see a clearer picture than when light is coming in from a larger area.

Ironically, the Blackfoot of southern Alberta used extracts from the spring buds to apply to the eyes of those suffering snow-blindness. The spring buds combine with blood to produce a permanent black dye. The Tsitsistas (Cheyenne) used the buds in spring as a dye fixative, as different colors—red, green, purple, and white—are preserved by the bud sap. They were scratched on sandstone and used to paint tipis.

The Ojibwe (Anishinaabe) boiled the spring buds of *man'asa'di* in bear or goose grease and used this mixture for wounds, sores, boils, eczema, rashes, rheumatism, and gout. The catkins of spring contain around 20 percent protein, richer than any cereal crop. The cotton fluff was sometimes mixed with buffalo berries.

The Cree call it "ugly poplar" or *mathamitos*. I have also heard it called *mayimiyitos*, meaning "rough looking." The punk from the inner bark was called *apustam* and used for the ceremonial lighting of pipes. The fresh roots are used for acne, according to Russell Willier, a Cree healer and friend from the Sucker Creek First Nation.

The newly sprouted aspen leaves are a main part of a bear's diet in late May and early June, at least in northern Alberta. Aspen poplar is called *meitos*, *miyotohs*, *mistik*, or *wapisk-mitos*, meaning "white tree" by many Cree. They traditionally shredded the bark, especially in spring, and made a liquid extract for coughs. Willier decocts a two-inch-long twig, about one inch wide, for diarrhea or stomach cramps. The inner bark was used as a nourishing food, either boiled or ground into flour. This flour can be used for food or mixed with the sun-dried leaves of bearberry and tobacco as a more mellow smoke.

The name Assiniboine is derived from Asinaan, meaning "stone Sioux." They are also known as Nakota and Hohe. One elder of the Assiniboine had this to say about the sweet-tasting cambium layer of aspen poplar: "We always call it ice cream trees, because they're sweet and they're juicy. 'Let's go and eat ice cream juice,' we'd say. It is sweet like honeydew melon."

Women in various indigenous communities steeped the roots of both poplar together as a tea to stop bleeding during pregnancy and prevent premature labor. The Blackfoot decocted the inner bark for women ready to give birth. Infusions were used for heartburn and general pain relief.

Aspen leaves (*mitosinipiah*) are chewed and applied to bee or wasp stings, mosquito bites, and cuts. The white powder on the south-facing side of aspen bark was mixed with fat and applied as a sun block, deodorant, and antiperspirant. It is scraped off and applied to cuts and deep wounds to coagulate and stop bleeding, or can be applied directly to bee stings to reduce swelling, or as a substitute for talcum powder. I will often rub the aspen bark for a sun block if I am outdoors for any length of time.

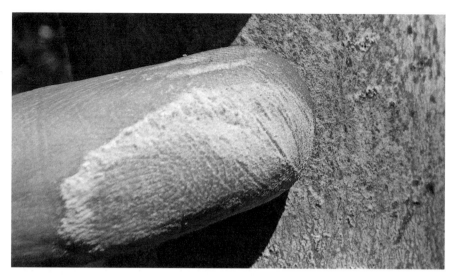

Aspen poplar bark yeast

This white yeast is reflective and protective for the poplar as well, preventing the premature flow upward of sap from late winter or early spring sunlight on the bark. Mors Kochanski once told me that native people traditionally mixed the white powder with vitreous humor of animal eyeballs as body paint or for marking artifacts. It was gathered and added to flour and water to produce a type of sourdough starter. It takes a few days to start working and then can be added to dough for bannock and such. Some form of sugar is needed to start the fermentation.

The Salish (Flathead) boiled the bark to repair ruptures and hernias. The cambium is boiled and then wrapped around fractures. This sets as hard as a cast when cooled. They made a poplar bud tea to calm bereavement and "opaque illness." The Dene (Chipewyan) know aspen poplar as *k'es* and the Balsam Poplar as *k'es t'ale*, meaning "poplar that has cracks." The Chippewa (Ojibwe) used either tree and steeped the root. This was used to relieve excessive menstrual flow or prevent miscarriage. On the other hand, the young seeds were chewed and swallowed to induce miscarriage. The young aspen poplar bark is cut into squares that are placed under the tongue for stomachache or for spitting up blood.

The Wood Cree of Saskatchewan would use the inner bark for heart ailments. It had to be cut at heart-height from the south side of the tree. The outer bark was combined with calamus root for diabetes. The eastern Mik'maq would roast the bark, from which they prepared a vermifuge tea. This is similar to the Gwich'in of the Mackenzie Delta, who burned poplar bark and mixed the ashes into dog food to kill worms and keep their hair in good shape. These ashes were mixed with caribou fat to make soap. Sophie Thomas, a Saik'uz herbalist, calls the tree *tl'ughusyaz*. The bark was chewed and applied to bleeding wounds, or boiled as a tea for intestinal parasites or cough syrup (Young and Hawley 2004). The Attikamek (Tête de Boule) of Quebec boiled aspen roots down to thick syrup for rubbing on painful joints.

The scent of balsam poplar reminds me of spring. Bees collect this balsam from new leaves, resulting in black spots produced by their vigorous tongues scraping on tender new leaves. This becomes propolis in the hive, used to protect the colony from infections.

Collect the buds when just opening, while the nights still freeze. The buds are often called balm of Gilead and used for cosmetics and cough syrups. Apothecary shops of old carried the buds under the name Oculi Populi. The European black poplar was used to make an ointment called Unguentum Populeon and an oil called Aegyrinum or Oil of Black Poplar. The buds are less useful when dried, and often become hollow or rotten. Collect and use them fresh. The Cree call the tree buds *osimisk*. The Anishinaabe (Ojibwe) use the pleasant balm to promote dreams. They are sometimes placed in hot bathwater and allowed to steep until a layer of extract forms on the surface. The patient with eczema or psoriasis then enters the bath. It is messy, leaving a ring around the tub, but effective. Teething babies have the buds rubbed directly on their gums, while for adults the buds can be placed in the nostril to stop nosebleeds.

The buds were heated and squeezed to make strong glue for feathers on arrow shafts and spearheads with sinew and for sealing cracks in birch bark canoes. While not as good as spruce gum for the latter, the bud resin makes a suitable temporary fix.

The Dena'ina of Alaska gathered the winter bud resin, called *k'elujiq'a*, "branch pitch," to treat frostbite, sores, and rashes. The buds are dried and ground into a powder and mixed with oil as a salve, or cooked with animal fat over low heat. This was used on a new baby's umbilical cord.

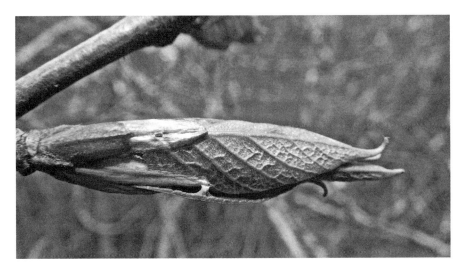

Poplar leaf buds

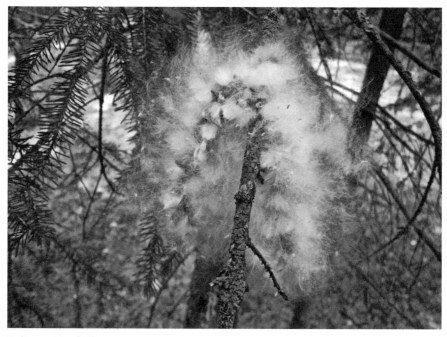

Balsam poplar fluff

The Dena'ina split the logs and removed the rotten inner part for a waterproof shingle that resembles adobe tile.

The cottonwood fluff gives a pleasant smell to blankets when used as insulation. It can be gathered by the handful in season. The dried inner bark of balsam poplar makes a suitable soap; as do aspen leaves and branches, when boiled in water. The ashes were used for cleaning buckskin or washing hair by soaking them in water overnight and straining off the upper part. The Hudson's Bay Company mixed the inner bark of balsam poplar with tallow to make a soap sold at their trading posts.

The larger balsam poplars and cottonwoods can be tapped like birch and the sap drunk fresh. It is ingested to treat diabetes and high blood pressure. Likewise, the buds and aspen bark are decocted for diabetes. The bark and sap together are boiled to make a tea given to children with asthma. It can be boiled down to a gooey consistency to serve as wood glue, tightly holding its bond under stress, and resisting cracking when dry.

The inner bark of Balsam Poplar was used at one time to make a cast for broken bones. The bark was slowly simmered for twenty-four hours, then the bark was removed and the liquid simmered down again to syrup. This was spread on a piece of cloth or hide and tightly wrapped around the affected limb and allowed to set. This thick sap or oakum is used by survivalists to trap roosting birds. Simply smear the branches liberally, and the next day they are helpless to fly away and make an easy meal. I have caught prairie chickens using this method. The sap helps de-scent traps and wire snares of human smell. Soak the traps in diluted sap and water overnight for best results. Treat your gloves, shoes, and clothes for added protection. In the boreal forest, wolves prefer underground dens for their cubs located under balsam poplar, due in part to the protective disguising balsamic odor.

The Chippewa (Ojibwe) combined balsam poplar buds, root, and blossoms with aspen poplar bark for heart and circulation issues; with snakeroot (*Polygala senega*) for excessive menstrual flow; and with the introduced Canada thistle for back pain and female weakness. The Wolastoqiyik (Maliseet) combined burdock leaf and balsam poplar buds for chancre sores. Their tribal name is derived from the Wolastoq River in New Brunswick and Maine; hence Wolastoqiyik, meaning "people of the beautiful river." *Maliseet* is the term given them by the Mi'kmaq, meaning "broken talkers" or "lazy speakers," suggesting they can't speak very well. Horses suffering colic chew on the fragrant leaf buds to self-medicate. The Gitksan of British Columbia used the bud gum as a hair perfume for young women. The young buds were boiled, put in bear grease, and kept in a bone with a hole in the side for later use. The Gitksan name for *P. balsamifera* and *P. trichocarpa* means "good for canoe." The Karok name for black cottonwood is *asappiip*, from *asa*, meaning "rock," and *ip*, meaning "tree." The buds were combined with mullein flowers and plantain leaves for indolent sores. A bark decoction was taken after childbirth if someone close had passed away. The bark and buds were used for sciatica (hip pain), whooping cough, tuberculosis, gonorrhea, and ringworm. Poplar wood headdresses dating to 3000 BCE have been found in grave sites in ancient Mesopotamia. In the Middle East, aspen poplar leaves were traditionally juiced for earaches.

Rahimi et al. (2008) found smoke of burned poplar leaves was more effective than cryotherapy on hand and foot warts. A trial of 60 patients conducted over 22 weeks found a 66% success rate using poplar leaf smoke versus cryotherapy and a recurrence rate of only 4.2% versus 32%, respectively. Poplar ashes are a good replacement for salt or baking soda in recipes. Simply double the amount called for. Charcoal from poplar is very absorbent and a good intestinal antiseptic. While traveling in Morocco, I noted the charcoal of black poplar was sold in markets for the same purpose. The herbalists in North Africa used the buds as a soothing and sedative balm for hemorrhoids.

Aspen branches, like willows, produce copious amounts of natural rooting hormone. Simply place a few branches in hot water for few days and use this for initiating root growth in transplants and cuttings. Fresh aspen leaves taste somewhat like spinach; contain 20 to 30 percent of their dry weight as protein; and contain eleven amino acids in larger percentages than oats or wheat. Research conducted in Ontario in the late 1970s found poplar leaves can be converted into a food concentrate for chickens. Whole aspen trees are chipped and turned into an animal feed called *muka*.

Russ Schnell, a summer student working at the Alberta Research Council, was looking for agents that cause water to freeze at higher temperatures. He came upon a mold growing on poplar leaves. In 1984 the lab began mass generation of the microorganisms from poplar leaves for the company Bio Frost, a California firm making snow for ski resorts.

Aspen poplar grows mainly from root suckering. In 1966, Burton V. Barnes found the clonal growth of a single aspen in Utah covering 43 hectares, with 47,000 stems, or trees. It is by far the most massive living organism known, weighing more than thirteen million pounds, and may be over eight hundred thousand years old. It is nicknamed "Pando," from the Latin meaning "I spread." The tree produces both male and female clones, the former favoring dry and high elevation and the latter found in lower wet conditions.

An unusual group of crooked aspen grows near Hafford, Saskatchewan. Based on work in Manitoba, these poplars are mutated, twisted, and contorted due to a gene variation. The twisted trees look like an enchanted forest, and due to recent popularity have a wooden boardwalk to help protect them. I could not resist producing a flower essence from this unusual tree.

Poplar possesses the ability to photosynthesize through its bark. This is why a few years without leaves due to forest tent caterpillars (*Malacosoma disstria*) or storms will not kill them. One year, the entire walls of my northern log cabin were covered top to bottom with tent caterpillars. They were falling down into piles several feet thick at the base, a writhing mass right out of a horror show. In fact, poplar will concentrate on growing either roots, leaves, or stems depending upon the time of year and circumstances. The caterpillars are attacked by parasites, the most common being a flesh fly that lays eggs in their cocoons. It has big red eyes and can be annoying in the woods. They only last a few days and help control the voracious tent caterpillars by laying eggs inside them. Tent caterpillar eggs prevent freezing by applying a coat of glycerol, similar to the chemical in a car's radiator.

A woolly caterpillar, *Gynaephora groenlandica*, has evolved to live within a hundred miles of the north pole. Temperatures of −94°F and thin snow cover are common, with short arctic summers allowing brief thawing and feeding. They are frozen solid most of the year, so it takes thirteen or fourteen years of growth until they are able spin a cocoon on an exposed rock to catch some directed sunlight. The butterflies are supplied by the rocks, a source of minerals and electrolytes, to brighten their wing color.

Beavers love aspen, consuming up to four pounds of bark daily, while ruffed grouse favor eating the buds at a rate of forty-five buds per minute. Aspen leaves, when damaged, will release methyl jasmonate from the wound, which in turn activates a proteinase response in other leaves and even trees. Insects are discouraged from eating more, and move on to other vegetation. Work by Baldwin and Schultz (1983) found damaged poplars send out signals to warn their neighbors about stressful situations, resulting in increased production of chemicals that help them combat stress. Salicortin and tremulacin content in leaves is quickly increased when munched on by insects. These compounds are toxic, and insects and herbivores move on to browse another tree.

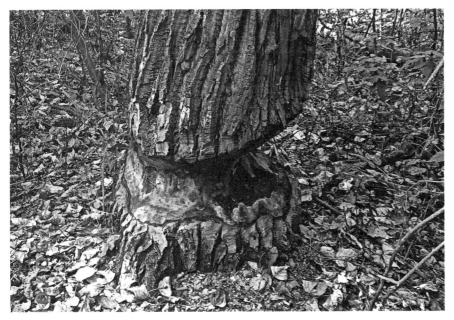

Beaver cutting down balsam poplar

Aspen leaves contain up to 22.6 percent benzoic acid, used for preserving foods and in the manufacture of dyes. Benzoic acid exhibits antifungal and choleretic activity. The buds contain the related p-hydroxybenzoic acid, used in organic synthesis and as an intermediate for dyes and fungicides. Deer, coyotes, wolves, and other animals eat the tasty leaves as an anthelmintic, to help kill and remove parasites. Poplar bark powder is fed to horses with worms, one handful in feed twice daily for up to a week. Catechol derived from aspen bark is used commercially in photography and dyeing, and exhibits anticonvulsive and antiseptic action.

In spring, when the sap is rising, poplar branches can be carved into pipe whistles. My good friend and world-class survival expert Mors Kochanski can make a nice-sounding flute from poplar in less than two minutes. I have watched him fashion as well a flute from cow parsnip stems.

Ozone is used on poplar to produce oxyaromatic compounds such as vanillin, syringaldehyde, catechol, and guaiacol, among others. These compounds are used by the cosmetics, food, and pharmaceutical industries for transformation into products of even greater added value, such as heliotropine, dopamine, papaverine, adrenaline, and others. Vanillin, for example, is used for flavoring and to synthesize L-DOPA, a drug used in Parkinson's disease. Vanillic acid is used to produce nontoxic fungicides and blood pressure medications (warfarin). Vanillin inhibits angiogenesis and prevents cancer metastasis through PBK inhibition (Lirdprapamongkol et al. 2009). Vanillin also enhances the antifungal effect of essential oils against gray mold rot *(Botrytis cinerea)* on commercial crops (Rattanapitig-orn et al. 2006). This sounds like a better source of vanillin than one recently discovered by Japanese researchers. Work by Mayu Yamamoto (2006) at the International Medical Center in Japan found a way to extract vanillin from cow dung by heating it under pressure. Disclosure of the origin of the ingredients would make it a hard sell for edible goods, but they hope to capture part of the cosmetic and aromatic candle market. Good luck with that!

Aphids are the tiny greenish-white sap-sucking insects on the underside of balsam poplar and cottonwood leaves. They are edible, and to the survivalist, a ready source of sweet sugar. They can be collected by brushing them from the branches or boiled with leaves, the insects serving as a sweetener in the tea. Ants will fold over a number of leaves to create an aphid house, where they keep their captives safe and raise them for their sweet nectar, similar to a human milking a cow.

Western cottonwood is found in the southern prairies, almost always on the edge of rivers and on gravel beds at the bends of slow-moving streams. The largest cottonwood in Manitoba, located on an oxbow on the Assiniboine River near Portage La Prairie, is 108 feet tall and nearly 7 feet in diameter. A plains cottonwood *(P. deltoides sargentii)* at Police Point Park in Medicine Hat, Alberta, is between 250 and 300 years old and has circumfer-ence of 17 feet. A grove of giant cottonwood trees, close to 400 years old, with trunks up to 30 feet in diameter, was recently found on the Elk River near Fernie, British Columbia. These are the largest and longest-lived specimens found so far in the world, according to Stewart Rood (2003), a tree specialist at the University of Lethbridge, Alberta.

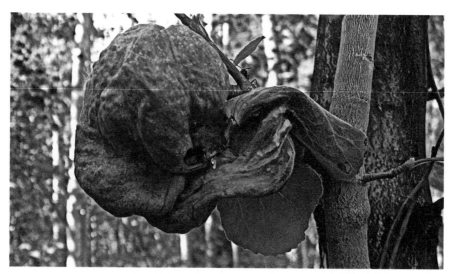

Aphid house formed and controlled by ants

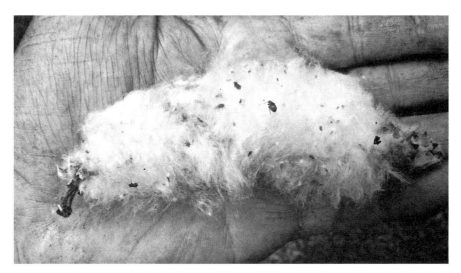

Cottonwood fluff and seeds

Cottonwoods produce huge seed crops. One forty-foot specimen discovered at the turn of the twentieth century was found bearing twenty-eight million seeds. These large trees really go through water, averaging 100 gallons per hour during summer heat. The Ojibwe made use of the fluffy cotton attached to the seeds for medicinal purposes, much as we used cotton batten today. The Lakota call the cottonwood *canyah'u*, meaning "peel away wood." The thick planks that easily peel away or eventually fall off make a great carving wood. The grain and smooth nature of the wood make it ideal for kitchen utensils, plaques, and such.

The Haida gathered the cambium of Black Cottonwood in spring and consumed it fresh. Known a cottonwood ice cream, it quickly sours so is not suitable for drying and winter storage like some coniferous cambium. The Mohawk (Kanienkehaka) and other members of the Iroquois (Haudenosaunee) Confederacy drank decoctions of the inner bark as a vermifuge cleanse. The name Kanienkehaka means "people of the flint." Haudenosaunee means "they made the house," symbolizing all nations coming together. The Tsitsistas (Cheyenne) of Montana used the gummy leaf buds as a fixative for different colors used to paint tipis and pictures of warriors' deeds on robes. The spring buds were combined with blood for an intense black dye. Black cottonwood bark fiber was prepared into skirts by the Chumash of California. They would strip the bark from a green tree, dry it, and then soften it by bending and rubbing it with their hands. This fiber skirt had a front flap and back flap attached to cordage from cottonwood fiber. Similar skirts were made from tule (*Scirpus*) or willow (*Salix*) species. To carry objects on their head, the Chumash fashioned the bark into a ring.

The plains cottonwood is the state tree of Nebraska and Kansas. The expression "cottonwood blossom" was used in the Old West to describe outlaws hanged from any tree limb. It is believed individual sensitivity to propolis, gathered from various poplars by bees is due to the pentenyl caffeates and 1,1-dimethylallylcaffeic acid esters, derived from cottonwood poplar.

Narrow-leaved cottonwood is found along streambeds and river valleys from southern Alberta to Arizona. Farther south, the ripe fruit, full of cotton, was dipped in water and placed on swollen gums or ulcerated teeth. The fresh flowers were steeped in cold water for several hours, strained, and drunk as an infusion to purify the blood in spring. The related valley cottonwood (*P. deltoides* ssp. *wislizeni*) leaves were traditionally decocted in the Southwest as a beverage to relieve dropsy.

Medicinal Uses

Constituents: aspen poplar (*P. tremuloides*) bark: populin (salicin-6-benzoate), salicortin, salicin 2.4%, salireposide, triploside, glucose ester of coumaric acid, pyrocatechol, tremuloidin (salicin-2-benzoate), tremulacin (salicortin-2-benzoate), grandidentotin, riciresinol-B, bisabol, trichocarpin, mannitol, and arachidonic acid. Various steroids include citrostadienol, stigmasta-3,5-dien-7-one, and tremulone. Alpha- and beta-amyrins, tannins, glucose, fructose, trisaccharides, fats, and waxes are also present. Cinnamrutinoses A and B are phenolic glycosides of the stem bark that has been infected with the pathogenic fungus *Hypoxylon mammatum.*

Buds: simple phenolics (up to 85%).

Male catkins: flavonoids including chrysin (5,7-dihydroxyflavone), chrysinic acid, ectochrysin, pinocembrin, and pinostrobin.

Leaves: five triterpenoids, including oleanic, ursanic, lupanic, lanostanic, and euphanic acid; butyrospermol acetate.

Cambium: up to 12% arabinogalactans (see "Tamarack and Larch" in Chapter 6), 1% glucomannan, 40% galacturonans, 6% xylglucan, 10% xylan, and a trace of 4-O-methyl-glucurononoxylan.

Balsam poplar buds: up to 36% phenylpropanoids, salicin benzoate, populin, benzoic and gallic acid, chrysin, tectochrysin, beta-caryophyllene, mannitol, trichocarpin, pinostrobin, apigenin, galangin, pinocembrin, bisabolol, curcumene, humulene, resins, tannins, essential oils as well as carboxylic, coumaric, gallic, malic, and cinnamic acids. Also contain cineole and alpha-bisabolol, and phenolic resins such as salicaldehyde and 6-hydroxycyclohexane.

Bark: salicin, salicortin, trichocarpin, benzyl gentisate, 6-hydroxycyclohexenone, trichocarposide, populoside, salicoysalicin, dihyromyricetin, salireposide, fatty oil esters, 11-eicosanic acid, 2,6-dimethoxy-p-benzoquinone, azelainic, behenic, cerotinic acids.

Leaves: (10.7%) extractable from water and alcohol and composed of prostaglandins, proanthocyanidins, tannins, and phenolics.

Inner bark: 0.2% protein, 0.5% fat, 6.3% carbohydrate. Energy yield is 27 kcal per 100 grams.

P. trichocarpa: bark salicin, salicortin, salireposide, salicyloylsalicin, tremulacin, tremuloidin, trichocarpin.

P. angustifolia: bark: salicortin.

P. candicans: bark: salicin, salicortin, salireposide.

P. deltoides: bark: deltoidin, HCH salicortin, populoside, salicin, salicortin, salicyloylsalicin, tremulacin, tremuloidin.

Like willow, various poplars contain salicin and populin glycosides, which are converted in the large intestine by healthy bacteria to saligenin, and then conjugated in the liver to salicylic acid. These compounds are very effective at reducing pain, fever, and inflammation. This process of conversion takes from ten to fourteen hours.

The inner bark of aspen poplars contains the highest concentrations and can be used in decoction or tincture form for headache, arthritic and rheumatic pain, and urinary tract inflammation. Even black poplar leaves can be crushed with vinegar and applied as a poultice for relief of gout. Balsam poplar bark inhibits xanthine oxidase, suggesting its benefit in treating gout internally as well as cool footbaths (Owen and Johns 1999). Tamarack needles combine well with balsam poplar bark as a decoction for rheumatic and gouty conditions.

The buds and bark can be boiled and made into fomentations wrapped around swollen joints and sprains. The leaf buds can be eaten every day to help stave off degenerative gum diseases like gingivitis and pyorrhea. Leaf buds contain kaempferide, which inhibits inflammation caused by tumor promoters, and acacetin, an inhibitor of lens aldose reductase, iodothyronine deiodinase, and histamine release from mast cells. Another compound in the buds, trans-coniferaldehyde, inhibits prostaglandin synthetase and reduces edema, albeit in rat studies.

Bud tinctures reduce excessive lactation and thus are indicated when breast milk production is too plentiful or there

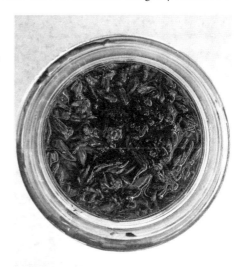

Sun-infused poplar bud oil

is a desire to wean. Tincture of balsam buds is very useful for colds, flu, and bronchial problems by increasing secretions when the mucous membranes are hot, dry, and inflamed. It can be taken internally to help lower cholesterol levels. The buds contain an antioxidant, and the tincture is used in natural cosmetics to prevent rancidity. For laryngitis with loss of voice, poplar bud tincture gargle is specific. For acute respiratory infections, poplar bud tincture could be combined with a cool, antiseptic expectorant such as pleurisy root. For more chronic conditions, combine with mullein leaf or coltsfoot root. For intestinal infections, combine the buds with plantain, calendula, purple loosestrife, echinacea, or horsetail, depending on the individual.

Salves can be made from sun-infused bud oil for burns, cuts, and numerous skin conditions, ranging from diaper rash to hemorrhoid swelling. A commercial pile ointment made from balsam poplar buds has been on the market in Europe for a number of years.

Poplar bud extracts have been extensively studied by Romanian scientists. They found 4–5% oil preparations and ointments help heal skin incisions, wounds, and burns. In the 1970s Soviet physicians used the extracts with great clinical success for bedsores, resistant infections, and postoperative abscesses. The bud oil helps soothe eczema and psoriasis when applied neatly to the affected area.

The mentholated aroma makes a great nasal and chest rub for sinus congestion and coughs as well as an anti-inflammatory component to relieve painful muscle aches and tension. Other herbs that complement poplar bud oil in ointments are sweet cicely root (*Osmorhiza longistylis*), chickweed, licorice root, and lobelia.

Work by Levin et al. (1983) has shown the living cambium as well as buds and leaves of balsam poplar contain prostaglandins (PGE1 and PGE2) similar to those found in animals. This may partially explain the hypotensive and anti-inflammatory nature of this tree. Balsam poplar buds contain tectochrysin, shown to induce apoptosis in colon cancer cells, including chemo-resistant cancer cell growth. Oral ingestion of the bud oil may be best for an adjuvant therapy (Park et al. 2015). Tectochrysin induces apoptosis in non–small cell lung cancer (Oh et al. 2014). Overexpression of the breast cancer resistance protein ABCG2 confers multidrug resistance to cancer cells. Work by Ahmed-Belkacem et al. (2005) found tectochrysin may be a useful inhibitor and may increase the potency of drug therapy.

Balsam poplar bud and bark tincture is used for lung, stomach, and kidney problems. The inner bark can be chewed for up to three weeks for those wishing to alleviate their addiction to chewing tobacco. Balsam poplar buds show a very low LC50 rate and yet possess potent antitumor activity against neuroblastoma cells. Mazzio and Soliman (2009) looked at 374 natural products for antitumor activity and rated the buds very high. Poplar bud extracts are similar in profile to propolis (see "Bees and Honey" in Chapter 6), containing pinocembrin, chrysin, and galangin. Propolis is sometimes adulterated with poplar extract, but the adulteration can be detected as it contains catechol.

The inner bark of balsam poplar shows antagonistic activity against peroxisome proliferator-activated receptor-gamma (PPAR-gamma), suggesting its beneficial use in treating obesity and other metabolic conditions (Martineau et al. 2010). Recent work found ethanol extracts of the bark mitigate development of obesity and insulin sensitivity in diet-induced obese and diabetic mice. Inhibition of adipocyte differentiation, decreased liver inflammation, and increases in hepatic fatty acid oxidation were found (Harbilas et al. 2012). The extract decreased glycemia and improved insulin sensitivity by diminishing insulin levels and the leptin-adiponection ratio.

Balsam poplar bark, like the bud oil, can be an extremely useful decoction for chronic constipation. It rarely causing griping and is mild and effective. A small amount of ginger root may be added if any irritation persists. Both chrysin and apigenin inhibit chymotrypsin and trypsin-like proteasomes that promote tumor growth (Wu and Fang 2010).

Aspen poplar tincture is made from the inner bark and is a bitter digestive tonic. It is an important ingredient in Dr. Thompson's famous debility tonic for restoring weight and appetite, especially in the elderly suffering chronic digestive complaints. The gallbladder may be involved.

Consider its use in cases of sympathetic nervous system excess, such as nervous shaking and tremor, or in cases of shivering associated with high fevers from influenza, with alternating chills and sweats. For chronic diarrhea, aspen inner bark blends well with sweet gale.

The British Herbal Medicine Association rates aspen poplar as a specific for rheumatoid arthritis. Keep in mind that the process of salicin or populin to salicylic acid can take 8–14 hours and relies on healthy intestinal bacteria to cleave the molecule and the liver to conjugate the compounds. Only then is salicylic acid released into the bloodstream without the stomach bleed associated with ASA or aspirin. For chronic arthritis, there is no better or safer remedy than poplar or willow bark. A combination of aspen poplar bark 90 mg, feverfew 110 mg, and yarrow 60 mg (Gitadyl) proved as efficacious as 400 mg of ibuprofen in one blinded study on osteoarthritis. A three-week double-blind randomized cross-over study by Ryttig et al. (1991) on 35 subjects found analgesic benefit equal to ibuprofen, but with fewer gastro-intestinal symptoms.

The leaves contain various triterpenoids, including ursanic, oleanic, and lupanic acids. Also found in apple peel, these compounds reduce various marker genes associated with inflammatory bowel disease (IBD) (Mueller et al. 2013). Dry leaf infusions may be trialed for treating this issue. The bud resin, extracted from *P. tremuloides* with alcohol, can be used sparingly as a kidney tonic. Populin relaxes the nervous system and relieves headaches due to liver or stomach acidity and gas. Populin is licorice-tasting, and its glycosides influence stomach and digestive tract health.

Aspen poplar helps correct lack of urine flow due to prostate or kidney inflammation. This may be due in part to the zinc lignans or flavonoids in the bark and leaves. It may be useful in enlarged prostate (benign prostatic hyperplasia), combining well with stinging nettle root and fireweed. Dribbling and irritating urination, especially with atonic bladder, call for aspen poplar bark, combined with bearberry (*Arctostaphylos uva-ursi*) leaf. Cystitis of a recurring nature may be helped when combined with couch grass or corn silk. It helps restore urogenital function, assists urinary incontinence, and may be especially useful to those individuals who have suffered a stroke and required catheterization. The damaged epithelial tissue is soothed.

According to Matthew Wood (2009), "poplar is beneficial in conditions where there is fear, hyperadrenalism, hyperthyroidism, and overactivity of the sympathetic branch.... It reduces fever and heat, and establishes groundedness and strength in people who are nervous." He has used the tincture successfully in cases of asthma associated with hyperthyroidism. Matthew mentions an external wash of poplar bark and rose thorns for wounds that are healing slowly, or serious wounds that need immediate regrowth of tissue. Fungi associated with rose thorns can be a significant problem, and untreated, may develop into conditions that require surgery.

It is worth noting a flavonoid from *Populus nigra* contains delta-4-3-ketosteroid, a 5-alpha-reductase inhibitor. These compounds are also found in various pine heartwoods and inhibit conditions of androgen-dependent prostatic hypertrophy and cancer as well as frontal hair loss associated with excessive androgenic effect.

The European *P. tremula* knot wood has been found to possess a high ORAC value, indicative of antioxidant potential (Neacsu et al. 2007). Tremulacin is weakly active against herpes simplex-1 and 2, as well as HIV-1 (Ishikawa et al. 2004). Poplar pollen is one of the eight original plant pollens composing Cernilton, a commercially available product for benign prostatic hypertrophy.

The fresh flowers (catkins) are steeped in cold water and taken as a spring blood purifier. The male catkins are rich in flavonoids including chrysin, which helps prevent

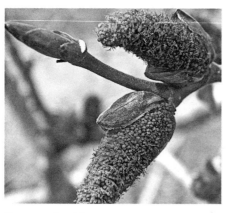

Cottonwood catkins

testosterone converting into progesterone. Small amounts of chrysin can make herbs such as puncture vine (*Tribulus terrestris*) more effective for bodybuilding and sexual stamina. Work by Dhawan et al. (2004) found 1 mg/kg of chrysin given to rats increased libido and sperm count and improved fertility rates. Chrysin is an aromatase inhibitor, preventing aromatization of testosterone to estrogen by inactivating the enzyme responsible. When compared to Cytadren, a strong antiestrogenic drug, it shows nearly identical activity. This is remarkable for a natural compound, as the drug inhibits estrogen production by up to 92% in human trials.

Chrysin reduces anxiety without inducing sedation or muscle relaxation. It may be a partial agonist of benzodiazepine receptors and is found in scullcap species (Paladini et al. 1999). Work by Wolfman et al. (1994) found chrysin has strong antianxiety properties, with effects on anxiety equal to prescription sleeping pills. Chrysin is present in passion-flower leaves, for those herbalists living in a more temperate climate.

Zanoli et al. (2000) found chrysin activates receptors of GABA(A). Chrysin down-regulates FCER1, suggesting a role in IgE-mediated allergic reactions such as atopic derma-titis, allergic rhinitis, asthma, and various food allergies (Yano et al. 2005). The compound reduces hypertension and relaxes the aorta after noradrenaline stimulation and may help suppress cortisol production. Chrysin ameliorates diabetic-induced cataract formation, at least in animal studies (Patil et al. 2016). Chrysin is cytotoxic to esophageal and adenocar-cinoma cancer cell lines, with G2/M arrest and apoptosis (Zhang et al. 2008). It appears to inhibit the growth and metastasis of cancers through the lymphatic system. It may play a positive role in bilirubin gluconoconjugation caused by an enzyme deficiency in cases of Crigler-Najjar syndrome. This condition is the result of an autosomal recessive trait, with death usually occurring within fifteen months of birth. Chrysin, as an aside, helps protect adult orchids from fungal attack.

Both poplars are superior to willow, alder, and even quinine in the treatment of inter-mittent fevers. The bisabolol in the young shoots of balsam poplar has been found active against tuberculosis. I find this interesting, as derivatives of salicylic acid (p-aminosali-cylic acid) inhibit the growth of tuberculosis bacilli. Known as PSA, it was one of the first important drugs in the treatment of tuberculosis before the discovery of streptomycin.

Another constituent found in the bark, trichocarpin is also an antifungal. Aspen poplar branches showed activity against eight of nine fungal species tested by McCutcheon et al. (1994). Experiments in Russia found aspen poplar bark extracts exhibit marked antiul-cerative properties with stress-induced, resperine-induced, and acetylsalicylic acid-induced ulcers. Sawicka et al. (1995) found water-soluble extracts from poplar buds increased immunotropic activity, while the leaf extracts did not. Sokolnicka et al. (1994) discovered bud extracts inhibit both lymphocyte and granulocyte migration; while leaf extracts only inhibit lymphocyte migration. Conclusion: the leaf buds are more potent. Amoros et al. (1994) found aspen poplar leaf buds contain a compound with antiviral properties. Salicin and salireposide, derived from black cottonwood, were found active at 25 mcg/ml against poliomyelitis and Semliki forest virus (Van Hoof et al. 1989).

The sap derived from poplar trees is also useful. Although present throughout the year, glutathione is particularly high in sap before the flowering of catkins. Cysteine and gamma-glutamylcysteine are present in reasonable amounts. Methionine content becomes more prominent into May and June. Glutathione is one of nature's most powerful antioxidants and is needed by the liver to detoxify organic material and help neutralize heavy metals. In fact, glutathione is so important to the body that a full 7 percent of the energy created by the body is utilized to produce this important compound. Balsam and aspen poplar contain Kunitz serine protease inhibitors, involved in reducing inflammation.

Carbonized poplar wood is called Carbo Ligni and is used as an antiseptic for the intestinal tract. William Cook (1869) considered aspen poplar one of the best woods for producing charcoal, which is generally taken dry in gelatin capsules for maximum benefit. A patent was obtained in Canada in 1996 for a medicinal composition for diabetes that includes extracts from aspen poplar and cow parsnip.

Homeopathy

Both aspen and balsam poplar have been proved for homeopathy use.

Aspen poplar is useful for gastric and bladder problems, especially in elders. It works well on bladder problems related to surgery or during pregnancy. There may be night sweats, cystitis, and a sensation of heat to the surface of the skin. Indigestion with acidity and gas is common. There is often a painful burning behind the pubis after urination and prostate inflammation. Cystitis is relieved after ovariectomy or hysterectomy.

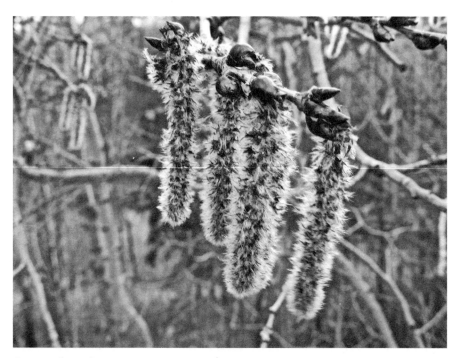

Aspen poplar seeds

There may be aversion to everything, with lots of cursing and swearing. There is a fear of losing direction or that one's memory will fail. Vertigo, upon looking down, may be present. General nervous excitement may combine with the delusion of being old. Aversion to bread, coffee, or wine may exist. Red blotches and spots on face, as well as swelling above eyes may be present. Throat pain is better from cold drinks, but nausea after excessive coffee is better from warm drinks.

Dose: Tincture to 30th potency. For prostatitis, bladder infections, pus in urine, and pregnant women, use the 2nd potency. The mother tincture is made from equal parts of the fresh leaves and fresh inner bark of the young twigs. Paine self-experimented with effects of 5–50 grain doses of populin; clinical observations were made by Hale and Farokh Master; and proving was done by Den Hartog with three provers at 30c in 1996. Hale reported several cases of bladder and prostate issues cleared with 1X–3X dilutions. Three cases of inflammation of the neck of the bladder (vesical tenesmus) in women were relieved with 2X doses.

Balm of Gilead poplar (*P. candicans*) has a pronounced effect on acute colds, especially when there is a deep hoarse voice. One peculiar symptom of this remedy is skin surface anesthesia, with or without numbness. The fingertips actually thicken and do not feel any sensation. There may be a hot head, with cold extremities, cold sores on the lips, or the tongue may feel thick and numb. There is burning of the eyes, nose, throat, and air passages. The lungs have acute hoarseness, with dry cough, loss of voice, and raw feeling in the chest. Dry asthmatic breathing is present. The patient is apprehensive, expecting death. Frightful vivid dreams of dead people may be present. They feel unable to do anything. Voices sound distant. There may be aversion to meat. Exhaustion is associated with hot sultry weather. The skin is harsh and dry. Vertigo may be present, as if from sunstroke. There may be sensation of vaginal burning, as if scalded. Large skin blisters are filled with water.

Dose: Mother tincture doses. Haworth self-experimented with tincture and 30c between 1870 and 1882. A woman was poisoned when preparing freshly gathered buds for domestic use in alcohol in 1875. Symptoms were observed by Allen (*Handbook of Materia Medica*), and additional clinical observations were made by Clarke, who cited a case by Stilson in which one evening a man drank rum into which balm of Gilead buds were placed to make liniment. A few hours later his wife found him breathing heavily, and on waking him, found he could not speak. He later could only speak in hoarse whispers and would forget what he was going to say in middle of sentence.

Salicylicum acidum (2-hydroxy-benzoic acid) patients have a disposition to regard things in a gloomy light. There may be the delusion of hearing music that wakes them. Mistakes in spelling and writing are noted, as well as dreams of being pregnant, not getting married, or a child dying. Profuse perspiration is present, with a longing for fresh air, and craving for wine and salt. There is pain in the head, vertigo, sounds in the ears, and imaginary odors like the smell of musk.

Dose: 1st to 30th potency. Lewi self-experimented at first trituration in 1875; Chase self-experimented at 3rd dilution; and Reinke at 10c and 30c in 1886. Proving was by Lesignang and Kuhnen with 13 provers at 30X in 1987. Clinical observations were made by Romer with eight cases of Ménière's disease successfully treated with LM 6, 30c, or 200c in the 1980s.

Salicylicum acidum (2-hydroxy-benzoic acid) is irritating to skin and mucosa and used for bunions, corns, warts, and dandruff shampoos as well as tinea and other fungal infections. In large doses it can impair hearing and the optic nerve. The cerebral symptoms resemble atropine, producing the so-called salicylate jag. The patient is talkative and very cheerful and may pass on to delirium with hallucinations, motor activity, and attempts to get out of bed. Very large doses produce weakness of heart and depression of respiratory and vasoconstrictor centers, with collapse.

Essential Oils

In early 2000 I became research chair for the Alberta New Crops Network. With government assistance, we were able to build a portable distillation unit. It traveled from one end of the province to the other and steam-distilled over 70 experimental plants one summer. The next year, Heather Kehr distilled aspen branches, including young buds, in the early spring. This produced a good yield of a sweet balsamic oil. We sent the oil, in November 2002, to the LASEVE lab at the University of Chicoutimi in Quebec for analysis. The thick oil was composed of 25.08% alpha-bisabolol, 2.87% beta-bisabolol, 16.06% alpha-eudesmol, 17.79% beta-eudesmol 9.59% gamma-eudesmol, and trace amounts of minor constituents.

A pleasant, somewhat balsamic and chamomile-like essential oil is produced from the balsam poplar buds. The yield is 0.3–0.6% of a pale yellow to light brown oil. It contains various sesquiterpenes, alpha-caryophyllene, with arcurcumene, humulene, cineole, alpha-bisabolol (27.4%), (e)-nerolidol (5.8%), gamma-curcumene, alpha-eudesmol, bisabolene, farnesene, and acetophenone. It distills best at 435–450°F and has a specific gravity of 0.89–0.910. Studies in Russia indicate balsam poplar bud oil exhibits pronounced antimicrobial activity. The bisabolol is a stereoisomer with a different configuration than that from German chamomile. In the latter, the configuration is 4S, 8S, and 68.4, while poplar bud oil is 4R, 8R, and 51–54.

A study to compare the anti-inflammatory potential of poplar bud oil should be undertaken. This would help determine the commercial viability of this product for worldwide application in a variety of cosmetic and pharmaceutical products. Alpha-bisabolol and n(e)-nerolidol demonstrate antitumor activity. Personal experience suggests the poplar and chamomile essential oils are synergistic in nature. Laurie uses the tenacious balsamic essential oil from poplar in some of her blends, developed for Scents of Wonder.

Balsam Poplar bark and twigs yield around 0.5% essential oil consisting of nearly 27% (+)-alpha-bisabolol, 11% each of alpha- and beta-eudesmol, and the minor constituents above. Aspen poplar buds yield an essential oil yielding a high 3.2% of the fresh weight. It is composed mainly of (+)-alpha-bisabolol, cineole, benzyl alcohol, arachidonic acid, and malic and citric acids.

Ceratocystis populina is an ascomycete fungus living on aspen poplar. When steam-distilled, it produces a pleasant fruit-like essential oil that includes various fruit esters, acyclic mono- and sesquiterpenes, terpenoids, and 2-phenyl-ethyl acetate (Hinds and Davidson 1967). Steam distillation of 17 day old culture of *C. populina* show an oil with 45% muurolol, 13% gamma-cadinol, 9.6% alpha-amorphene, 7.3% gamma-amorphene, 6% isoamyl alcohol, and minor components.

Various *Ceratocystis* species offer different scents. *C. moniliformis* has a fruity, peach-pear odor and contains 3-methylbutyl acetate, delta- and gamma-decalactone, geraniol, citronellol, nerol, linalool, and alpha-terpineol. The related *C. virescens* is rosier and fruitier and consists of 6-methyl-5-helten-2-ol acetate, citronellol, linalool, geraniol, and geranyl acetate. *C. variospora* is more fragrant and geranium-like, with geraniol, gernayl acetate, linallo, geranial, neral, and citronellol as major volatiles.

Aspen bark extracted with benzene yields a yellow-green fat of pleasant odor with an iodine value of 70–109, depending upon the age of the tree. The yield also varies with age: 12% for trees 10–15 years old down to 4% at age 60.

Gum resins are extracted from the balsam poplar buds and exported to Europe under the name *tacamahaca*. The word is of Aztec or West Indies origin, later becoming *hackmatack*. An oleoresin is prepared by simply heating five parts of good quality vegetable oil to near simmer in a low-temperature crock pot and then adding one part by weight of fresh buds. This is slowly simmered, lid off, for four to six hours, then cooled, strained, and bottled. It is a wonderful remedy for long-standing constipation where the use of chemical laxatives has debilitated and dried out the mucous membranes of the bowel.

According to Eclectic physician Edward Shook (1978), it is a remarkable

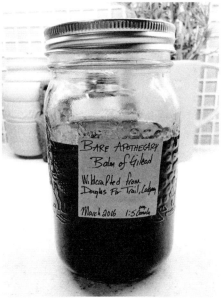

Sun-infused poplar bud oil

dissolver of cholesterol and uric acid. Not only does it dissolve the excess, he suggests, but the diuretic effect carries it out of the system. The oil makes a suitable salve for lung and respiratory congestion, and for the swelling and pain of rheumatism.

I love preparing this oil in the spring. The hands will become resin-coated, but the scent is a true sign of impending spring. I can never make enough, as once they have used it, people will ask where they can get more. It relieves muscle pain almost immediately. Culpepper (2009) wrote, "the ointment called Populneon, which is made of this Poplar, is singularly good for all heat and inflammations in any part of the body, and tempers the heat of wounds. It is much used to dry up the milk of women's breasts when they have weaned their children."

The buds contain a large set of carboxylic acids, which may be useful to both the food and medical industries. Some acid derivatives and oil content (in % mg/kg) are malic (6.56), malonic (2.3), citric (1.99), ketoglutaric (1.95), adipic (1.33), oxaloacetic (1.51), succinic (0.33), and butyric (0.32). Ingest 1 tablespoon with equal amounts of honey three times daily between meals for obstinate constipation. Otherwise use externally.

Balsam Poplar bark and twigs yield a fixed oil consisting of approximately two-thirds polyunsaturated, 25% saturated, and 9% monosaturated fatty acids. This is composed mainly of over 47% linolenic acid, 18% linoleic acid, 13% palmitic acid, 5% stearic acid, 7.2% eicosenoic acid, 3.1% docosanoic acid, and 2.2% tetracosanoic acid.

A commercial oleoresin is prepared from the balsam poplar buds. It is a yellow-green viscous liquid with a sweet balsamic odor reminiscent of cinnamon. An essential oil can be prepared from the oleoresin using vacuum distillation in the presence of ethylene glycol. The main constituents are salicin, chrysin, tectochyrsin, populin, and small amounts of gallic acid and tannins. Both the essential oil from distillation and the oleoresin are used in perfumery and liqueurs.

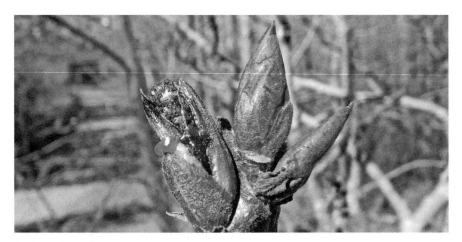

Spring poplar buds

Gemmotherapy

Poplar buds are collected in early spring and macerated in alcohol and glycerin. Black poplar buds act upon the arterial system of the legs and relieve spasms. It favors the establishment of the collateral circulation and aids in the treatment of associated nutritional disturbances. In arteriosclerosis, with a tendency to thrombophlebitis, it is effective, but should be taken slowly and not be used for more than four weeks.

Dose: Take 10 drops three times daily in water of the 1D vegetable macerate. This product is available commercially, or you can make your own.

Medicinal Mushroom

In my part of the world one important medicinal mushroom is found on older balsam poplar. The artist's conk (*Ganoderma applanatum*) is a close cousin of the famous *reishi* (*G. lucidum*) mushroom. Both are important adaptogens, like roseroot, helping modify response to stress, modulating the immune system, and reducing inflammation. More information can be found in my book on medicinal mushrooms and lichens, *The Fungal Pharmacy: The Complete Guide to Medicinal Mushrooms and Lichens of North America* (2011). They can be sizeable: one fruiting body discovered on an Aleutian Island in the 1950s was sixteen feet in diameter and weighed over 110 pounds.

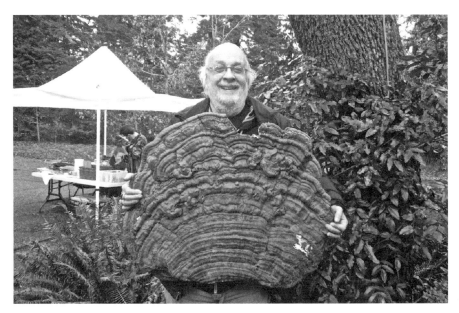

The author with a twenty-two-pound artist's conk

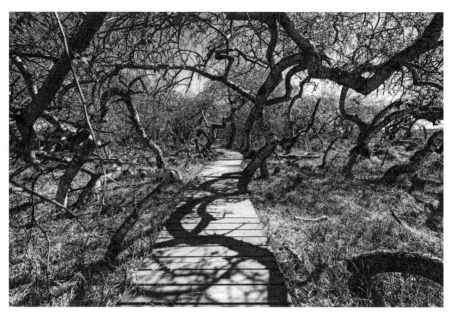

Crooked aspen (courtesy of Jason Schultz, www.schultzphoto.ca)

Flower Essence

There is a small forest of crooked aspen in Saskatchewan that is unique in the world. The research essence is available from Prairie Deva Flower Essences. Crooked Aspen flower essence is associated with the formation and deformation of the spinal column. It represents a structural quality with fixed or imbalanced beliefs surrounding ideas, motivations, or experiences. It may be helpful in any number of arthritic or rheumatic complaints, including autoimmune responses related to bone, ligament, and cartilage in the body.

On an emotional plane, the essence may be helpful in those individuals suffering from distortions of paranoia or feelings of imbalance from drugs or early childhood trauma and training. On a spiritual level, crooked aspen essence helps separates religion from spiritual growth and alleviates experiences associated with cults and distorted belief systems.

Spiritual Properties

Pamela Chase and Jonathan Pawlik (1991) describe the spiritual properties of aspen poplar and both eastern and black cottonwood. Aspen can give a sense of safety, an anchoring in times of change. It becomes easier to affirm that everything is going to be all right. When we feel like the bottom has dropped out from under us, or we are troubled with anxiety and fear about an upcoming experience, aspen restores our sense of perspective. When we see more possibilities for learning and growth, then it is easier to move with a sense of anticipation. The leaves of the aspen enjoy the wind from all sides, and they speak of the exuberance of living fully in the face of challenge.

The cottonwood family teaches us about the sacredness of our physical body. When we have been wishing that we had someone else's physical characteristics, black cottonwood (*P. trichocarpa*) reminds us of the joy and beauty of the physical forms on this planet, especially our own. With eastern cottonwood (*P. deltoides*), we can learn to see our bodies as more than a machine that we can order around. Its energy supports us in learning the patience and acceptance that is the foundation for a more intuitively complete connection with our physical bodies.

Trees have a personality that one can tune into with relative ease. It takes time and patience, but trees and the dryads associated with them will speak to those open to the experience.

Personality Traits

Gina Mohammed (2002) offers her insight:

One of [poplar's] secrets—and one shared by many northern plants—is that it focuses its energies and emphasizes one thing at a time. It concentrates either on growing roots, or leaves, or stem, as dictated by the time of year. If we could focus on one thing at a time and do it well, how much more peace, energy, and satisfaction we would have. We could enjoy a sense of accomplishment instead of merely stumbling from task to task. In today's challenging world, we have a great advantage if we can simplify and focus.

Laurel Dewey (2001) looked at aspens from a different point of view:

Aspens can be a bit aloof in their nature. Some observers of aspens often say that this trembling reveals a deep-seated nervous character trait. However, aspen never seems too nervous to me. With its tall, outstretched trunk arching far into the blue sky, aspen has always acted more "above it all" rather than some frightened forest tree. Aspens can definitely be standoffish in character and suspicious of anyone new venturing into their domain. However, if you befriend them and they take you in, the aspen can help guide you on your path as they communicate with your spirit on incredible levels.

McFarland (2003, 189) wrote:

Aspen is a name for someone who is trying to face up to his or her own fears. It is a transformative name leading from fear into a fiery burst of courage. People who are shy, naive, or inexperienced could wear Aspen well. It could also be a good name for a dancer, drummer, or anyone working with movement and rhythm. This is a mountain person's name. Aspens have a lot of potential.

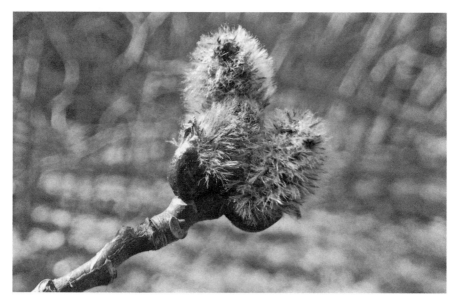

Poplar catkin

Beresford-Kroeger (2010) offered her take on aspen:

Trembling aspen was also used as a treatment for serious heart conditions.... This process was modified for the Boreal world, where a length of aspen bark was cut the same size as the human heart. This was taken from the south side of a mature tree. It was removed at the height of the beating heart. The bark was chewed to solubilize the medicine and the juice was drunk. This simpler form was also an effective heart medicine.

Myths and Legends

Michael Mucz (2012) collected stories and wrote a book on Ukrainian-Canadian folk medicine. Here is one excerpt on aspen:

An Indian once told me that to have healthy teeth (zuby), you had to chew on wood from a poplar tree that you saw being hit, and split open, by lightning (blyskavka). I actually saw this happen to a tree and took some of the wood splinters home for such use. Over the years, every month or so, I cut off (vidrizav) some small pieces and chewed on them for a couple of hours. I am ninety-one years old, have never had a toothache, and still have all my teeth except for a broken one. —J. P., Two Hills

Guillet (1962) collected and recorded this myth about poplar:

Jupiter did not think so highly of the white poplar. One day he lost some of his spoons and bade Ganymede search through the woods for them. All the trees disclaimed any knowledge of them, and so did the white poplar, but very guiltily. When Ganymede questioned her, she tossed her branches in disdain and said, "Why should I be charged with keeping the goods of Zeus?" At that, she tossed her branches still higher. But she had not stowed the spoons securely, and they came rattling down on the ground. Ganymede caught them up and sped with them Jupiter while the poplar trembled and paled with fear. As punishment, Zeus condemned the tree to hold up its arms forever and show pallor beneath its leaves.

Jenifer Morrissey (2000) wrote this beautiful tribute to the cottonwood:

Storms will tear off large branches, leaving a star-shaped formation on bark. The Arapaho Indians of present-day Colorado believe that cottonwoods are fundamental to the creation of the star-studded night skies. When the night spirit needs stars, it asks the wind spirit to blow, and blow hard it does, until cottonwoods shed some of their branches. At the broken places is left a star-shaped pattern in the wood, where a new star was born into the sky.

Astrology

Hageneder (2005) writes his astrological take on aspen:

Aspen leaves enjoy the wind more than any other tree and are therefore a channel for the voice of Mercury, the messenger of the more subtle spheres. Like an emblem of tolerance and flexibility, Aspen can accept impulses from all directions of the wind, and make them a harmonious part of its own movement and being.

RECIPES

Tincture: 10–20 drops as needed. Fresh leaf bud tincture is made fresh at 1:4 (1 part leaf by weight to 4 parts 75% alcohol). The dry buds are produced at 1:5 in 90% alcohol. A tincture of the inner bark is also prepared fresh at 1:5 and 40% alcohol.

Dose: 6–30 drops three times daily. For chest colds take 1 teaspoon in 1 cup of warm water three times daily. Honey is a good addition. Bud tincture is specific for laryngitis with loss of voice, and for chronic bronchitis. Combine with a chest rub of bud oil externally.

Decoction: Take 1 ounce of aspen inner bark or twigs to 1 pint of water. Simmer for 20 minutes. Drink 4 ounces, cool, up to four times daily. You can add this to children's baths lasting 5–15 minutes for fever reduction.

Decoction: Take 1 pound of dried, cut balsam poplar bark to 1 gallon of water and slowly simmer for half an hour. Strain off the liquid and return the bark to glassware and cover to 3 inches above bark. Reduce with a slow simmer until the water is just above the bark. Strain and combine the two liquids and then reduce to 1 pint. Add an equal amount of vegetable glycerin, cool, bottle, and label. Keep in the fridge. Dose is 1–2 teaspoons before bedtime for adults.

Infusion: Steep the dried leaves and drink up to 3 cups daily.

Oil: Add beeswax and other carrier oils, such as fireweed, for hemorrhoid suppositories or arthritic salves.

Balsam bud oil: Add 1 part buds to 4 parts of canola oil and heat in a double boiler for at least 24 hours at 115–120°F. Strain. Make sure buds are at room temperature before putting in oil. A crockpot with a low-temperature setting will work wonderfully. Leave the lid off to allow any moisture to evaporate. An alternate method is to freeze the buds overnight. Then take four times the weight of buds in canola oil by volume and place both in a blender. Liquefy until a beautiful, thin, runny combination is obtained. To make a salve, add some melted beeswax. Do not try this without freezing the buds. Trust me!

Caution: Poplar bark preparations are contraindicated in those patients allergic to salicylates. Poplar buds should be avoided by those allergic to salicylates, propolis, and balsam of Peru.

Do not use chrysin derivatives in hormone-sensitive cancers in both sexes, or in pregnant women. It may interfere with breast-cancer therapies such as Femara. Balsam poplar use can reduce breast milk production.

Many herbalists note that clients who have taken aspirin over a period of time do not receive benefit from aspen poplar bark decoctions or tincture.

6

Leaf-Budding Moon Herbal Allies

Bees and Honey

Last night, as I was sleeping, I dreamt—marvelous error! That I had a beehive here, inside my heart. And the golden bees were making white combs and sweet honey from my old failures.

—Antonio Machado

Hope is the only bee that makes honey without flowers.

—Robert Green Ingersoll

In the mid-1970s I was living in a small log cabin, without electricity, running water, central heating, and other luxuries of modern life. My good friend and neighbor Terry Anderson had several beehives, and I became instantly excited about these amazing insects. I bought four used hives, stacked five high, from a neighbor. In late April, Terry and I drove to Edmonton and returned with our boxes of imported bees. In those days, it was less expensive to winter over, and beekeepers started with a new colony each year. This is no longer the case, but it was pretty standard practice forty years ago, even among the large commercial beekeepers. In fact, the town of Fahler, two hours northwest of my place on the south shore of Lesser Slave Lake, calls itself the Honey Capital of Canada.

Alberta is the fifth largest producer of honey in the world, so there was lots of expertise to draw upon. The transition from small box went well, including the release of the queen bee. I had saved some money and invested in a bee suit, a helmet with a veil, long leather gloves, a smoker, and so on. All summer I checked on their health and watched in amazement as they filled the hive with honey. I had a sting here and there but learned that slow and gentle movements were important aspects of the relationship. It was a good summer, with lots of sun, timely rains, and a long fall.

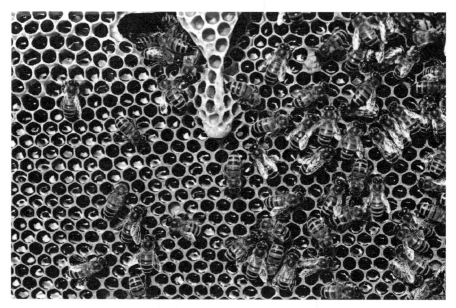

Bees and honey

Terry had built a shop and bought a used four-frame extractor. We helped each other with the day-long process, and one year my four hives yielded just over five hundred pounds of fresh honey. I would have said organic, but there is no such thing as organic honey. The beekeeper can practice organic husbandry, but the bees go where they wish. Fortunately I had no commercial farmland in my area, just miles and miles of forest and lakeshore.

As I studied more, I became fascinated with the life cycle of bees and the other products they produce, like royal jelly, and I began to gather propolis and pollen as new herbal allies. The medicinal use of any of these bee products would take up an entire chapter. I have included abbreviated findings.

The word honey is believed derived from the Hebrew *ghoneg*, which means literally, delight. Theodore Zeldin (2012, 95) said, "Once a rare and divine medicine—honey was called the perspiration of the sky, the saliva of the stars...."

Traditional Uses

Native peoples made infusions of wild honeybee and gave it to those suffering from suppressed urine. The same remedy assisted those needing to suppress sexual over-indulgence. Ironically, in Europe, newlywed couples drank a honey wine called *hyromel* every night during the first lunar month of marriage; hence the term *honeymoon*. The Cherokee used bees in times of difficult labor. Alder bark was scraped upward from the root and a weak decoction made with a pint of water. A small amount of dried, powdered bumblebee was added to half a cup of the above tea. A single tablespoon was taken and seldom needed repeating.

The Cree of Northern Alberta refer to the bee as *amo*, and the honey from the hive *amomey*. The Dene of northern Canada burned bee and wasp hives into ash for application to swellings, boils, and skin rashes. Celine Eyakfwo writes:

> *They light the beehive and burn it when it turn to ashes. When they burn it really good, then they add a little bit of water into ashes. When they smear it on our swollen part it feels like burning. It just feels like burning and hot. When they do that then it would go away. If it would go away, then it goes away. And if it has to break open, it would break open.* (Rogers 2014)

For newborn anuria, pour boiling water over angry bees (if they weren't already, this should do the job), and give the strained water to infants. In seventeenth-century Europe, bees were killed with sulfur fumes, baked and powdered, and given in water for urinary stones and related obstructions. The ash of bees was added to oil of rose to cause rapid hair growth. In Syria, bees were roasted in olive oil and applied on scalp to turn gray hair black.

It is worth noting that beekeepers have the lowest incidence of cancer of all the occupations. It is widely believed beekeepers live longer than the average human. A study by Nasir et al. (2015) on thirty male beekeepers and 30 male non-beekeepers looked at telomere length and found the former significantly longer than the control group. Both raising bees and consuming bee products is associated with increased telomere length. Telomeres are the caps on the end of each strand of DNA that protect our chromosomes, like the plastic tips on the end of shoelaces. Without a coating, they become frayed, the DNA strands become damaged, and telomeres become too short, causing cells to age.

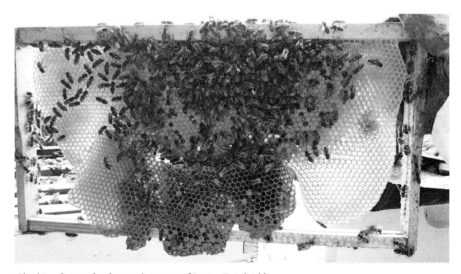

Checking frames for disease (courtesy of Jessica Friedrich)

103

Those handling bees have long known that the insects dislike alcohol and will attack keepers who have ingested any amount. I learned the painful way that a beer after checking hives was good, but beforehand, not so much.

It is worth noting various substances from the beehive are mentioned in religious texts, including the Bible, the Koran, the Torah, the Book of Mormon, and the Scrolls of the Orient. Throughout history, humans have been functional kleptoparasites of honeybees. That is, we have enslaved them for our purposes. The first beekeeping images were put on cave walls in Valencia, Spain, around 7000 BCE. The Bee goddess, representing the mother and the hive representing her womb, was found painted on a vase dating to around 6000 BCE. The bee appears quite frequently as a symbol of the soul. In the Orphic teachings of Greece, the bee was the emblem of the soul. Priestesses at Eleusis were known as bees and Essence priests. In the Christian tradition, the term *beehive* is used to describe either the church or monastic communities.

A bee's honey and sting represent sweetness and pain. In Siberia, the Buriats depicted the soul as a bee visible when issuing from the mouth of a sleeping person. In Hittite mythology, the bee saved the world from drought by finding the lost son of the weather god. Indo-Malaysian and Muslim traditions also speak of the soul as a bee. In India, a blue bee on the forehead symbolizes Krishna; on a triangle, Shiva; and on a lotus, Vishnu.

The Mayans used the same word for "the world" and "honey." Ah Muzen Cab was the Mayan god of bees, who the books of the Jaguar Priest say created the world. They would sometimes add a toad (*Bufo marinus*) to their honey mead. The toad's venom contained DMT, which added a certain psychedelic twist to the drink. The honey was produced from the flower of the *Turbina corymbosa*, in itself a powerful hallucinogen. Mayans still collect this honey to make *balché*, a narcotic mead. This honey was used to induce labor during childbirth due to ergoline alkaloids stimulating uterine contractions.

In early Christian mystical writings, the bee came to symbolize virginity, perhaps because no one ever saw them mating. In Slavic folk tradition, the bee is linked with the Immaculate Conception. The feast of Saint Anne, mother of Mary, is held on July 26, the time for beekeepers to pray for the conception of healthy new bees. Hildegard of Bingen, the twelfth century mystic and priestess, wrote:

> For anyone on whom ganglia grow, or who has had some limb moved from its place, or who has any crushed limbs, take bees that are not alive.... put a sufficient amount on a linen cloth, and sew it up. Soak this cloth, with the bees sewn within, in olive oil, and place it over the ailing limb.... A person whose eyes are cloudy should take the small bladder from between the head and stomach of the bumblebee. One who has deep scabies on his head should often smear the same liquid over his head and he will be cured. (Throop 1998, 200-201)

Bee larvae are a popular cooked food in Thailand, Japan, and Korea. The honeybee larva is a richer source of protein than pork and is similar in vitamin and mineral content to chicken and shrimp. Oven dry at 160–175°F or simply fry up in butter; they're delicious.

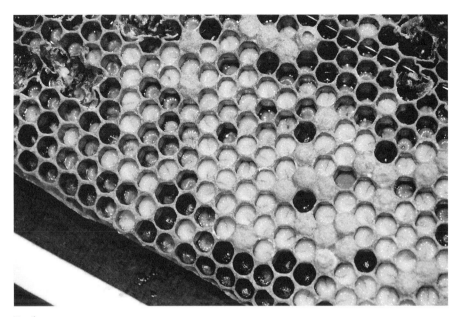

Bee larvae

The leafcutter bee (*Megachile* species) is a typical solitary. There are no workers, and all the females are capable of motherhood. She will cut neat round or oval pieces from rose leaves and fashion cylindrical cells in a tubular hole in rotted wood. When complete, it is filled with a mixture of pollen and nectar, an egg is laid, and the mother bee puts on the lid and builds another cell on top.

The introduced honeybee is the official insect in twelve different U.S. states. It makes possible the reproduction of 80 percent of the world's grains, fruits, nuts, seeds, vegetables, and legumes.

The communal life of bees has inspired architects and artists. Several interesting people come to mind, including Juan Antonio Ramírez. He wrote *The Beehive Metaphor* (1998), a book that explores relationships of communal buildings and social creatures, such as insects and humans. Those interested in such connections may wish to look at the works of Antoni Gaudí, Mies van der Rohe, Le Corbusier, and Frank Lloyd Wright. The last three all lived in Berlin at the same time, and this may have set the inspiration for collective harmony in their future work.

The uncontrolled use of antibiotics is now creating overgrowth of candida fungi and other infections in beehives, causing high mortality rates among both pupae and larvae. The use of neonicotinoids is significantly affecting colony health. These pesticides are five to ten thousand times more toxic to bees than DDT, according to the Task Force on Systemic Pesticides. These pesticides were recently banned in Europe. In April 2016, Maryland banned their use, and in July of 2016 several environmental groups banded together to take the Canadian government to court over the approval of these toxic pesticides.

My medicinal mushroom colleague Paul Stamets recently released medicinal mushroom products to help bee colonies restore health. Between April 2014 and April 2015, Colony Collapse Disorder reduced by 41 percent the population of commercial bee colonies in the United States. The product contains extracts of chaga and *reishi* mushrooms and is put into feed water. Check out www.beefriendlyinitiative.org.

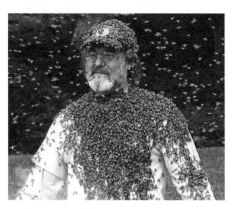

Paul Stamets and bees

Antibiotics, if used at all, should be discontinued at least fourteen days before the flow of nectar. New Zealand beekeepers do not use antibiotics to control American foulbrood, for example, because their residue-free products receive preferential access to Japan and other countries. *Varroa*-resistant bees may be part of the future, as the honeybee genome has been sequenced. In the 1920s, Rudolf Steiner (1933) warned that artificial breeding of queens would lead to dire effects. When a beekeeper in the audience objected, he said they should talk again in a century.

"Eat honey, my son, for it is good," was advice given by Solomon around 1000 BCE. Pliny could not decide whether honey was the sweat of the sky, the saliva of the stars, or a juice formed from the air as it cleared itself. Aristotle believed it was dew distilled from the stars and rainbows. In 1708 Saint Francis of Sales said, "All kinds of precious stones cast into honey become more brilliant thereby." Medicinal honey was extolled on Sumerian tablets carved over four thousand years ago. The ancient Egyptians, Assyrians, Chinese, Romans, and Greeks all used honey to treat wounds and diseases of the gut. An Egyptian myth recalls the sun god, Ra, crying. Tears dropping from his eyes turned into bees making honey.

The ancient Persians used honey to cleanse mortals of sin, because it came from sinless bees that created the precious fluid without touching the flowers. Honey was so highly prized by ancient Anglo-Saxon chiefs that portions were demanded for tax and tribute. It was prized for making mead, a honey wine, or metheglin beer. The Greeks made a kind of mead or *hydromeli*, as did the Romans, who called their honey and wine compounds *mulsum*. Galen mentions *oxymeli*, honey mixed with vinegar as a medicine, no fewer than 221 times. Attila the Hun drank so much mead on his wedding day that he suffered a heart attack, or so the story goes. A similar liqueur is today distilled in Georgia and known as *santlis*, while the national drink of Ethiopia, *tej* is made from fermented honey.

The Slavs used honey in love potions, and the Magyars of Hungary smeared honey on the genitals of young men and women to make them more attractive to the opposite sex. I bet that worked. Various Brazilian indigenous groups conduct fall honey festivals after gathering it in spring and hanging it in gourds from ceilings. A creation myth of the Caduveo of central South America tells of a falcon seeing honey forming in gourds and telling the creator god to place it in the middle of trees so that humans had to work to retrieve it.

Honey was considered in seventeenth-century medicine to be hot and dry and thus no good for the liver and spleen in individuals with hot temperaments. The Chinese believe crude honey is cool, and the purified product is warming and digestive. According to ancient Hindu medical writers, new honey is laxative, and honey older than a year is more astringent. Ancient Syrians mixed honey and hot water to inject into their nostrils to treat phlegmatic congestion or head pain. Honey has been used in Egypt as an embalming liquid, and Alexander the Great was buried with a honey coating. Mummies in Egypt were traditionally covered with beeswax, the name derived from the Egyptian name for wax, *mum*. The Talmud believed honey was a remedy for gout and heart trouble and would heal the wounds of both people and beasts.

Honey is gathered from the nectar of flowers and brewed around 86°F. To manufacture one kilogram of honey requires an average of two hundred thousand loads of nectar, or about ten million visits to individual flowers. A worker bee, during her entire lifetime, produces just one-twelfth of a teaspoon of honey. The average hive of 20,000 bees needs about fifteen kilograms of honey to overwinter. Bees reduce brain activity and the size of their brains in winter, and then enlarge brain activity when flowers begin to bloom in spring (Meyer-Rochow and Vakkuri 2002).

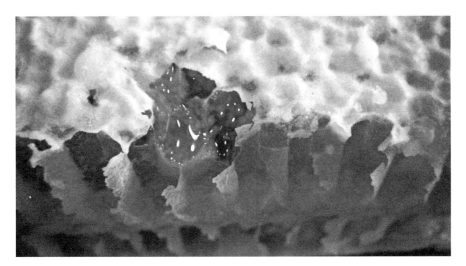

Honey in comb

Medicinal Uses

Today raw unpasteurized honey is prized for its nutritional and medicinal value. Containing fructose and laevulose, it is not metabolized through the pancreas in the same manner as refined sugar. When I lived up north and raised bees, honey and birch syrup were the only sweeteners I used.

Work in the 1940s suggested honey from high altitudes is a stronger antibacterial than honey produced in lower valleys. Polish research, and common sense, suggests organic honey may be more desirable for consumers' health. Work by Glinski (2000) looked at honey contaminated with sulfa drugs and its allergic and suppressive action on the immune system. A recent human clinical trial found daily consumption of honey helps prevent lipid peroxidation, the damaging effects of free radicals, and their negative influence on atherosclerosis and cardiac disease. In one trial, 25 men ages 18 to 68 drank a mixture of 4 tablespoons of honey in water daily for 5 weeks, with significant improvement in blood serum antioxidant levels.

Specialty honeys, of course, hold and transfer the energetics of specific flowers to the consumer. Sweet clover, fireweed, dandelion, buckwheat, goldenrod, and willow are a few available on the prairies. Sunflower honey is considered good for fevers, linden flower honey for insomnia, and thyme honey for stimulating digestion. Manuka honey produced in New Zealand is a strong antimicrobial, with a market share based on a few scientific studies. Honey collected from the high-aluminum soils of North Carolina has a bluish color, making for an unattractive food. The so-called pine honey is in fact honeydew, a sweet sticky liquid exuded by aphids living in pine forests and feeding on the sap of young shoots. This is collected and processed by bees in the manner of honey, as conifers do not bear nectar-producing flowers.

Honey derived from dandelions, canola, or members of the *Brassica* genus crystallizes in two to three weeks, often hardening in the comb. Linden nectar, while pleasant in honey form to humans, has a stupefying effect on bees. Honey from the nectar of belladonna, henbane, and members of the *Solanum* genus retains some of the plant alkaloids' psychoactive effect. Buckwheat honey has been shown in studies to contain high concentrations of kaempferol, making it high in antioxidant value. A study in China found buckwheat honey inhibited *E. coli* and *Salmonella* species at full strength.

Bee Well Laboratories from Israel have developed very unique medicines based on honey infused with therapeutic properties. Treatments for asthmatic bronchitis, gynecological problems, and even simple wounds and ulcers are produced by feeding their bees medicinal herbs as well as various ferments and microelements, which the bees turn into honey.

If you are interested in different honeys from around the world, you must visit Les Abeilles in Paris. The owner has a private collection of over two hundred honeys, and a vast number are for sale. The shop's owner is involved with a society for city beekeepers with some three hundred rooftop hives around the city. Medihoney is the only honey allowed for medical use in the United Kingdom. Revamil is a brand used in the Netherlands. Over thirty clinical trials using honey to treat surgical wounds and burns have been conducted in the United Kingdom. Another fun adventure is the annual Sagra del Miele festival, held each October in Sicily. Local varieties are on display for tasting and sale. Rose honey, tasting almost like licorice, sells for 136 euros per pound.

Honey is very useful in chronic bronchitis, and healing peptic and duodenal ulcers. A new study sought to determine if honey can kill the *Helicobacter pylori* bacterium related to gastric ulcers. One study involving 20 cases of ulcers showed complete healing in 15 patients, progress in 3 more, with pain completely disappearing in 18 and decreased in the other 2. Patients took ⅓ cup of honey three times daily before meals. That is a fairly high dose.

Honey helps clear the most chronic constipation with its laxative effect; as well as chronic diarrhea from bacterial or viral origin. It is safe during pregnancy. It is sedative and works well for insomnia. In moderation, it is healing to the kidneys. The Bible mentions honey as "healing to the bones," perhaps in reference to the stimulation of new white blood cell production. In cases of hypochromic anemia, take 2 to 3 ounces of honey in three divided daily doses to increase red blood cells and hemoglobin counts. Raw honey is alkaline and potassium rich and helps to counteract the acidity that accompanies arthritis. Burns of the skin heal with little scarring and quick pain relief.

In short, its properties are antiseptic, diuretic, and demulcent—perhaps helping to explain the use of honey for urinary problems. Honey is hydroscopic, meaning it dries the area around it. And its hypertonic effect draws water from the bacterial cells, causing them to shrivel and die. Both gram-positive and gram-negative bacteria are destroyed by unpasteurized honey. Inhibitory effect has been reported for *Salmonella typhimurium* (49 strains), *Staphylococcus aureus* (58 isolates), *Pseudomonas aeruginosa* (152 isolates), *E. coli* O157:H7 (25 strains), and various *Mycobacterium* species. Honey is effective against MRSA and in wounds infected with other multiresistant bacteria.

One active principle, inhibine, is secreted by the pharyngeal glands of the bee. Inhibine concentration controls hydrogen peroxide production but is destroyed by light and heat. Hence the importance of raw honey. Honey contains high levels of hydrogen peroxide, a natural antiseptic. Well, actually, glucose oxidase converts glucose to gluconolactate, which in turn yields gluconic acid and hydrogen peroxide. Catalase then converts peroxide to water and oxygen. Pasteurized honey contains no such enzyme. Cavanagh et al. (1970) found that raw honey, applied twice daily into extensive wounds following operations for carcinoma of the vulva, healed remarkably well. Fournier's gangrene, a rapidly spreading infection usually requiring aggressive surgery, has been successfully treated with raw honey. Labial and genital herpes respond well to honey—better than acyclovir in most cases.

In one clinical trial of 139 children, honey was found more effective than dextromethorphan or diphenhydramine in relieving nighttime coughs due to respiratory infections. In Canada, over-the-counter cough remedies are not recommended (and are labeled as such) for children under six years of age. Honey on wounds has a natural debriding effect on wounds, so surgical debridement is either unnecessary or only minimal removal of dead flesh is required. Honey promotes healthy granulation tissue, which helps the skin regenerate with little or no scarring. Stimulation of new blood vessels in the bed of wounds has been observed. A review of twenty-two clinical trials with more than two thousand patients concluded that honey cleans up existing wounds, protects against infection, reduces swelling, minimizes scarring, and speeds up growth of new tissue (Molan 2006).

Honey may give great relief in seborrheic dermatitis (SD), which responded to raw honey when used every other day for four weeks. The condition has a number of origins, including excessive protein intake, or inability to breakdown protein properly, leading to bacteria in the bowel metabolizing amino acids into cadavrine, putrescine, and spermidine. These enter the bloodstream and remove a brake on skin cell growth that multiplies and produces excessive amounts of sebum. Many medications are implicated in SD, including L-DOPA for Parkinson's, hydralazine for congestive heart failure and hypertension, isoniazid for TB, penicillamine for kidney stones, rheumatoid arthritis, Wilson's disease (hypothyroid), and oral contraceptives. Ironically, d-penicillamine is sometimes prescribed for SD. Holy contraindication, Batman!

Honey diluted in warm water was applied to 30 patients with chronic lesions of the face, scalp, and chest and left on for 3 hours. Itching and scaling disappeared in 1 week, and skin lesions healed in 2 weeks; 15 patients who followed up for 6 months had no relapses, while 12 of 15 who did not continue honey use had recurrence of lesions in 2 to 4 months (Al-Waili 2001). Honey is used in numerous cosmetics; including shampoos, moisturizers and skin masks, face creams, and hair conditioners. Research is currently underway to develop a process of using honey to create alpha-hydroxy acids (AHAs). Examples include Johnson's Baby Shampoo, Honey and Vitamin E, Avon Rare Pearls Eau de Parfum spray, and Revlon Professional Cuticle Massage Night Cream. Honey extracts are used in Suave shampoos, Salon Selectives Conditioner, and Happy Daisy Relaxing Baby Bubbles. This does not suggest that less desirable ingredients are not found in these products.

Local honey (raw and unpasteurized) taken 1 teaspoon daily for three months in advance of your regional hay fever season may reduce symptoms. It will diminish milk secretion in nursing mothers, and may be used for weaning when desired. Garden sage tea will assist this process as well. In 1936 Professor Haydak set out to subsist for three month's on a diet of unpasteurized cow's milk and honey (three ounces per quart of milk). His ability to work remained normal, and clinical work showed maintenance of weight, normal bowel movements, absence of protein or sugar in the urine, and a slight rise in hemoglobin levels. Only toward the very end of three months was a vitamin C deficiency noticed.

The work of Subrahmanyam (1991) is of interest. He found honey has an antiseptic effect, useful in connection with skin-grafting surgery. A trial compared honey and silver sulfadiazine, a common burn dressing, in 52 patients with partial thickness burns. They found 87% of those treated with honey healed in 15 days compared to 10% using the silver dressing. Another study looked at wound healing after cesarean section and hysterectomy surgeries. Compared to the group receiving iodine and alcohol, the honey-treated group was infection-free in fewer days, healed more cleanly, with reduced hospital stays.

Despite the historical and folkloric use of honey in medicine, it was not until 1976 that two physicians on two different continents conducted clinical trials on incurable bedsores and burn-related infections with a 98–99 percent success rates confirmed in both five-year studies. The sugars in honey create osmotic pressure, literally sucking the water from germ cells so they shrivel and die. And sugars retard collagen growth, which produces scarring. The acidity of honey prevents ammonia from bacterial metabolism becoming harmful to body tissues. And, of course, honey supplies a wide range of vitamins, minerals, and amino acids to the cells for healing.

A study by Cooper et al. (2000) revealed all 20 strains of antibiotic-resistant *Burkholderia cepacia* in the sputum of cystic fibrosis patients showed sensitivity to honey. This suggests honey may have a potential role to play in the clinical management of these infections. Keep in mind that children under one year old should not be given raw honey. Work at the University of Illinois found drinking honey water led to significant increases in blood antioxidant levels within sixty to ninety minutes. This same team discovered buckwheat honey increased serum antioxidant capacity in humans (Gheldof et al. 2003).

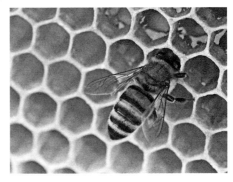

Bee depositing nectar

Work by Al-Waili (2004) found honey taken for 15 days by 12 adults positively lowered serum levels of thromboxane B_2, PGE_2, and PGF_{2a} by 48%, 63%, and 50%, respectively. It increased serum iron by 20%, copper by 33%, and decreased IgE by 34%. Immunoglobulin E is a marker of allergic response.

Honey serves to create a film of liquid between burn or wound tissue and dressing, which allows them to be lifted off painlessly and without tearing of regrown cells. It is superior to silver on wound healing (Lindberg et al. 2015). Honey applied to the oral cavity of patients undergoing radiation for neck and head cancer significantly reduces levels of oral mucositis. Honey is used to coat catheters and other medical devices before insertion. Pinocembrin, one antioxidant unique to honey, is currently being studied for its antibacterial activity. Honey is frequently recommended for feeding and medicating falcons: to make meat attractive to them, to revive tired birds, and to encourage the growth of new feathers in place of broken plumes. Of course, it is also a quick source of energy, passing into the bloodstream in about ten minutes. Jarvis (1960) wrote:

The taking of honey each day is advised in order to keep the lymph flowing at its normal tempo, and thus avoid degenerative disease which shortens life. The real value of honey is to maintain a healthy flow of the tissue fluid called lymph. When this flow rate slows down, then calcium and iron are precipitated as sediment. When the lymph flow is stagnant, then harmful microorganisms invade the body and sickness appears.

A recent study of thirty-nine weight trained athletes, both male and female, who underwent an intensive workout and then immediately ingested protein as well as sugar, maltodextrin, or honey found the latter group maintained optimal blood sugar levels throughout the two hours following a workout. Muscle recuperation and glycogen restoration was most favorable in those taking the protein-honey combination.

Fifty-eight boys were divided in two groups, one taking 2 tablespoons of honey daily and other none. All received the same diet, exercise and rest. After one year, the honey group showed an 8.5% increase in hemoglobin and overall increase in energy, vitality, and general appearance.

Studies suggest honey is of benefit to cardiovascular health. Al-Waili and Haq (2004) looked at diabetic, high-cholesterol, and healthy subjects for 15 days, giving them either dextrose, artificial honey, or the real thing. In healthy subjects, plasma glucose was elevated at 1 and 2 hours and decreased after 3. Honey levels elevated for 1 hour and decreased after 3. Elevation of insulin and C-peptide was significantly higher after dextrose than honey. Honey consumed by healthy subjects for 15 days lowered cholesterol by 7%, LDL by 1%, triglycerides by 2%, C-peptide by 7%, homocysteine by 6%, and plasma glucose by 6%. HDL, the good cholesterol, increased 2%. In high-cholesterol subjects, it decreased cholesterol 8% and C-peptide by 75%. In diabetic subjects, honey caused significantly lower plasma glucose.

Mesaik et al. (2008) found honey taken internally helps modulate immune function during phagocytosis. And honey appears to induce apoptosis in human renal cancer cells (Samarghandian et al. 2011). Bee bread, a mixture of pollen and honey fed to bees in the hive, has been found to contain antioxidative properties and inhibit ACE, associated with cardiovascular risk (Nagai et al. 2005). A 1976 editorial in the *Archives of Modern Medicine* suggested honey is in a category of "worthless but harmless substances." Ho hum!

Caution: Honey may contain *Clostridium botulinum* spores, harmless to adults and children over age one. It should never be given to babies, either raw or pasteurized, as these spores may produce a toxin that causes infant botulism. For medicinal benefit, it should not be heated above 100°F. It deteriorates in sunlight, and should be kept dark and cool. When replacing sugar in recipes, use 20 percent more and reduce water by the same amount.

BEE VENOM

Constituents: over 40 components, including 11 peptides (melittin, apamin, adolapin, and mast cell degranulating peptide or MCDP); five enzymes, the most important being phospholipase A. Eighteen pharmacologically active components have been found.

When attacked, bees release an alarm substance called isoamyl acetate, detectable over considerable distance. Beekeepers avoid this alarm pheromone by using a smoker that generates clouds of smoke. The bees gorge themselves on honey, producing a narcotic, tranquilizing effect. Otherwise, the potential for a barbed venom attacks is quite high.

Bee venom therapy (BVT) was first described by Hippocrates nearly two millennia ago. The first modern report was in the medical journal *Lancet* in 1910. In 1888, an Austrian physician, Phillip Terc, advocated deliberate bee stings to treat rheumatism. In the 1930s a German firm, Mack, began commercial bee venom production. They worked out a system where the bees were gently shocked and stung a piece of paper. A Czech company in the 1960s developed a material so thin that the bees can withdraw their stinger and live. Bees could then inject venom into the paper ten times in only fifteen minutes, and the venom could then be safely collected.

Many people now practice BVT for relief of symptoms from arthritis, lupus, cancer, and MS. In this therapy, the live bee is pinched and placed on the skin until it stings. In the United States alone, an estimated five to ten thousand sufferers of MS use BVT to ease their painful symptoms. Some practitioners use injectable venom extracted from the honeybee by electric shock; others use the live bee. The injection is generally applied to the same trigger points used in acupuncture. Some therapists combine bee venom with procaine for injection into scar tissue, painful joints, and into the scalp to prevent hair loss. Clinical observations include relief of chronic herpes zoster neuralgia, post–third-degree burns, fibromyalgia, bursitis, kidney failure, chronic fatigue, depression, and temporomandibular joint (TMJ) facial pain. Over one thousand papers on this therapy have been produced in the last hundred years, mostly from Europe and Asia. No one knows how or why it works, but it appears to stimulate the immune and endocrine systems. Bee venom is a hundred times more anti-inflammatory than hydrocortisone or adolapin. It is thought to affect the transmission of messages of pain along the nervous system.

Melittin is a molecule that kills cells by slicing through the cell membranes. A research project in Australia hopes to modify the structure of the molecule to remove the part that causes allergic reaction while still maintaining the ability to kill cells. Another problem they face is targeting the killing activity only to cancer cells and not to normal healthy cells. They plan to achieve this by attaching the modified melittin to an antibody molecule that specifically recognizes cancer cells. This combination of a toxin and antibody is known as an immunotoxin. Melittin binds to calmodulin, associated with inhibition of superoxide production. German research has shown melittin exhibits antitumor activity.

Melittin is used in the treatment of hepatocellular carcinoma, but its mechanism of action is not well known. Wu et al. (2015) have found a signaling pathway to understand how melittin inhibits cell proliferation. Melittin suppresses HIV-1 gene expression and inhibits infection in both acutely and persistently infected T-lymphoma and fibroblastoid cells, at an IC_{50} of 0.5–1.5 µM. It may well inhibit cells associated with HIV-1 production at the transcription level.

The therapy has shown improvement in cases of rheumatoid arthritis, MS, depression, chronic fatigue, shingles, skin tumors, and premenstrual syndrome. One study of BVT on fifty sufferers of arthritis showed 84 percent benefit. Another study used either bee acupuncture or indomethacin on forty rheumatoid arthritis patients. After three months, the bee acupuncture group showed better results than those taking 50 mg of the drug daily. Another study looked at ten patients with MS, four quadriplegics and six paraplegics. The patients all received honey, pollen, royal jelly, and propolis as well as bee acupuncture for six months, starting with one and moving up to twenty-five stings per session. Four out of six paraplegia patients showed improvement in gait, control of the bowels, constipation, and urination; three of four quadriplegia patients found improved movement in bed, bedsores, bowel control, motor power improvement; and two cases were able to stand for a few minutes. Both vision and sleep were improved.

In all, bee venom is anti-inflammatory, antifungal, antibacterial, antipyretic, stimulates ACTH, and improves vascular permeability. It obviously stimulates the adrenal glands to produce cortisol, but much more remains unknown. Melittin is highly active against both gram-positive and negative bacteria. It also strongly inhibits the Lyme disease spirochete at very low doses (Lubke and Garon 1997), which then cannot replicate and is more susceptible to other medications. VeneX-10 contains 1 mg/ml of bee venom, approximately the same as one bee sting. It is available through prescription. Adolapin is a painkiller and anti-inflammatory. Apamin enhances nerve transmission, and is believed to be a mood elevator.

The Canadian firm Micrologix Biotech fused melittin from honeybee venom with another peptide—cecropin—from the giant silkworm moth and created a whole new class of antibiotics. These bug drugs function differently and may prove useful in treating drug-resistant bacteria. MCDP is said to rival the effectiveness of hydrocortisone as an anti-inflammatory agent. Hyaluronidase augments the permeability of the sting site, enhances blood flow, and provides some pain relief.

Plaque psoriasis is a difficult medical condition for both patients and practitioners. A double-blind randomized clinical trial by Eltaher et al. (2015) found apitherapy effective and safe for treatment of recalcitrant localized plaque psoriasis when other topical or physical therapies have failed. In the apitherapy group, complete response was achieved in 92 percent of patients, with a significant decrease in tumor necrosis factor-alpha (TNF-alpha) serum levels.

M. J. Kim et al. (2002) found aqua-acupuncture utilizing bee venom helped rheumatoid conditions and the production of osteoblast cells. Bee venom induced apoptosis in human

U937 leukemic cells via activation of caspase-3, 6, and 9. It down-regulates antiapoptotic protein such as Bcl-2. Bee venom acupuncture was found effective in alleviating post-stroke shoulder pain, in a systematic review by Lim et al. (2015). And one animal study found bee venom suppressed the development of benign prostatic hyperplasia (BPH) (Chung et al. 2015).

PROPOLIS

Constituents: Up to 55% resin and balsam, up to 30% wax, and 0.3–1.5% fragrant essential oils (eugenol, guaiol, anethole, pinene). It is rich in fatty and amino acids, especially proline and arginine; beta-eudesurol, benzyl benzoate, 3-methyl-but-2-enyl caffeate, caffeic, ferulic and coumaric acids, benzyl-trans-4-coumarate, cinnamyl alcohol, 7-methoxyquercetin, luteolin, apigenin, hydroquinone (0.1%), acacetin, esculetol, zinc, aluminum, manganese, iron, copper, silicon, tin, nickel, and vitamin B. Also contains flavonoids including chrysin, galangine, pinobanksin, pinocembrine, quercetin, iso-kaempferol, kaempferol, iso-quercitrin, and iso-hamnetin. Caffeic acid phenethyl esters (CAPE) have been determined to be the strongest antioxidant. Caffeic acid and its esters make up 2–20%.

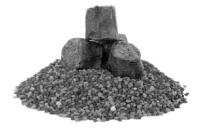

Propolis on top of bee pollen

Propolis is derived from the Greek *pro*, meaning "before" or "protect," and *polis*, meaning "city," here referring to the hive. In the Bible's Old Testament it was known by the Hebrew name *tzori*. Bees do not make propolis—they gather it. In the north, it is collected from poplar buds and cracks in the bark of poplar, willow, birch, and pine trees. The resins are mixed with saliva and placed near the opening of hives to sterilize and protect from infection. Propolis and wax are used to encase any small animal misfortunate enough to enter the hive. Each hive produces three to six ounces of propolis annually. Hives set under the influence of power lines have been shown to increase propolis production, helping counteract the negative effects of radiation.

Historically, propolis was used for skin ulcers and sores by Hippocrates and others. Pliny, the Roman, wrote, "Current physicians use propolis as a medicine because it reduces swelling, soothes pains in the sinews, and heals sores where it appears hopeless for them to mend." In Rome, every legionnaire carried a small amount of propolis into battle to help speed wound healing and for its analgesic effect. The Inca of South America used propolis for febrile infections.

Today, it is used in the republic of Georgia for buccal and dental infections, and in numerous veterinary medicines. It is added to toothpaste and dental floss. Topical applications to dental sockets show enhanced epithelial growth. Propolis has been used in treatment of over three hundred conditions, too numerous to list. Those interested are referred to the Apitherapy Reference Database, which contains over nine hundred titles on the scientific research surrounding propolis.

In a double-blind placebo-controlled trial of 40 patients with chemotherapy induced oral mucositis, 65% of the 20 patients using propolis mouthwash were completely healed in seven days (Akhavan-Karbassi et al. 2016). Burdock (1998) gives a good summation of the various health benefits of propolis. Matthew Wood (2009) considers propolis a specific therapy for dust and mold allergies, laryngitis, and hot raw bronchitis. Simply place a small piece in the mouth and slowly swallow along with saliva.

Recent investigations show propolis is effective against bacteria, protozoa such as giardia, and fungi. Cuban studies found propolis more effective than tinidazole in treating giardiasis, a common intestinal parasite, also known as beaver fever. One study showed a 52% success rate in children, and a 60% rate in adults given propolis extracts. Propolis with Oregon grape root may be a good combination. Freitas et al. (2006) found propolis at 125 mcg/ml inhibits 50% of giardia organisms, and plays a role in the parasite's detachment from mucous membrane walls. Propolis, in lab studies, kills viruses responsible for influenza, hepatitis B, and recurrent genital herpes.

In various studies, propolis shows cholesterol-lowering effect, helps impotence, relieves depression, and suggests strong immune-enhancing properties. It appears more effective against gram-positive than gram-negative bacteria, and shows activity against persistent *Trichomonas vaginalis*. Dalben-Dota et al. (2010) tested propolis against ninety-seven strains of *Candida*, compared it to nystatin, and found it strongly inhibits vulvovaginal *C. albicans*. Propolis significantly decreases toxic side effects of the cancer drug doxorubicin (Tavares et al. 2007). Another study found propolis provides liver protection in a manner similar to silymarin, derived from milk thistle seed.

CAPE inhibits two enzymes involved in formation of eicosanoids. Produced in excess, these can worsen arthritis, asthma, psoriasis, and allergies. Propolis inhibits glycosyltransferase, myeloperoxidase, ornithine decaboxylase, lipoxygenase, tyrosine protein kinase, and arachidonic acid metabolism. Since CAPE's enzyme inhibition selectively killed precancerous cells mutated by viral infections and left healthy cells alone, more research is warranted. Ether extracts possess cytostatic activity against cultured human nasopharynx, uterine, melanoma, and glioblastoma multiforme cancer cell lines. One study found artepillin C reduced tumor multiplicity by 72%, when lung tissue was exposed to one of the most powerful carcinogens associated with tobacco smoke. Researchers have found various CAPE compounds prevent colon cancer in animals by shutting down the activity of two enzymes, phosphatylinositol-specific phospholipase C and lipoxygenase. Both are involved in the production of cancer-causing compounds. Work in Croatia found CAPE and caffeic acid possess pronounced antitumor activity, due in part to immune-modulating activity. Water-soluble derivatives of propolis are potent inhibitors of metastasis formation in lungs.

Apigenin, also found in chamomile, plantain, echinacea, and other herbs, inhibits hyaluronidase, an enzyme that stops the breakdown of hyaluronic acid. This acid is an important part of the extracellular matrix that holds cells together, preventing invasion of bacteria, viruses, and tumors that depend upon this breakdown of tissue for opportunistic growth. Arginine stimulates mitosis and enhances protein biosynthesis, while proline promotes buildup of collagen and elastin, two major components of connective tissue.

The work of Dr. Lavie has found no propolis more potent than that derived from balsam poplar. He discovered bee propolis from around the world does not possess equal antibiotic effect. He then discovered chrysin, common to both poplar and propolis. He made extracts from the buds and found the activity almost identical, proving this theory. See "Poplar" in Chapter 5.

Propolis tincture is invaluable for reducing inflammation of mucous membranes of the mouth and throat, including tonsillitis. Clinical trials in Austria have confirmed the efficacy of propolis in treating stomach ulcers. For this treatment, fill 00 capsules with propolis tincture and take two immediately before each meal. This works well for irritable bowel or spastic colon, again taken before meals.

Studies in Russia show propolis ointment effective in acne, gum infections, and shingle pain. One randomized double-blind controlled trial by Bretz et al. (2014) found a 2% propolis rinse comparable to sodium fluoride and cetylpyridinium chloride in the treatment of gingivitis. Romanian clinical trials suggest benefit in wound healing, treating tuberculosis, and treating various fungal infections. Japanese researchers have found 3-methyl-but-2-enyl caffeate isolated from poplar buds and propolis reduces herpes simplex virus (type 1 or cold sores) replication by thirty-two fold. Propolis combined with bioflavonoids is even more effective. Work by Vynograd et al. (2000) found propolis more effective than acyclovir or placebo in treating genital herpes. Bankova et al. (2014) found a propolis extract, collected from two species of poplar in Canada, active against herpes simplex virus types 1 and 2. Israeli scientists believe propolis stimulates interferon production. They postulate that when propolis is taken up in the human body, the phenolic part of the caffeoylic compound in propolis is oxidized to a quinone structure. This forms covalent bonds with amino acids from either structural or functional proteins, and the resulting compound gives it antiviral and anticancer properties. Isolated compounds from propolis do not work as well as the synergistic effect of whole product. This should come as no surprise to herbalists.

Prostapin is a suppository based on bee products such as pollen, royal jelly, propolis, honey, and wax. A clinical trial involved 36 male patients suffering acute and chronic prostatitis, 24 males with prostate enlargement, and 22 female patients with vaginitis. Suppositories were administered once a day for 30 days, with control groups administered a placebo. Nearly 90% of the first group had significant change, with pain relief, urethral excretions removed, and the function and secretion of prostate, basic blood, and urine values normalized. Prostate size and improvement was noted in only 67% of the second group, while vaginal inflammation in female patients showed 82% improvement.

Song et al. (2002) found propolis produces estrogenic effect through activation of estrogen receptors. The implication for use during menopause or hormonal cancers in humans has not been determined. The study found propolis induces estrogenic effect via receptors and increases uterine weight in lab animals. The effectiveness of antibiotics tetracycline and penicillin increases synergistically by ten to one hundred times when combined with propolis. Early work estimated its analgesic strength at three times greater than cocaine and fifty-two times more powerful than novocaine. Propolis is a surface anesthetic with peripheral action on the mucous membrane of the eye, greater than the activity of cocaine, and with infiltrative action equal to procaine. Its anti-inflammatory properties have been tested successfully in Poland, where it is used to treat rheumatism. In particular, consider propolis if a viral component is aggravating polymyalgia rheumatica, or if joint pain becomes progressively worse after a viral lung infection.

Propolis has been shown effective in promoting regeneration of bone and dental pulp, collagen, and cartilage. This may be due in part to the large amount of proline in propolis that combines with vitamin C to form collagen. This is an elastic tissue that attaches bone to cartilage, and gives elastic tone to arterial walls. Other compounds in propolis protect against the deposit of cholesterine crystals, and lipofuscins that accelerate the aging of heart muscles, liver, and nerves. Dentists in the former Czechoslovakia used propolis to provide temporary pain-free dental fillings. A double-blind study with 5% propolis vaginal dressings for ten days had significant positive effect on women suffering acute cervicitis relative to controls (Santana Pérez et al. 1995).

Recently, the popular press has reported the successful use of propolis to treat Alzheimer's disease. Sister Carole, an English nun, used propolis to help clear up a bacterial chest infection that did not respond to antibiotics. Not only did the infection clear up after five days, but the Alzheimer's patient became more alert and responsive. Studies on twenty-two other patients are showing good results. This is not unusual. Residents of long-term care facilities often suffer undiagnosed bladder infections that, left untreated, severely affect mental capacity and memory. It is often written off as early dementia, but once the bladder infection is treated, the brain regains its previous health.

A human study found propolis extract reduced respiratory infection in young children. In a double-blind study of fifty subjects, the propolis group became symptom free more quickly than control group. Cyclophosphamide is widely used to treat Hodgkin's and non-Hodgkin's lymphoma, Burkitt lymphoma, chronic lymphocytic leukemia, Ewing's sarcoma, breast and testicular cancer. Side effects are common. Work by Akyol et al. (2016) found propolis and CAPE promising agents to help reduce toxicity. Propolis is an emerging adjuvant therapy for cancer and shows efficacy against brain, head and neck, skin, breast, liver, pancreas, kidney, bladder, prostate, colon, and blood cancers (Patel 2016). Most importantly, propolis shows no observed adverse effect level (NOAEL), meaning it has no known toxic levels. In studies on calves with neonatal diarrhea, propolis was as effective as enrofloxacin in reducing symptoms. Propolis is used in some soaps and cosmetics and in varnishes for high-quality violins—or at least that is what Antonio Stradivari believed. It is used to repair accordions.

Dose: Raw propolis the size of a corn kernel is chewed for sore throats or upper respiratory complaints. Saliva activated by the resins moves throughout the entire region. For tinnitus, take 4 parts olive oil to 1 part propolis tincture. Soak a plug of cotton batten and insert into the ear for 36 hours.

Propolis differs greatly between fresh and aged product. For example, it takes a minimum 80 µg/ml fresh propolis of to inhibit *Bacillus subtilis* and *Staphylococcus aureus*, but 100 µg/ml in aged. The flavonoid content is 20% less in older propolis. Propolis from cottonwood poplar appears to be more highly sensitizing and capable of allergenic reactions. The scent is due to the content of cinnamyl cinnamate. Pure propolis from poplar contains no catechol, an adulterant found in poplar bud oil.

Tincture: make at 1:4 and 95% alcohol. Use 5–20 drops as needed.

Caution: Jeananne Laing, noted herbalist, found taking propolis tincture before working on beehives provokes a surprising and nasty reaction from the bees.

FLOWER POLLEN

Constituents: amino acids, enzymes, every known vitamin, rare trace minerals, and more than 5,000 enzymes and co-enzymes. It contains up to 23% protein, is rich in pantothenic acid (B_5) and B_{12}, and has a a pH of 6. Flower pollen is gathered by bees in the process of gathering nectar. Back at the hive it is shaped into grains and used as nourishment for young larvae. When fed pollen, the larvae increase their weight by 1,500 times in less than one week. These small grains, upon closer examination, exhibit every color of the rainbow. Fireweed pollen is turquoise, snowdrop pollen the color of a chicken egg yolk, red dead nettle pollen is blood red, asparagus pollen is bright plastic orange, raspberry is gray, and Oriental poppy, bright blue. It is nutritious for humans and contains all five major tastes—sweet, spicy, salty, sour, and bitter. More chemical constituents are found in pollen than any other concentrated food on the planet.

The 1948 *Journal of the National Cancer Institute* noted that "the development of mammary tumors in mice can be decreased by the ingestion of pollenized food." More clinical research has been done over the past seventy years. Recent experiments with pollen have shown incredible potential for the production, or superoxide dismutase (SOD). This free-radical quencher is useful in reducing inflammation and prolonging the aging process. It is, however, destroyed by stomach acids. This is significant. In one study at Long Island University, 189 patients with rheumatic knees and elbows received significant relief with bee pollen poultices. Pollen is used for impotence, and prostate inflammation. Habib et al. (1995) found one fraction of pollen extract, designated FV-7, to inhibit growth of prostate cancer cell lines. After all, pollen is the male reproductive substance of plants. Bee pollen from *Brassica campestris* triggered apoptosis in human prostate cancer (PC3) cell lines (Wu and Lou 2007).

It is rich in aspartic acid, helping rejuvenate the sex glands. Other content includes gonadotrophic hormones similar to those produced by our pituitary. Acetic, butyric, and propionic acids provide energy for the liver. Bee pollen extracts show significant improvement in menopausal symptoms, including headache, urinary incontinence, vaginal dryness, and decreased vitality in various double-blind studies. Münstedt et al. (2015) found bee pollen and honey improve menopausal symptoms in breast cancer patients receiving tamoxifen and aromatase inhibitors. The symptoms included hot flushes, night sweats, pain during sexual intercourse, hair loss, forgetfulness, depression, and insomnia.

Pollen possesses antibiotic effect, as well as allergy relief. Flower pollen allergies in your own region can be effectively neutralized by ingesting small amounts of local pollen four to six weeks prior to your personal allergy season. Leo Conway, a medical doctor in Denver, has compiled over 60,000 documented cases of the successful use of local pollens for treating allergies. Ishikawa et al. (2004) found bee pollen inhibits the IgE receptor–mediated activation of mast cells, suggesting a pathway for alleviation and prevention of allergies. Asthmatics should approach the use of all bee products with some caution as they are powerful foods. It can, however, be used in cases of chronic fatigue syndrome with good success.

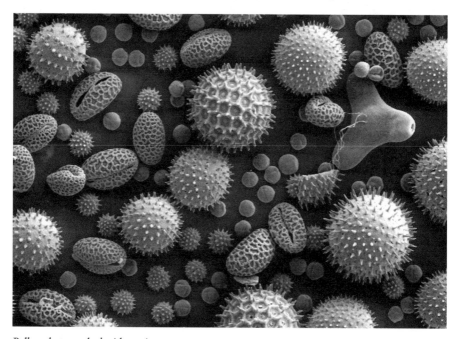

Pollen photographed with a microscope

Bee pollen supports low blood pressure, but it is contraindicated in cases of hypertension. Recent German studies report a lowering of cholesterol and triglycerides with regular daily intake of pollen. It has been shown by Kilmer McCully, a medical doctor from Harvard Medical School, that heart disease is often initiated by B_6 deficiency and increased methionine. It follows that foods with a high B_6/methionine ratio may help prevent heart disease. Carrots have a ratio of 15 to 1, bananas 40 to 1, and bee pollen 400 to 1. A recent study found bee pollen, taken before meals, reduced food consumption by 15–20%, assisting in weight reduction.

It allays depression, and increases hemoglobin and calcium retention. It boosts the immune system and is helpful in reducing the side effects of chemotherapy and radiation, including of cervical cancer. It helps sleep disorders, nausea, and urinary tract and rectal dysfunction. When pollen was taken three times daily with meals for three days before, during, and following radiation treatments, patients did not suffer side effects such as hair loss. Bee pollen contains as-yet-unidentified compounds that slow the growth of breast cancer.

There is one note of caution. Insulin and bee pollen should probably not be used at the same time. That is, bee pollen is contraindicated in cases of diabetes. Use local pollen, as imported pollen is sterilized and radiated, and therefore lacking many enzymes and nutrients. It may contain heavy metals, particularly when derived from China. Sulfonamides and other nasty herbicides have been found in trace amounts. Bee pollen has a hard membrane that cannot be broken down or digested by enzymes in the human body. Therefore it must be well chewed, or crushed into a very fine powder and then put in capsules.

Bee pollen is used in cosmetic applications due to its restoring, dissolving, softening, anti-infectious, anti-inflammatory, and tissue-repair properties. It is useful in formulas for skin ulcers, scabs, sores, boils, and abscesses. In concentrations of 0.0008–0.004%, pollen extracts significantly improve cell proliferation.

Bee pollen may have some application in treatment of autism spectrum disorder. Propionic acid is a metabolic product of intestinal dysbiosis and is a commonly used food additive. A study by Al-Salem et al. (2016) on animal models found propionic groups showed multiple signs of brain toxicity, as indicated by depletion of serotonin, dopamine, and noradrenaline, along with increase in IFN-gamma and caspase 3. Bee pollen was effective in ameliorating the neurotoxic effects. Bee pollen, added at the rate of 1.5% to the rations of broiler chickens, promotes earlier development of their digestive systems. The villi, for example, increased in length by 37%, suggesting an investment would lead to increased nutrient absorption in later life (Wang et al. 2007).

Royal Jelly

Constituents: water (66%), protein (12%), royalisin, lipids, thiamin, riboflavin, niacin, pantothenic acid, B_6, biotin, inositol, folic acid, vitamin C, gamma globulin, acetylcholine, and up to

15% of HDA or 10-hydroxy-trans-(2)-decanoic acid, methylparaben, 3-hydroxydodecanedioic acid, sebacic acid, and neopterin.

In the larval stage, there is absolutely no difference between a queen and worker bee. In the first three days of life, the larvae are fed special milk by the nurse bees, secreted only from the sixth to the tenth day of life from their hypopharyngeal gland. This is called royal jelly. It is similar to the beebread that is a mixture of pollen, honey, and worker-bee secre-

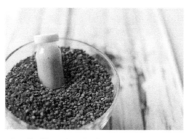

Royal jelly in bowl of bee pollen

tions, but contains ten times more pantothenic acid and biopterin as well as secretions. Royal jelly is milky looking, acidic, protein-rich, and possesses the highest natural source of pantothenic acid (B_5): 20 times the amount found in liver. The supplement B_5 is invaluable in certain forms of asthma and prevention of hay fever. It is so potent that only the next queen continues to be fed this special delight. She continues to grow 50% larger and lives forty times longer than worker bees.

China is the world's largest producer of royal jelly, accounting for 90 percent of market, with approximately five hundred tons exported annually. It was French beekeepers in the 1950s who pioneered its commercial use by creating artificial queen cells and sucking out the royal jelly with small pumps. One hive produces just 7 ml, hence its high price.

Besides B_5 and B_6, royal jelly is one of the richest natural sources of acetylcholine. This compound allows nerve impulses to pass from one nerve to the next. Deficiency is often found in the tangled nerve bundles of patients suffering Alzheimer's disease and other nerve-related disorders. Royal jelly does essentially four things. It strengthens the body, builds up immunity to disease, treats anemia, and increases personal stamina. It has been found to possess antitumor activity in experimental laboratory mouse leukemia due to medium-chain hydroxy-fatty acids.

Some menopausal women find royal jelly and bee pollen a potent combination for smoothing their hormonal transition. Mishima et al. (2005) found royal jelly's estrogenic activity was due to interaction with estrogen receptors followed by endogenous gene expression. Royal jelly improves hair, nail, and skin health. Vasilisa, a cream with 0.5% propolis and 2% royal jelly, showed good results in one study, treating skin conditions after just 5–7 days. The component 3-hydroxydodecanedioic acid (HDA) is active against *Staphylococcus aureus*, *S. epidermidis*, *Streptococcus mutans*, and *S. viridans* in the low range of 0.17–0.36 mg/ml. HDA is 25% less active than penicillin, and seems to be pH dependent. Sebacic acid shows moderate antifungal activity. Royal jelly accelerates bone tissue formation, lowers cholesterol, and regulates and normalizes blood pressure by making arteries more flexible. It inhibits ACE, associated with cardiovascular risk (Takaki-Doi et al. 2009).

In one human study, a dosage of 50–100 milligrams daily decreased total cholesterol levels by 14% in patients with moderate to severe elevations ranging from 210–325 mg/dl. A better-quality product may have produced even more significant benefit. It may be useful in treating type 2 diabetes. A double-blind randomized placebo-controlled trial of 50 patients, conducted by Khoshpey et al. (2016), gave one group 1,000 mg of royal jelly or placebo three times daily for eight weeks. A significant difference was found in serum glucose and apolipoprotein levels and ratios. Royal jelly regulates low blood sugar and encourages the breakdown of fatty adipose tissue, thus aiding weight-loss regimes. Royal jelly may be useful in the treatment of BPH. In a study by Pajovic et al. (2016), forty men were given 38 milligrams of royal jelly for three months. PSA levels reduced and the International Prostate Symptom Score improved. Hidaka et al. (2006) found royal jelly prevents osteoporosis by enhancing intestinal calcium absorption. Although it was a rat study, royal jelly was 85% as effective as 17beta-estradiol in preventing femur bone loss. 10-hydroxy-2-decenoic acid (HDA) appears to benefit rheumatoid arthritis (Shang et al. 2012).

Apinhalin is a suspension inhalant containing royal jelly and propolis, used in Russia for bronchitis and bronchial asthma. Royal jelly is used in cosmetic skin diseases, blackhead rash, herpes, and dermatitis, along with more serious conditions like diabetic foot and leg ulcers. Neopterin, also known as 2-amino-6-(1, 2, 3-trihydroxypropyl)-4(3H)-pteridinone, is found in both royal jelly and humans, where it appears to play an important and as yet unexplained role in the immune system. Increased levels have been observed in the plasma of patients with recurrent atrial fibrillation, but the relationship is not fully known. Neopterin increases in patients with pediatric burn wounds post-infection, and is present in athletes following intense exercise. More research would be welcomed.

Royal jelly protects against radiation-induced apoptosis in human peripheral blood leukocytes, suggesting adjunct therapy for radiation patients (Rafat et al. 2016). Both honey and royal jelly reduce cisplatin-induced kidney toxicity in animal studies (Ibrahim et al. 2016). Apalbum 1 from royal jelly exhibits antihypertensive activity.

Note: Because of its volatility, royal jelly must be kept chilled, frozen, or freeze-dried to retain any potency. It should be stored fresh at 40°F or frozen at 0°F to retain any nutraceutical or functional value.

It takes the contents of one thousand three-day-old queen cells to harvest a pound of royal jelly. Furosine is the marker associated with freshness and quality; the lower the number, the better the quality. Highest antioxidant levels are noted in royal jelly harvested twenty-four hours after larval transfer (Je-Ruei Liu et al. 2008). There has been one case of fatal royal jelly-induced asthma, reported in the *Medical Journal of Australia* in 1993–1994. Allergic reactions are generally rare; in fact, one study suggests pure natural royal jelly should not cause allergic reaction. F.C. Thien et al. (1996) found nearly half of patients with food or respiratory allergies demonstrated IgE antibody cross-reactivity to royal jelly proteins.

Dose: 0.1 ounce daily.

Bee Larvae

People in various parts of the world use bee larvae for food. They contain more vitamin D by weight than fish oil. In Chinese medicine they are considered good for the stomach and spleen and reputedly beneficial for leprosy. Bumblebee larva, known as *tu feng*, is indicated for swollen, infected boils. In Romania, two patented products called Apilarnil and Apilarnilprop are produced from the drone (male) honeybee larva. The adult honeybee contains potent antibacterial peptides, apidaecins, and abaecin (Casteels et al. 1990). Bee larvae, *feng zi*, are used in traditional Chinese medicine (TCM). They are a sweet, balanced medicine, useful for head wind, eliminating toxins, and supplementing for vacuity and languor.

Beeswax (Cera Flava)

Constituents: myricin (up to 80%), cerolein, myricyl alcohol, fatty acids, cerotic and aliphatic acids, lactones, pollens and resins, cholesteryl esters. It melts at 144–148°F, with a saponification value of 87–104, ester value of 70–80, and acid value of 17–24. The specific gravity is 0.967.

Wax is secreted from the abdominal rings or scales of the bee and used to form cells where food or eggs are kept. It is extracted by boiling honeycomb in water and skimming wax from the surface. An estimated ten pounds of honey are consumed to produce one pound of wax, leading to the hexagonal frugality of the comb.

Virgil noted that Pan made his pipes by "joining with wax the unequal reeds." The ancient Egyptians used wax to ensure an airtight seal on urns, jars, and coffins. The Persians and Syrians covered the bodies of important people with wax before burial. A cerecloth was wax impregnated and wrapped tightly around bodies to keep out air. The Romans found wax-covered wooden tablets were ideal for writing notes and letters. They used the wax to seal legal documents, as official seals are used today. Throughout Europe, beeswax has been used during birth, circumcision, and marriage. Later, wax was used for casting molten metal statues, and eventually, for the famous Tussauds wax museums.

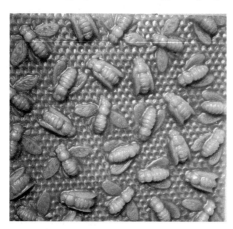

Beeswax

Ceromancy is the art of divination by dropping melted wax into water and reading the future by observing the shapes formed. Traditionally, wax was much used for eye salves, and today for ointments and salves. In China, beeswax is dissolved in hot wine and is drunk for diarrhea, hiccups, and inflammation. It is considered a great vaccine against hay fever. The antibiotics present in beeswax are active against certain types of enterobacteria.

In the West wax has mainly found use as an emulsifier and thickener in cosmetics or candle-making. It is used for dressing and polishing leather and furniture, modeling fruits, transparent papers, engraving and lithography, chewing gum, food products, and finishing textiles. Revlon, Cover Girl, Aussie, Avon, Ponds, and, of course, Burt's Bees use the wax in a variety of personal-care products, including mascara, lip-liner, lipsticks, night creams, and moisturizers. In Persia, Avicenna used beeswax for ulcers of the bowels and to increase the flow of urine and semen.

It stimulates the stomach and relieves heart pain. Honey and wax are both yin and considered restorative to the spleen. Dogs, given the opportunity, choose beeswax as a natural antibiotic and will eat it. Caroline Ingraham (2006) wrote, "I have noticed that dogs with ear infections and gastrointestinal problems relating to infection (indicated by diarrhea) frequently choose beeswax, especially with rosehip extract added." Myricyl alcohol, a wax constituent, is a plant stimulant, increasing yields of tomato, cucumber, and lettuce.

Beeswax has long been praised for slowing the aging process, increasing potency and desire for love, and invigorating physical and mental capacity. Beeswax is the only fuel that can be burned safely in closed quarters, and is the only fuel on the planet that emits negative ions. Originally, the mass candles used by the Roman Catholic church were 100% beeswax. In 1851, this was reduced to 65%, later to 51% and now to only 25%, corresponding, some would say, in direct proportion to church attendance.

German artist Wolfgang Laib sculpts with slabs of beeswax, building thirteen-foot towers, such as the ziggurats of ancient Assyrian temples. He uses the wax to build narrow chambers with an electric bulb to warm the wax and release the honey scent. His works sell for up to $150,000. His most ambitious project is a beeswax chamber tunneled forty feet into the Pyrenees near Marcevol, France.

Closer to home, Aganetha Dyck is an artist from Manitoba who collaborates with bees to produce art. She places objects into hives and then waits for the bees to transform them by building cells of wax and honey. Some projects take several years to complete. *Working in the Dark*, produced in 2000, is a poem by Di Brandt put into Braille and placed in a beehive. When the fifty-four lines of poetry came out, the bees had created a new language of this translation. More recently, she is working with her son, Richard Dyck, a multimedia computer artist, recording the sounds within beehives.

In Ukrainian folklore, bees were believed to have a special relationship with God. Beeswax ceremonies were traditionally performed by *babas* (grandmothers) who poured molten wax into cold water held over the patient's head. When the dish was overturned, the wax formation was interpreted to find the source of the health issue. Among the Kayapo of

Brazil, a ceremonial hat is formed from beeswax to symbolize the universe. These hats are worn by young men when they receive their ceremonial names.

Policosanol is a very effective plant wax derived from sugarcane. Extensive studies, from Cuba, suggest it can reduce both total and LDL cholesterol by 10–20%, as well as modestly elevate HDL. Policosanol can be derived from beeswax, and because sugarcane wax is less available to U.S. companies and is patent protected, the beeswax derivative may be a good substitute. No studies have yet been conducted, but the supplement company Hauser has recently purchased the rights to policosanol-isolating technology. Policosanol is composed of long-chain primary aliphatic-saturated alcohols, the main one being 28-carbon 1-octanosol. This product may reduce total serum cholesterol and LDL levels in some people. It may also help reduce platelet aggregation and benefit those suffering intermittent claudication. In one recent human study, LDL cholesterol was reduced by 24% compared to 22% for lovastatin and 15% for simvastatin. The HDL level increased in the policosanol group, but not with the two drugs, suggesting a "safe and effective cholesterol reducing agent" (Prat et al. 1999).

Beeswax alcohols (D-002) help protect gastric tissue while reducing inflammation in joints in a COX-2 manner (Molina et al. 2015). This is important, as COX-2 drugs increase cardiovascular risk, and aspirin and other COX-1 type mediations cause stomach bleeds. At a dose of 20 mg daily, policosanol appears as effective as 100 mg of aspirin in reducing blood platelet aggregation.

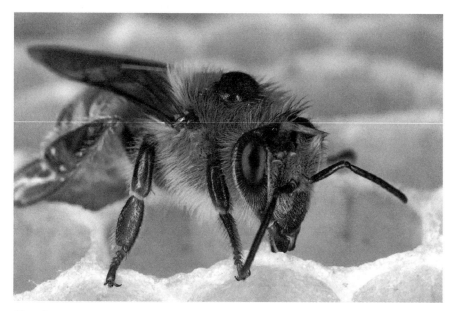

Honeybee

Homeopathy

The venom of the honeybee has been long utilized in homeopathic medicine. The familiar stinging, burning pain of a bee sting, along with the live welt it produces, are the key symptoms to using Apis. Any acute inflammation accompanied by stinging and burning, marked redness, swelling, and heat calls for this remedy. Lupus erythematosus, chronic nephritis, pharyngitis, and right-sided ovaritis are some examples of inflamed and swollen conditions relieved by Apis. Painful urination may be present, with the final drop the most painful.

Medical doctor Eli Jones suggested this remedy in treating breast cancer where there is induration and the skin is dark purple with light yellow discharges. Sore throats, hives, conjunctivitis, sties, as well as insect bites and stings are relieved with Apis. The most typical swellings have a puffy, water-filled appearance. The inflamed eye with a sty looks like a red bag of water—as if stung by a bee. The throat may appear red, sore, and puffy.

Those requiring Apis generally have little thirst, although some crave milk. They may be sad, depressed, or weep constantly for little reason. Females are busy as a bee and overly protective of their immediate and extended family.

Ovarian inflammation may be worse on the right side, with swollen and red labia that feels better from cold application. Children that can benefit from Apis cannot easily urinate and are anxious, mutter in their sleep, or are restless, and suddenly awaken from sleep. Apis may be helpful in severe reaction to vaccination, such as high fever, convulsions, and the brain feeling inflamed. For left-sided ovaritis, try homeopathic Tiger Lily.

Dose: Tincture to the 30th potency. In edema, the lower potencies are best. Sometimes the action is slow. For breast cancer indicated above, use 3X at rate of 20 drops to 4 ounces water. Give 1 teaspoonful every hour.

Apis mother tincture is created in one of two ways. Live honeybees are put in a bottle and irritated by shaking. For eight days the bottle is open long enough to add diluted alcohol. It is then shaken to anger the bees and get them to emit venom. When they die, the alcohol is poured out, strained, filtered, and is the mother tincture. The other method involves a drop of bee venom secreted with help of tweezers.

This drop is then added to dilute alcohol. In a sense, the remedy is a sarcode (made from a live animal) first created in 1852 by Dr. Frederick Humphries.

Mel cum Sale (Honey with Salt)

This homeopathic remedy is specifically for prolapsed uterus with inflammation of the cervix. The special symptom is a feeling of soreness across the hypogastrium from ileum to ileum. Accompanying this is a sensation as if the bladder is too full, with the pain moving from front to back.

Dose: 3rd to 6th potency, as needed.

Materia Poetica

Honeybee so busy
I hope you will not sting
Puff me up with redness
Swollen painful thing
Heated like a fire
Give me something cool
To settle down this burning pain
Inflamed, out of control
Active little worker
Buzzing round the hive
I hate to make you angry
I think I'd rather hide
You've got a robust way
Of taking full control
A swelling up with vigor
Your stinging takes a toll
I've never seen you drinking
You certainly lack thirst
And when I think of anaphylaxis
You're practically the worst
Oh Apis, go ahead
I'll stay out of your way
I'll never make you jealous
You can work away your day!

—Sylvia Chatroux (1998)

Essential Oils and Absolutes

Honey oil is an absolute produced by extraction from the honeycomb. The best solvent is 95% ethanol, which leaves no toxic residue. It contains palmatine and hydroxy-palmatine acids. Honey essential oil has a fragrance that is mild, warm, and sweet. It is calming, relaxing, and balancing. It may be added to a therapeutic bath for relieving colds. Laurie used both honey and apple absolute in a popular blend called Honey Bear. It was a best seller for our company Scents of Wonder while on the market.

Beeswax absolute is made from the fresh wax by an alcohol washing. It is mild, oily, and coumarin-like. It yields about 0.1–0.2%. It is reminiscent of good cold-pressed linseed oil with a honey trace. In perfume work, it is used to mellow and modify harsh synthetics and

128

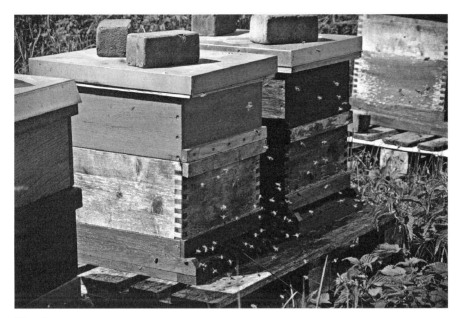

Hives buzzing in summer

is called *absolue cire d'abeille*. It contains cerolein and cerotinic acid. A good aromatherapist or perfumist can tell what country or harvest of what flowers are associated with production of the beeswax absolute.

It blends well with orris, violet, and some meadow-like blends. The absolute is used as flavoring in some alcoholic beverages. Given the magnitude of the honey industry in Alberta, particularly in the Peace Country, a good-quality product that can compete on the world market would seem to be a good value-added venture.

Propolis essential oil is obtained from steam distillation and yields from 0.3–1.5%. Composition varies according to the vegetation of the surrounding area, but generally is composed of 40–60% sesquiterpene alcohols like beta-eudesmol, quaiol, farnesol, and nerolidol; 20–40% of benzyl benzoate as well as beta-bisabolene, patchoulane, and thirty other compounds. The first dominates in poplar forests; the second in pine regions. Propolis oil shows good to moderate activity against both gram-positive and negative bacteria and various fungi.

Hydrosol

Honey water is left over from the steam distillation described above. It has a limited, but steady, retail aromatherapy market. Dr. Fernie mentions that honey water is an excellent wash for promoting the growth of hair, either by itself or mixed with spirit (hydrosol) of rosemary. A toilet water very popular in England and France during the eighteenth century, known as Aqua Mellis, contained honey water, coriander, rose water, and other exotic spices.

Brunschwig, in his 1530 *Book of Distillation*, mentions honey water for restoring and growing hair, old sores and holesunclean wounds, and soothing the eyes." "Put as much as you will in a crooked glass named retort, and stop it well fast and leave forty days in horse dung that is changed every week. Then put the glass in a wand and distill.... The first water is white and clear, put away. The second is yellow, and that we shall keep."

Personality Traits

"Wax is an important element in Ukrainian folk rituals. Its special symbolism is related to its production by bees, sometimes affectionately called "God's birds" or "God's flies." Beekeeping has a long history in Ukraine, where wax and honey have historically been important commodities. "In most descriptions, melted wax is poured into cold water.... Although the wax ceremony is said to cure many different maladies, it is most commonly used as a cure for fear.... Untreated fear is thought to manifest itself in emotional and mental illness" (Hanchuk 1999).

Elder Simon Inuksaq spoke about using bees to help a woman in labor: "I had mittens when I was a child and I had a pouch in each mitten. There were two adult bees in each, and baby bees were put there as well. These were there so that when a woman in labor has complications I could help ease the delivery." (Van Deusen 2009)

The bee is an incredibly restless insect that reacts instantly and angrily to any outside interference. It is sensitive to heat and has elaborate systems for cooling down a hive. In fever, a person may be weepy for no apparent reason. They may be restless and fearful regarding death or the fear of being left alone. Generally, the Apis personality is quite jealous. A child in a family with a new baby exhibits many of these symptoms. Ironically, they also dislike being touched. Barbara Walker (1988) writes :

The honeycomb is perfect six-sided hexagon. To the early Pythagoreans, the hexagon was an expression of the spirit of Aphrodite, whose sacred number was six (dual Triple Goddess). They worshipped bees as her sacred creatures, as they made perfect hexagons. In Aphrodite's temple at Eryz, the priestesses were melissae, or bees. The goddess was also called Melissa, the queen bee who annually killed her male partner, and a golden honeycomb her symbol.

As the Pythagoreans meditated on the 60-degree angles, they continued the lines until they met in the center of adjacent hexagons. This signified, to them, the underlying symmetry of the cosmos.

Honey cakes formed like female genitals were prominent in worship. This led to medieval hymns that addressed the virgin Mary as a "nest of honey," and "dripping honeycomb."

> *Bees are Hymenoptera, or "veil-winged," recalling the hymen or veil that covered the inner shrine of the goddess's temple, and the officiating nymph called Hymen who ruled over marriage rituals and the honeymoon.*

There is a certain sense, said Rudolf Steiner (1933), in which the individual bee, whether it is a worker, a drone, or even the ruling queen, is not an organism in its own right. It is a constituent element of the true organism, the hive as a biological entity. Save in exceptional circumstances, its temperature is maintained at a constant level that approximates the 98.6°F of the healthy human being.

Steiner's intuitive faculties induced him to attach significance to this fact. He taught that the coincidence of temperature between the hive and the individual human being indicates a certain relationship between the latter and the ego. Another subtle relationship discerned by Steiner was based on the similarity between the regular six-sided cells of which the honeycomb is made up and the hexagonal crystals of various naturally occurring mineral substances. Anthroposophical medical practitioners see the polarity of the hive as reminiscent of the polarity tendencies of the ego in the human biosystem—a hardening, mineralizing, sclerotic tendency

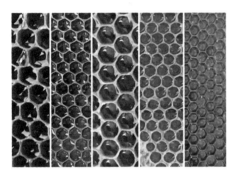

Hexagonal honeycomb

manifesting itself as the cephalic pole; a softening, warming tendency manifesting itself at the motor-digestive metabolic pole (Felter and Lloyd 1898).

> *The symptoms of a bee sting—burning, stinging, redness and swelling—and the activities of bees—collecting nectar, converting it into honey, living in hives, building exactly similar honey combs, all serving the queen and the whole family working in harmony, stinging with poisonous venom in defense, flying about slightly erratically—all point to its people picture.*
>
> *Family orientation is number one, so love of family is the first idea. They are busy looking after the family and love them all "to bits." It's just natural for them to be busy looking after and controlling and defending the family.*
>
> *She is a straightforward person with straightforward sets of activities or tasks. The busy-ness can move toward workaholic tendencies, and they can also be frivolous and fruitless in their family-oriented activity. There is awkwardness, especially dropping things and restless activity. Dreams of flying are typical, but more likely it's an indication for one of the bird remedies. The mother is protective jealousy and irritability, and you can expect to be stung if you cross this person.... The golden threat of this remedy is caring for family, the spiritual core is love, the emotion is caring love, and the defense of this by stinging in*

some way; that's how it feels to the recipient. The physical result is busy activity in support of the family and the physical pathology is immune-protective swelling and inflammation that is caring and protecting on the cellular level. (Chappell 2003)

Silvertown (2009) wrote:

Male bees hatch from unfertilized eggs, so they have no father and carry only a single set of chromosomes, derived from mom. All a male bee's sperm are therefore identical, and when he mates with a queen bee, all of their female offspring get an identical set of genes from him. The result is that sisters in a beehive share not only just half their genes (as in human families), but three-quarters of them.

Spiritual Properties

The holy bee-maidens, with their gift of prophecy, were to be Apollo's gift to Hermes, the god who alone could lead the souls of the dead out of life and sometimes back again. The etymology of the word *fate* in Greek offers a fascinating example of how the genius of the Minoan vision entered the Greek language, often invisibly, as well as informed its stories of goddesses and gods. The Greek word for "fate," "death," and "goddess of death" is *e ker* (feminine); the word for "heart" and "breast" is *to ker* (neuter); while the word for honeycomb is

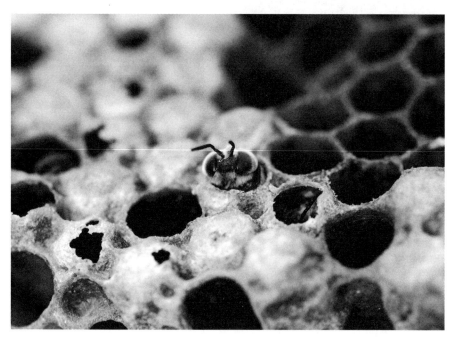

Male drone emerging from a cell

to *kerion* (neuter). The common root *ker* links the ideas of the honeycomb, goddess, death, fate, and the human heart, a nexus of meanings that is illumined if we know that the goddess was once imagined as a bee.

> *In the Ukraine, bees are the tears of Our Lady, and the queen bee of any hive is called Queen Tsarina, a name associated with Mary, Queen of Heaven. Throughout Eastern Europe, Mary is the protectress of bees and beekeepers, and consecrated honey is offered on altars on the Feast of the Assumption of the Virgin Mary on August 15, the date linked with her ascension into heaven.* (Eason 2008, 77)

RECIPES

Propolis tincture: Take 1½ ounces of dry propolis and macerate for 3 days in 3½ ounces of 96% alcohol. Shake daily. Use 4–20 drops three times daily. Use more frequently in acute cases. Commercial products standardized to 1.8–2.2% total flavonoids (galangin) are available from European firms.

Note: Urban beekeeping is increasingly popular. Propolis collected from urban sources may contain petroleum derivatives obtained from asphalt. Caution is advised.

Ointment: 5 parts of propolis powder and olive oil. Combine with 2 parts lanolin in top of a double boiler. Stir until smooth. Remove from the heat. Use for burns, shingles, ear infections, and skin problems. Do not use on wet eczema.

Bee pollen poultice: Dissolve 1 tablespoon of crushed pollen in warm water. Place a cotton towel in water. Wring out and apply to the affected joint.

Bee pollen: ¼ to 1 teaspoon daily as indicated. Should not be taken in cases of hypertension, pregnancy, breast-feeding, or by diabetics taking insulin. Grind well, or chew thoroughly to break the cell walls.

Scrambled brood: Squeeze freshly sealed brood comb through a colander to obtain a puree of the larvae and pupae of honeybees. It looks and cooks up like scrambled eggs, only whiter.

Steamed bee brood with chili: Cut three-inch squares of fresh sealed brood comb. Use new combs to avoid pollens or cocoons from previous generations. Wrap in aluminum foil and steam for 7–10 minutes. The brood will cook and the wax will melt and mix. Add chili sauce for dipping.

Recommended reading: *The Sacred Bee* by Hilda Ransome is a 2004 reprint of the classic 1937 history on this fascinating insect. The International Bee Research Association in Cardiff, Wales has a library of 60,000 papers, 4,000 books, and 130 journals on the subject of bees.

Spruce

Black Spruce—*Picea mariana* (Mill.) Britton, Sterns & Poggenb. ◆ *P. nigra* (Ait.) Link.

White Spruce—*Picea glauca* (Moench) Voss ◆ *P. canadensis* (Mill.) Britton, Sterns & Poggenb. ◆ *P. albertiana* S. Br.

Engelmann Spruce—*Picea engelmannii* Carrière ◆ *P. latifolia* Sarg.

Norway Spruce—*Picea abies* (L.) Karst. ◆ *P. excelsa* (Lam.) Link

> *Gum, the gum of mountain spruce.*
> *He showed me lumps of the scented stuff,*
> *like uncut jewels, dull and rough.*

—Robert Frost

> *All day the sun has shone on the surface of some savage swamp,*
> *where the single spruce stands hung with* Usnea *lichens …*

—Henry David Thoreau

To me, spruce epitomizes the boreal forest. Both black and white spruce are widespread and plentiful in the northern forests of North America. Spruce may come from *prusse* or

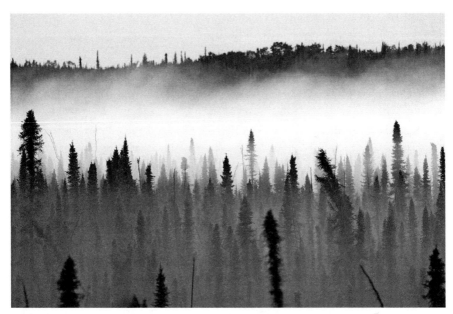

Spruce forest

pruce, from the French word for Prussia. To spruce up, meaning a dapper, smart appearance, stems from the courtiers of Henry VIII dressing like Prussian noblemen, appareled in a spruce fashion. Spruce leather was a sixteenth-century term for fine soft leather sewn into jackets.

Picea is from Latin *pix*, meaning "pitch." *Mariana* is named in honor of Maryland by an eighteenth-century botanist who felt the region epitomized North America. It is ironic that not a single black spruce grows in that state. *Glauca* is derived from the Greek *glaukos*, meaning "gray," in reference to the bloom on the foliage. Engelmann Spruce is named after the German botanist and physician George Engelmann, who moved to St. Louis to study plants, especially conifers, in the mid-1800s. His personal herbarium initiated the incredible Missouri Botanical Garden Herbarium. It is truly worthy of a visit.

The odor of spruce gum takes me back to early childhood memories. Start out chewing a small marble-size piece, and after an hour of spitting, you are rewarded with a pinkish gum that does not lose any flavor on the bedpost overnight. Today it remains a favorite of athletes who want to keep their mouths moist without the harmful side effects of chewing tobacco. In 1848 the State of Maine Pure Spruce Gum began selling the product commercially, and two years later changed its name to American Flag. I remember seeing the commercial spruce gum when our family went to visit relatives in Bangor, Maine. In its commercial prime, chewing gum from *P. rubens* or red spruce was selling at rate of forty-eight million pounds a year. Of course, that was in the days before chewing gum was manufactured from petroleum by-products.

Mors Kochanski once told me that Ingalik women believe chewing spruce gum increased their breast size.

Traditional Uses

The spruce gum or pitch collects on trees in a form reminiscent of brittle tears. It is collected and burned in the same manner as frankincense. The northern Cree call this *sihtipikow* and used the softened resin for waterproofing baskets, canoes, and cooking pots. Russell Willier, a noted Cree healer, cuts a small white spruce and stands it near his house to protect the surrounding land from curses. This is changed every year.

Spruce pitch is known as *dze* to the Dene (Chipewyan). The gum is pounded

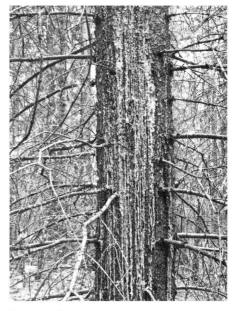

Spruce pitch

together with charcoal to make glue that sticks when hot in order to set arrowheads and spear points before binding. It is smeared on burned pine torches for greater efficacy and waterproof strips of hide for snares and snow shoes.

It is a good medicine for infected wounds and stomachaches. When boiled with spruce cones, water, and lard, the mixture turns pink, and when cooled, it makes an ointment the Cree call *pikim*. This is used to draw infection from cysts or to soothe various itchy skin rashes, including chicken pox. Russell Willier uses black spruce cone decoctions for stomach problems.

When speaking generally about white spruce, the Cree will call it *siyihtah*. The black spruce is *minahyik* or sometimes *wapasiht*. The northern Cree made use of the strong and pliable roots to weave baskets and set snares. Black spruce is known as *itinatik*, the people tree; *napakasihta*; or sometimes swamp spruce, *maskekosihta*.

The long roots will sometimes yield knotless, straight-grained wood that is cut green. When split 90 degrees to the grain, it will yield very thin plies that can be woven into waterproof baskets for cooking. It is often twisted, but experienced eyes can spot the straight ones. I have pulled roots up to forty feet long that split perfectly equal and thin for their entire length. The split roots of black and Engelmann spruce have been used traditionally for basketmaking and fishnets. The Cree call the roots *watubiah*. The roots, when gathered in sphagnum moss, are long and thin. Remove the bark as soon as possible. These roots can be used right away or stored for later use and rehydrated in water. The roots are easily split and have a multitude of uses. One great advantage is that the root is very pliable but dries to shape.

If a tree leans or falls over and then rights itself, it produces annual rings that are wider on the outside curve. These are redder than the rest of the wood and highly prized for making strong wedges. In the past, native people would limb a growing spruce that was straight so that their children or grandchildren would inherit knot-free wood.

White Spruce is known to the Dene as *ts'uchogh*, meaning "big spruce" or "big brother." It is sometimes known as skunk or cat spruce due to the unpleasant scent of the needles when crushed. Black Spruce is simply *el*, or branch. This may be related to the relatively larger size of white spruce.

The inner bark and needles were traditionally boiled for tuberculosis and other lung complaints by several tribes. The inner bark was even used as a survival food, the thin layers eaten raw, cooked like spaghetti, or dried and later ground into flour. The small immature cones were chewed by the Cree for sore throats, while the tender young tips were peeled and eaten to prevent shortness of breath, or held in the mouth to treat hypertension and heart problems.

The Dene (Chipewyan) boiled the young cones, *najuli*, for mouth infections, sore throats, toothache; or to clear mucus from the throat. The small green cones of black spruce provided a red dye for porcupine quills. They decocted a fomentation from the boughs, and wrapped it around a mother's waist to ease afterbirth pain, speed labor, and later loosen and remove any retained placenta.

Snow-blindness results in a whitening of the affected pupil. If allowed to develop unhindered, sight will be lost. Balsam of young black spruce tops is produced by cutting the upper shoots of the sapling and then bending them over and splitting them in two. These are left beside a fire, and after the resinous liquid is heated out, the ball of the eye is gently coated using a bird quill. The Koyukon of Alaska call it *ts'ibaa*. The Saulteaux boiled the green cones and drank the liquid for dry scaly skin. The Abenaki (Alnombak) infused the green cones and gum resin to treat frequent urination. The dried, rotted spruce wood was finely ground and used as a baby powder.

The boughs make great mattresses for those who enjoy the vigors of winter camping. The wood is harvested for construction purposes due to its flexibility and relative strength. Cree and Chipewyan people used spruce for traps, snares, meat-drying racks, snowshoes, hide-stretching frames, and the frame of spruce bark canoes.

The inner bark is scraped out and chewed for colds, or dried for later use. The outer bark is stripped off large trees in spring when sap is running and used to make smokehouses to dry fish. This is preferred to plastic or canvas due to the constant inside temperature that is maintained. The rotten wood is used to smoke tanned moose, deer, or elk hides. Splints for broken limbs are made from the outer bark. The bark is high in tannin and is still used in parts of the world for tanning leather.

Spruce beer was very popular and was rationed on sailing ships in the 1800s to prevent scurvy. *Sapinette*, from sapin du Nord, was decocted from various conifers, including spruce, to prevent scurvy. Spruce beer was used by James Cook on his second Pacific voyage to British Columbia. Is it tasty? Some reviewers think not: "The flavor, if that is the right word for self-inflicted torture of this depth, is pine and menthol. If you ever wanted to lick a pine tree, here is your chance." Another reviewer wrote. "If ever offered a bottle, save yourself the trouble and drink some paint thinner." Henry David Thoreau (1848) was kinder, describing the taste as if "sucking at the very teats of Nature's pine-clad bosom … a lumberer's drink, which would acclimate and naturalize a man at once—which would make him see green, and, if he slept, dream that he heard the wind sough among the pines." British Admirals fancied a cocktail of rum, molasses, and spruce beer in a drink that was called calabogus. See below for a recipe, remembering that the young soft tips of spring contain more vitamin C and possess a distinct citrus flavor that makes it more enjoyable. Several microbrews now produce spruce beers as a seasonal beverage. In Quebec, a carbonated drink called *bière d'epinette* is widely available in supermarkets.

Don Durzan (2009) wrote an interesting article about Jacque Cartier's "tree of life" or Annedda. It has been suggested in popular literature that this was a pine, fir, spruce, or eastern cedar, and the content of vitamin C helped relieve scurvy for his ill ship crew in 1536. Durzan suggested the content of arginine and guanidine compounds may be even more important than ascorbic acid in helping restore balance to the immune system.

Engelmann spruce is found on cool, moist slopes from southwestern Alberta all the way to New Mexico. It is a very cold-tolerant tree, surviving temperatures of −76°F. They live up to one thousand years. The wood is used by piano makers for sounding boards and violins, as it is lightweight, fine-textured, and straight-grained. Larger trees are used for utility poles, as the tree can reach up to 150 feet. The record living specimen is 179 feet tall, with a diameter of 92 inches, or nearly 8 feet. Various native communities prized the bark, using the inner side for canoes and baskets. Bark infusions were taken for tuberculosis and other bronchial complaints.

The Norway spruce is a very popular tree for ornamental purposes and may be the most planted conifer in North America. There is only one tree in Antarctica, a Norway spruce. It is believed to be the remotest tree in the world, living on Campbell Island. Norway Spruce symbolizes kindness, and is associated with November 25. In the Nordic Runes, it represents the 24th symbol, *dag*. A tea of the needles is good for healing wounds and ulcers and good for stones in the kidney and gravel in the bladder. It will cut phlegm in the lungs and helps open lung alveoli. The knot wood is rich in up to 10% lignans, particularly 7-hydroxy-matairesinol (HMR) as the predominant source. The knots are not used in pulp nor in lumber. White spruce contains almost the same amounts of lignans as Norway spruce, with hydroxy-matairesinol accounting for 40–80% of the lignans. Black spruce contains much less, and the relative amount of HMR is also lower.

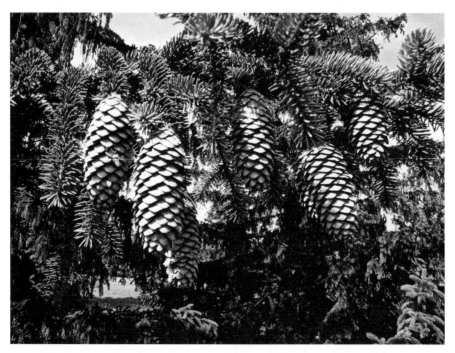

Norway spruce

White spruce branches contract with atmospheric changes, bracing for the weight of heavy snows. The dried branches, trimmed of needles, bow or straighten with barometric pressure and are a very accurate measure of upcoming weather. The liquid within the needle cells flows out so they can freeze without damage, even to −60°F. Black spruce is the provincial tree of Newfoundland, white spruce is representative from Manitoba, and blue spruce is the state tree of Colorado.

Bits and Pieces

During infestation by insects, spruce forests contain trees that do not change their terpene chemistry. Researchers have found these trees can change their chemical makeup, but they do not. These are not the weakest trees, falling prey to Darwin's survival of the fittest theory. These are strong, healthy trees that intentionally do not produce deterrent chemicals. Why? Because in the long term, the production of antifeedant compounds in *all* trees, would ensure that insects develop resistance in the same manner that crop pests develop resistance to pesticides. As Stephen Buhner (2002) points out, "plant communities literally set aside plants for the insects to consume so as to not force genetic rearrangement and the development of resistance."

Researchers working in the Sierra Nevada of California found 120 chemical compounds in the mountain forest air and could only identify 70 of them. We are literally breathing things we know little about. The Japanese have a term, *shinrin-yoku*, meaning forest or wood air bathing, for aromatic walks. Researchers found that when diabetic patients walk through the forest, their blood sugar drops to healthier levels (Ohtsuka et al. 1998). Ants use spruce resin for medicinal purposes. A Swiss study found deposits, some as large as forty-five pounds, in ant mounds, scattered around the living quarters to protect from microbial disease.

Medicinal Uses

Constituents: *P. glauca*: beta-sitosterol, alpha-keto-delta-guanidinovaleric acid.

Needles: shikimic acid (up to 4%); 120–160 mg/kg free arginine N.

P. abies bark: various stilbene glucosides, including isorhapotin, piceid and astringin, pinocarvone, fenchol, O-methythymol, myrtenal, trans-pinocarveol, trans-verbenol, verbenone, L-carvone, cuminal, alpha-terpenylacetate, 8-hydroxy-p-cymene, alpha-pinene-oxide, pinocamphone, isopinocamphone, and cuminol.

Twigs: mycrene, limonene (150 ppm).

P. engelmannii: astringin, iso-rhapontin.

Spruce buds and tender new shoots can be gathered in early spring and made into a brisk herbal tea. The early needles have a somewhat pleasant lemon citrus taste. The needles contain shikimic acid, the starting point for the production of Tamiflu, a pharmaceutical antiflu drug. Many plants contain the compound, but not all are commercially as viable as the needles of spruce, fir, and pine trees. Shikimic acid inhibits fibrin formation in a manner similar to aspirin. It disrupts the cell membrane and integrity of *Staphylococcus aureus* bacteria. Shikimic acid is a major phytoconstituent in coconut water.

Needle tea can be used for steaming in cases of bronchial or sinus congestion. The female cones can be decocted and the water used as a mouthwash for canker sores, gum-boils, infections, and toothaches. Spruce resin was used for centuries as a less expensive incense and was previously called common frankincense. Older herbals mention placing the resin in anthills to improve the scent. It was believed that formic acid, secreted by ants, produced a chemical transformation in the resin. The incense was burned to cleanse and protect against disrupting influence and to enhance inner peace.

The pitch or sap can be used on burns and sores and is most effective as part of an ointment, tincture, or salve. Spruce gum can be applied directly to wounds, or decocted for a stomachache. Spruce gum, according to Diana Beresford-Kroeger (2010),

> *when used as a chewing gum, is a cardiotonic and helps the oxygenation of the blood as it circulates, especially during exercise. The gum, when used as a tisane, is antihypertensive and will reduce blood pressure. It is antianginal and will help with the circulation within the beating heart as it oxygenates its own musculature and enabling it to act as a more efficient pump. The resin gum of spruce is also antiarrhythmic and will help the individual myocardial cells with their electronic message system of communication, one area with the other in the different geographic regions of the heart. In the past and in the present time, spruce gum has been used as an aboriginal endurance medicine for running or other tasks that physically stress the physiology of the body.*

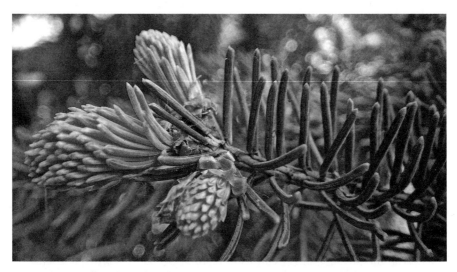

Young spruce needles

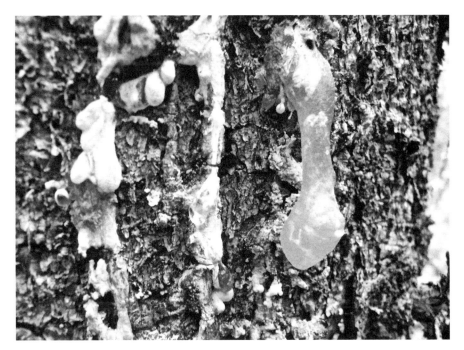

Spruce pitch

Ritch-Krc et al. (1996) found white spruce pitch active against *E. coli, Staphylococcus aureus, Pseudomonas aeruginosa, Candida albicans*, and *Aspergillus fumigatus*. For cuts, sores and skin irritations, take 1 tablespoon of dry resin, along with equal amounts of dried bugle (*Ajuga reptans*), calendula, and hound's tongue. Place in a jar with 4 ounces of ethanol. Shake daily and strain in 2 weeks.

A salve for more severe wounds or burns requires 1 teaspoon of spruce gum with 1½ ounces each of sumac and St. John's wort flowers, and 4 ounces of vegetable oil, slowly simmered for half an hour, then strained and cooled. A salve from the oleoresin has been found superior for treating burns and surgical wounds. Work by Sipponen et al. (2012) found 0% allergenic response in 23 patients with skin burns. A popular cough syrup from 1930 to 1950, available in most drug stores, was Dr. Gray's Syrup of Spruce Gum. See the "Recipes" section below.

An essence of spruce is made from a decoction of young branches that thickens and concentrates as it boils down. This viscid, molasses-like liquid is bitter and astringent in flavor. It is terrific for vaginal discharge, prolapsed uterus, or hemorrhoids, administered as a douche or enema. Tinctures of the gum are a useful diuretic and stimulant.

White spruce needles and stem extracts by water and ethanol possess activity against gram-positive bacteria and mycobacteria. Conifer bark infusions are antifungal and used to treat yeast infections. This suggests using cooled, strained tea in the form of a vaginal douche or retention enema.

White spruce needle extracts show protection against glucose toxicity and glucose deprivation, suggesting use in blood sugar regulation (Harbilas et al. 2009). *Gaultheria hispidula, Rhododendron tomentosum,* and *Vaccinium vitis-idaea* showed anti-diabetic potential in the same study. Black spruce extracts contain an insulin sensitizer that exerts effect through PPAR activation. PPAR agonists, such as rosiglitazone, increase the sensitivity of muscle and adipose tissue to insulin (Spoor et al. 2006). Recent work in this field, looking at seven traditional Quebec Cree plants for diabetes, found the activity is analogous to metformin, and not via an insulin pathway. Rather it is AMP activated by a protein kinase pathway (Martineau et al. 2010).

Hot water extracts of black spruce bark show benefit in psoriatic keratinocytes, suggestive of psoriasis relief (García-Pérez et al. 2010). Fomentations or gentle bathing of affected areas may be helpful. Norway spruce shows lipase inhibition associated with weight loss and other digestive issues (Slanc et al. 2009). Norway spruce contains isorhapontin, which possesses antileukemia activity (Mannila and Talvitie 1992).

A U.S. patent (#6,271,257) was granted to a Finnish nutraceutical company for an extract from Norway spruce. The lignan hydroxy-matairesinol A is a novel enterolactone precursor with antitumor properties. It is specifically aimed at those individuals with increased risk of developing colorectal cancer; the lignan is used as a supplement or ingredient in functional foods. The product, called HMRlignan, cleared FDA approval as a dietary ingredient in May 2004. At low doses of 10–30 mg/day, the lignan is an effective precursor of enterolactone, a compound derived by healthy gut bacteria from compounds in flaxseed, but seventy times more effective.

About a decade ago, I was hired to formulate a line of herbal supplements, including one for breast health. One of the ingredients was 10 mg per capsule of HMRlignan. A placebo-controlled double-blind clinical study conducted in 2010 found a positive link between this supplement from femMED, and better breast health in 96 perimenopausal and postmenopausal women (Laidlaw et al. 2010).

Enterolactone levels are related to prevention of cardiovascular disease and hormone-related cancers such as breast and prostate. In one Finnish study of 68 premenopausal and 126 postmenopausal breast cancer patients, an inverse association was found between serum enterolactone and the risk of breast cancer in both groups (Pietinen et al. 2001). In one clinical trial, doses of 10–30 mg were sufficient to raise enterolactone to levels research has shown as beneficial. In another study, the lignan inhibited tumor growth and reduced tumor formation rates (Kangas et al. 2002). Vanharanta et al. (2003) found an association between coronary heart disease and low serum enterolactone levels. This may be due to enhanced lipid peroxidation, as noted in an earlier study. Unlike other lignans, this one is not attached to sugar molecules that need to be cleaved in the intestinal tract. Work by

McCann et al. (2008) found enterolactones from HMRlignan restrict the proliferation of human prostate cancer cell lines in vitro. It appears that the antiproliferative activity is a consequence of altered expression of cell cycle–associated genes. The product, HMR, at 50 mg daily, dramatically reduced the number of hot flashes experienced by menopausal women in a study by Medicus Research.

Norway spruce salves show activity against MRSA and vancomycin-resistant *Enterococcus* (VRE) bacteria (Sipponen et al. 2007). An interesting study by Legault et al. (2013) found white and black spruce bark extracts possess higher antioxidant activity than Pycnogenol, a well-researched bark extract from *Pinus maritima*. Work by Klippel et al. (1997) focused on the use of beta-sitosterols from *Picea* and *Pinus* species for the treatment of benign prostatic hyperplasia. In a double-blind placebo-controlled trial with 133 patients, significant improvement over control was noted using 130 mg of beta-sitosterol daily.

Fresh organic Norway spruce bud juices and extract are combined with sundew (*Drosera rotundifolia*) in a popular herbal product for respiratory conditions, including whooping cough and bronchial asthma. Black spruce is often a great source of *Usnea* lichen species. This particular herb has a multitude of usage in herbal medicine, especially for *Streptococcus* and *Staphylococcus* bacterial infections and drug-resistant tuberculosis. See my book *The Fungal Pharmacy: The Complete Guide to Medicinal Mushrooms and Lichens in North America* (2011) for more complete details on *Usnea* and related lichens.

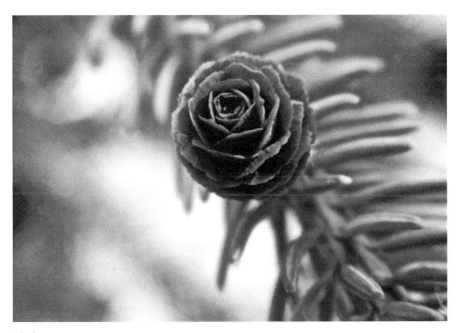

Black spruce young cone

Homeopathy

Black spruce has been used in homeopathy for nearly 150 years. Black spruce's main identifying characteristic, especially in elderly people, is a sensation that something is lodged in the esophagus. The person may have digestive system weakness as a result of excessive tea or tobacco intake. At night the person wakes up hungry or is restless with unpleasant dreams. During the day they are sleepy and may alternate between hot and cold intermittent fevers. They always feel worse after eating, but are ravenous at noon and night, with lack of appetite in the morning. Bulimia and religious affections may be present. Symptoms are worse from cold wet weather. Constipation is chronic, especially after abuse of alcohol, tea, and coffee.

Dose: 10–20 drops, as needed. 1st to 30th potency of the mother tincture, made from the gum of the tree. Proving by Leaman with three provers with tincture in 1867. Bell also experimented with various potencies from tincture to the 30th potency.

Essential Oils

Constituents: Black spruce: needles: camphene, beta-pinene (14%), 3-carene, longifolene, bornyl acetate (42–52%), camphene (19%), alpha-pinene (15%), camphor (4.9%), santene, myrcene, limonene, longiborneal, and sesquiterpenol. Yield, about 1.4%, is highest in April needles in my part of the world.

Buds: over 50% 3-carene, with over 25% alpha- and beta-pinene, as well as terpinolene (4.7%), Yield 0.2%.

Twigs: nearly identical to buds with less bornyl acetate, and limonene. Yield 0.2%.

White spruce: needles: camphor (2.8%), limonene (15.3), bornyl acetate (12.1–14%), and smaller amounts of camphene, mycrene, alpha-pinene, and beta-pinene. Yield is about 0.2–0.5%, highest in April.

Buds: contains over 40% alpha- and beta-pinene, over 30% mycrene, and 9% 3-carene, not present in needle oil. Yield about 0.5%.

Twigs: rich in limonene (37.5%), alpha-pinene (22%), mycrene, and beta-pinene. Yield is 0.5–0.7%.

Cones: 14.4% borneol, 9.1% bornyl acetate, 3.1% citral, 1.8% carvone, with a yield of 0.154%.

Engelmann spruce: 8.5% bornyl acetate.

Norway spruce needles: beta-pinene (4–32%), camphene (7–26%), alpha-pinene (14–21%), (+)-limonene (9.5–16%) and minor amounts delta-3-carene, beta-mycrene, bornyl acetate, beta-phellandrene, 1,8-cineole, borneol, tricyclene, camphor, and others.

The essential oils of spruce needles are antispasmodic, antifungal, and antiparasitic. They can reduce inflammation and act hormone-like, stimulating the thymus gland and adrenals. It is a tonic in general, but also a good recharger of the nervous system and solar plexus.

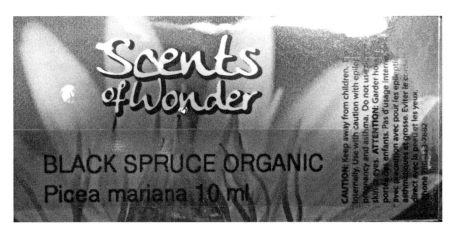

Organic black spruce essential oil

Wonderful oil is steam-distilled from the branches and needles of black spruce. It is fortifying and invigorating oil, having the constituents to regenerate exhausted adrenals. The oil is applied directly to the adrenal area in the lower back. Daniel Pénoël, a French physician and medical aromatherapist, uses a hair drier to drive the oil into the affected area more efficiently. Prostate inflammation can be reduced by massaging the surrounding area externally with black spruce oil diluted to 5% in a carrier oil. A pessary with the same ratio can be formed using coconut oil and inserted rectally for similar benefit. It may be used to fight internal fungal infections like *Candida albicans* as well as parasites. It is healing to acne and dry eczema. It slows down a hyperthyroid condition and generally boosts the immune system. The essential oil can be rubbed directly onto the thyroid region once or twice daily.

Bornyl acetate potentiates the anticancer activity of 5-fluorouracil (5-FU) in human gastric cancer cells by inducing apoptosis and other pathways (Li and Wang 2016). Kurt Schnaubelt suggests combining pine, black spruce, and black currant essential oils for exhausted adrenals. Black spruce essential oil is approved by the German Commission E for the treatment of colds, cough, bronchitis, fevers, stomatitis, pharyngitis, muscular and nerve pain, rheumatism, and proneness to infection.

North Americans have normalized the magnificence of black spruce. But as my wife and I discovered on a recent trip to Grenada, the powerful grounding scent of spruce is valuable and exotic to those living in a different climate. It is estimated five million pounds of black spruce essential oil could be produced annually in Ontario alone.

White spruce essential oil has similar properties, but contains less bornyl acetate and more limonene. This is a basic ingredient of most perfumes with a pine scent, and used for synthetic camphor production. Gall formations on white spruce contain more essential oil than the healthy shoots, with a slight variation of the constituents. White spruce oil from twigs and leaves is relatively constant throughout the year, but the spring buds change significantly. The relative amounts of beta-pinene, limonene, and mycrene change during fall and winter. In May, substantial amounts of sesquiterpenes are present in the new growth, but this moderates during the summer.

The adulteration of black spruce with essential oil from white spruce can be easily spotted by percentage of camphor. The former has less than 0.5%, while the latter can be up to 38%, making for easy detection. The essential oils from white and black spruce possess antimicrobial activity similar to exotic oils like eucalyptus, cinnamon, and clove (Poaty et al. 2015). Spruce oils are used in the food industry for chewing gum, ice cream, and soft-drink flavoring. Branches from sun-exposed white spruce yield 20% more oil than dense bush. And work by Duke (1983) found 25-year-old trees yield twice the essential oil of a 45-year-old.

Colorado blue spruce yields an essential oil containing over 37% limonene, 7% camphene, 7% alpha-pinene, 7% myrcene, 6% camphor, and 12% bornyl acetate. Engelmann spruce oil has a distinct odor of camphor, yields 0.895%, and has a saponification value of 24.15. The oil contains 8.5% bornyl acetate.

At one time, a spoonful of the oleoresin obtained from a bark blister of Engelmann spruce was used to treat cancer. Norway spruce shoots yield an essential oil effective against *Staphylococcus aureus*, *Streptococcus faecalis*, and *Bacillus subtilis* as well as strains isolated from patients of beta-hemolysing *Streptococcus aureus*, *S. pneumoniae*, *S. milleri*, *Staphylococcus* strains, *Corynebacterium diphtheriae*, and *Candida albicans*.

The tree yields a resin called burgundy pitch, used as a varnish for musical instruments and a chest plaster for chronic pulmonary affections. It may be applied in a 10% dilution to buttocks and thighs for sciatica or neuralgic pain and various rheumatic and muscular conditions.

Hydrosol

Black spruce hydrosol is at once reminiscent of the air around lumber mills in northern Alberta, a kind of resinous, cool, and evergreen scent. It has a cat urine–like scent, unpleasant to some. The new growth buds of spring, which are almost citrusy and lemon-like, make a superior hydrosol. The pH is 4.2 to 4.4.

Suzanne Catty (2001) suggests consuming up to 1 ounce of the hydrosol daily in 1 quart of water for adrenal benefit. She mentions that placing one drop of the hydrosol on acupuncture points for the adrenals has an extraordinary effect. She writes that an odd effect of both the oil and hydrosol is sprucing up the bust line, both in size and tone of tissue.

Florentine water, or needle water, is produced from fir or spruce needles during distillation. The colorless bitter liquid contains vitamin C, pro-vitamin A, and trace elements. It is presently discarded in Canada but is used in parts of Russia (up to one million tons annually) for livestock enterprises and medicine. Florentine water, rich in mono- and sesquiterpenes, if used in steam distillation, increases the yield of essential oils from pine, fir, spruce, and larch, as compared with fresh water.

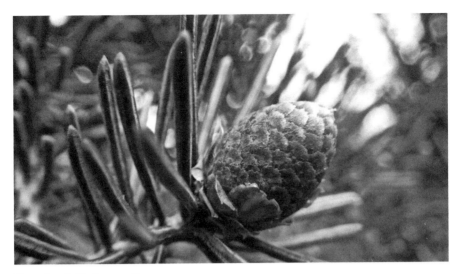

Young female black spruce flower cone

Flower Essence

One of the first flower essences I worked with was the beautiful pink cone of black spruce. Here is what I perceived about the essence, now part of our Prairie Deva Flower Essence line.

Black spruce flower essence allows us the clarity to see our own shadow. It also ignites our inner wisdom by letting some of our shadow qualities come to light and be accepted or dissipate. This is a grounding essence that helps us be more realistic. Visiting this essence is like taking a voyage to a monastery. It gives us strength during times of frustration and helps bring clarity to those involved with addictions.

Used in psychotherapy or with dream work, this essence works to regenerate or patch our wounds. It may increase emotional stamina and strength to discard old patterns that no long serve us. It allows us a glimpse into how our personal power has been tied up in repressing our shadow. It is a useful essence for practitioners working with addictions, helping them see more clearly through the double-speak and confusion presented by individuals suffering alcohol and drug dependency.

Spiritual Properties

David Suzuki is a famous scientist who has been championing the need for environmental stewardship for over fifty years. In this book co-authored by Peter Knudtson (2006), they write:

> *White Spruce harbors within it a potent spirit known as* biyeega hoolanh, *an expression of its mythical Distant Time connections. Most plant spirits are viewed as relatively minor*

forces in nature, but biyeega hoolanh *rivals the strength even of some of the most spiritually potent game animals, such as bears and wolverines. To Koyukon sensibilities, the spiritual powers of a mature white spruce tree tend to be concentrated in its boughs and top, or crown.... It was traditionally employed by shamans during healing ceremonies to "whisk" away a patient's illness.*

Myths and Legends

Grinnell (1905) collected and recorded the following legend: When a young man was in love, he gave spruce gum to his potential lover if she did not care for him. If he could get her to chew it, her thoughts would constantly be directed toward him.

Bits and Pieces

The most famous use of spruce wood is due to its resonant qualities. For this reason it is used in the manufacturing of guitars, mandolins, organ pipes, piano sounding boards, and the top plates—or bellies—of violins. Foremost among violins are the acoustically exquisite three-hundred-year-old instruments of Antonio Stradivari, topped with Norwegian spruce. The secret of these violins has eluded musicians, craftspeople, and scientists for centuries.

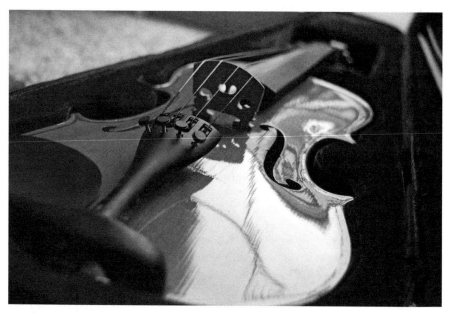

Violin

Research at Texas A&M by Joseph Nagyvary et al. (1984) found the wood is full of distinctive open holes—the result of microbial degradation. It seems that the Italian loggers floated green logs down from the Alps by river. In the warmer Italian water, the logs were invaded by bacteria and fungi, producing batteries of cell wall–dissolving enzymes. This destruction increased the wood's permeability without altering its strength. Once dried, the fungi-chewed wood is lighter and more porous, and hence the tone is richer and warmer.

Astrology

All living beings are influenced by the placement of the sun and the planets. Astrological influence comes to bear on the growth of plants including conifers. Hageneder (2005) expounds:

> Conifers are completely dominated by Saturn, and the forces that inhibit growth processes, contract substance, and harden form. The way in which the branches of a conifer focus tightly around the central trunk, just as the needles do around the twig, are further expressions of these forces.… The very needle shape only allows the smallest possible contact with the environment. Saturn governs the conifers, and many of them reach sexual maturity only after the planet has performed one full cycle (twenty-eight years). Saturn's long rhythm also grants them long life. With their confined, hard shapes they can venture deeper into the winter, into the mountains, and into the north than any other tree or shrub.

RECIPES

Infusion: Place 1 handful of new spring buds in 1 pint of boiling water. Let gently simmer 10 minutes. Drink 1 cup daily. The spring needles are fresh and citrus-like, and easy to discern due to their soft texture and lighter color of green.

Tincture: Take 2 parts by weight of spruce gum and dissolve in 9 parts of 95% alcohol. Filter. This is a sticky product that will turn cloudy when added to water. Take 10 drops in water as needed for bronchitis and other respiratory conditions.

Spruce beer: Boil 2 gallons of water and 6 ounces of spring tips for 1 hour. Take from the heat and remove the spruce. Add 2 pounds of molasses and stir well to dissolve. Cool to 70°F and pour into a fermenter with yeast. When complete, prime bottles, fill, and cap. It's ready in 10 more days (Buhner 1998, 255–56).

Spruce essence: Take the new green shoots of white or black spruce, cover with water, and boil until pungent, reddish brown, and reduced by half. Bottle and save for year-round use. It requires refrigeration.

Tamarack and Larch

Tamarack ◆ Eastern Larch—*Larix laricina* (Du Roi) K. Koch

Western Larch ◆ Western Tamarack ◆ Hackmatack—*Larix occidentalis* Nutt.

Subalpine Larch ◆ Wooly Larch—*Larix lyallii* Parl.

Siberian Larch—*Larix sibirica* Ledeb.

European Larch—*Larix decidua* Mill.

Dahurian Larch ◆ Kurile Larch—*Larix gmelinii* (Rupr.) Rupr. ◆ *L. gmelinii* var. *japonica* (Maxim. ex Regel) Pilg.

Parts used: bark, needles, resin

> *A fool sees not the same tree that a wise man sees.*

—William Blake

> *In winter, it is still more lamentably distinguished from every other deciduous tree of the forest; for they seem only to sleep, but the Larch appears absolutely dead.*

—William Wordsworth

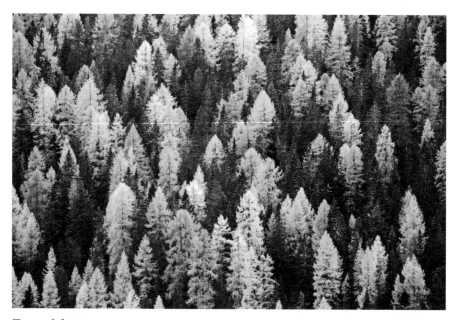

Tamarack forest

I first became acquainted with tamarack in my early twenties. I noted how entire bogs and swamps would turn yellow-gold in the autumn, unlike the other evergreens like fir, spruce, and pine. I later learned they are known as deciduous conifers, something I was not taught about in my botany courses at university.

My neighbor John was fencing a small pasture for goats and asked me for help cutting wooden posts. Off we went one cold December morning to the nearby muskeg forest, he with his chainsaw and me with a sharpened ax. The tamarack were relatively immature, probably twenty to thirty years old, measuring four to six inches in diameter at the base. Fortunately the snow was not that deep, so walking was fairly easy. John fired up his chainsaw and felled the first, and then another and another. He cut them into eight-foot lengths, and I trimmed off the sporadic branches. It was −8°F, so they snapped off very easily. After a few hours we stopped for some hot soup from a thermos, and then hauled the poles and tops to the pickup. John got quite excited when he took a closer look at the poles and noted a green-blue stain on many of them. He explained that for some reason, the posts with this fungal infection lasted a lifetime. We stopped at my cabin and dumped off the wood too small for fence posts but perfect for woodstove kindling.

Tamarack may derive from the French-Canadian *tamarac*, perhaps based on an Algonquin name. Another route of origin is from the Abenaki of eastern Canada, who called the tree *akemantak*, "wood for snowshoes." This was pronounced "hackmatack," and then "tamarack." *Abenaki* means "dawn people." They refer to themselves as Alnombak, meaning "the people." According to Geniusz (2015), "The Hebrew name Tamara means 'medicine woman.'" *Larch* derives from the Latin *lar*, meaning "fat," in reference to the resin produced. Think *lard*. Another possibility is from the French *l'archer*, the bowman, in reference to the wood's flexibility. In German, the tree is called *Larchen*. *Lyallii* is named in honor of David Lyall, a nineteenth-century Scottish botanist.

Tamarack is a very common tree in the muskeg of northern areas. Western larch is a much larger tree, particularly in British Columbia, where it can grow to 150 feet, as opposed to the 60-foot average of a mature tamarack. One exception is a tamarack found near my hometown of Edmonton that is 152 feet tall. Both are unique in being deciduous conifers that drops needles in fall after turning a brilliant yellow.

An insect pest destroyed nearly all the large tamarack in my province in the 1930s. The larch sawfly is still the most destructive of the forty insect pests that attack this tree. They literally devour one branch and then another until the whole tree is defoliated. Females, accounting for 98 percent of the population, do not require mating to lay fertile eggs.

Traditional Uses

The Cree of northern Alberta used the strong pliable wood as a birch substitute for snowshoes, toboggans, and canoes. The long thin roots were split and used as wrapping material, like rope. The Dene (Chipewyan) call the tree *nidhe*, and made toboggans with the wood *beth chene* or "load stick." The Dena'ina name for tamarack is *ch'dat'an denlzuya*, meaning "grayling's rattling noise." The wood was widely used in south-central Alaska for boat ribs and sled runners. The dry root was used to carry fire, according to Mors Kochanski, a good friend and survival expert. The director of the film *The Revenant*, Alejandro González Iñárritu, insisted on hiring Mors for technical advice to ensure wilderness authenticity in the film.

The root, when lit at one end, burns like a fuse without flame until all of the root is consumed. This property should be noted when using tamarack for campfires, making sure the coals are completely doused before leaving. Tamarack makes great walking sticks, something that Dennis Purschke has turned into a full-time commercial venture. The Tamarack Hiking Stick is now the official walking stick of the Trans-Canada Trail, the American Discovery Trail, and the Lewis and Clark Bicentennial Path.

The knees of the original *Bluenose*, a schooner built in Lunenburg, Nova Scotia, and featured on the back of the Canadian dime, were fashioned from tamarack roots grown at right angles. The wood is ideal for railroad ties, being disease-resistant, straight, and strong. Tamarack is used in the pulp-and-paper industry to make the transparent windows in business envelopes. In Quebec the tree is known as *violon*, or "violin wood," from its early use making musical instruments. The James Bay Cree know it as *waachinaakan*. As late as the 1840s, the city of Detroit used hollow tamarack logs for its water piping system.

The long split roots were used to sew birch bark, especially in areas where black spruce

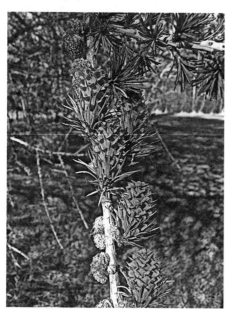

Young tamarack cones

was not available. They were pulled up and split lengthwise. The Cree made tea from the inner bark for washing sores, burns, frostbite, and wounds, as well as hemorrhoids, ear and eye inflammations, jaundice, colic, and melancholy. It is known to the Woods Cree of Saskatchewan, and the northern Cree of Alberta as *wakinakun* or *waginatik*, meaning "bends easily." The western larch in the mountains is known as *waskwayahtik*.

Russell Willier calls it *wakanakahn*, meaning "Bendable Stem." He uses bark decoctions in combinations to help cleanse the blood and throat, and when cooled, he applies it to open sores to suck out the poison and infections. He uses the bark to treat tuberculosis (Young et al. 2015). The Woods Cree of Saskatchewan used the inner bark as a poultice to heal frostbite, hemorrhoids, boils, burns, and deep infected wounds. A tea of the inner bark is used as an eyewash or ear cleanser, or combined with other herbs as heart medicine. The Gwich'in of the Mackenzie River Delta decocted a tea made from four or five tamarack cones for colds and headaches. They call the tree *ts'iiteenjuh*. Small branches were boiled and cooled and the tea taken for tiredness or upset stomach. The sap gum was chewed for indigestion or sore throat. Sophie Thomas, Saik'uz elder and herbalist, calls this tree *netsi'ul*. The whole branches are boiled and used for hypertension and diuretic (Young and Hawley 2004). Her book mentions the female cones are red, so she may be referring to western larch, a closely related tree. Tamarack has both red and white female cones. The rotten wood, when found, was used for smoking tanning hides, while the bark contains tannins needed to treat the leather.

Tamarack bark was decocted and used to dye porcupine quills red by the Northern Saulteaux, while the Kanien'kehá:ka (Mohawk) fashioned snowshoes from the flexible wood. The term *Mohawk* was derived by Dutch settlers from a word spoken by the neighboring Muh-heck Heek Ing, an Algonquin tribe called Mohican or Mahican. The Mohican called their neighbors *Maw Unk Lin* (Bear Place People), and the Dutch turned this into "Mohawk."

Other tribes shaped the branches and twigs into large decoys resembling geese to use during hunting season. The trunk near the top of the tree was chopped into small pieces and boiled for ten minutes. This liquid was drunk and the sticks saved. This process was repeated every two days for a week using the same pieces for "sore bones" or arthritis. At the end of the week, the sticks were buried. Other tribes dried the needles, inhaling the powder for colds, bronchitis, and urinary-tract infections. As the needles are high in tannins and vitamin C, this makes good sense. The Potawatomi used bark extracts for bronchitis and chronic urinary tract inflammation, while the Mi'kmaq steeped it as a tea for colds, consumption, or general debility. The Potawatomi also mixed shredded inner bark with oats for horses to make their hide loose and slip around when pinched. For tuberculosis, the bark was decocted with skunk cabbage root and taken in small amounts. The Ojibwe steamed the fresh needles over hot rocks for lung congestion; while the Abenacki combined the bark and fireweed roots as an infusion for persistent coughs. The Anishinaabe name for tamarack is *mashkiig-mitig*, meaning "muskeg tree" or "swamp tree." The Eastern Cree used the young branches or inner bark of *watnagan* as a tea with laxative and diuretic effect. Geniusz (2015, 106) explains:

> *Tamarack also is beneficial for a hardened condition of the liver and spleen. When a person's personality changes, the mental condition may be a result of a sluggish, underfunctioning liver and/or spleen. This medicine from the tamarack was traditionally used to treat postpartum melancholia and for jaundice, when the whites of the eyes have a yellowish cast, or in viral infections like mononucleosis, where the spleen and liver are affected.*

The gum resin was chewed and the juice swallowed for sore throats and indigestion. It is one of the better-flavored gums from coniferous trees. When dried and powdered, the gum was used as a type of baking powder. The Dene (Chipewyan) called the soft inner bark of tamarack *nidhe k'a*, meaning "tamarack fat." They applied the inner bark to burns and boils to draw out poisons and promote healing. A tea was prepared from the young branches of *diweh* for stomach problems, or the bark was chewed and applied to boils, mastitis, and other breast infections.

Early people considered larch a symbol of new beginnings, spontaneity, luck, and renewal. The wood, needles, and resin were all used as incense to help free blocked energy and stimulate renewal. Larch was considered the home of friendly elves or plant devas, and thus the connection between worlds.

Western larch is a much bigger tree, growing up to 200 feet tall and 3 to 4 feet in diameter. One specimen in Montana is 177 feet tall and nearly eight feet in diameter. Western larch was highly prized by various native tribes like the Salish (Flathead) and Ktunaxa (Kutenai). They hollowed out the trunks and allowed the sweet sap or syrup to accumulate. This could be further evaporated or eaten straight like a mild, bitter birch sap. A good tree might yield as much as one gallon of the liquid a year. I have come upon such trees in British Columbia, with large hollowed bases, long ago deserted. The accumulation of dried sap in some cases is over twenty pounds, easily chipped out with a hatchet. The inner bark is sweet, the pitch is used as a chewing gum, and a baking powder substitute is derived from the sap. A small amount of resin was chewed to increase or quicken menstrual flow.

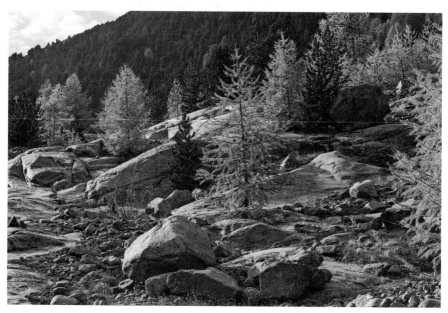

Western larch

The bark tea was drunk for tuberculosis, dry coughs and colds. See the "Recipes" section below. The Nlaka'pamux decocted the bark, sometimes combined with squaw currant (*Ribes cereum*) twigs as a wash to ensure healthy, strong babies. It was taken internally for broken bones and to treat breast cancer. It was said to stimulate appetite and heal stomach ulcers and was combined with saskatoon (*Amelanchier alnifolia*) inner bark for birth control.

Arabinogalactans, in larch and tamarack, are involved in plant growth and development and possibly in signal transduction. Larch arabinogalactans are used in the food industry as emulsifiers, stabilizers, binders, and bodying agents for essential oils, dressings, and pudding mixes as well as industrially for paints and inks. It may be used as a 1% additive to flours for bread making. Larex is the primary producer of eight million pounds of arabinogalactans annually at its plant in Cohasset, Minnesota. Today, arabinogalactan is used in blood cell separation and personal care products, with a FDA generally recognized as safe (GRAS) status. This is partly due to the fact that the compounds are easily extractable by water in a pure form. In comparison with gum arabic, a highly branched source of arabinogalactan, the larch compound possesses higher solubility and lower viscosity.

The gum resins from *Larix* species prevent concrete from curing, so don't use its wood for cement forms. European larch symbolizes daring or deceitful charms and has two birth dates, April 27 and February 12. It is widely planted in northern urban centers. Larch and alder piles support much of the city of Venice, Italy. In Russia, larch oleoresins are used to manufacture larix-aroma, used in perfumery as a substitute for ambergris. The Japanese larch (*L. kaempferi*) is hardy to zones 3 and 4 and is found in a number of forms, including several beautiful weeping specimens. Dahurian Larch (*L. gmelinii*) is a very hardy native of eastern Siberia. It will grow up to 100 feet tall and 30 feet wide in optimal conditions but becomes quite shrubby in extreme cold and wind. In Siberia, the larch is associated with the shamans of the Tungus tribe. In the *Primitive Mythology: Masks of God*, Joseph Campbell (1991) notes the larch poles are used in a sacred ceremony. They are an earthly symbol of Tuuru, a mythical tree, where the souls of all shamans develop before coming to earth. When the Tungus shaman is working, his soul is symbolically climbing the Tuuru tree's larch pole, which extends into heaven. His drum has a rim of larch bark taken from a living tree.

The Ostiaks of Siberia consider a group of seven larch trees to be a sacred grove. Larch is described as the abode of the *saligen*, the blessed ones. Spirits called the *salgfraulein*, blessed maidens, were said to sit under an old larch dressed in white or silver and sing the sweetest music through the valleys. Larch was considered a male tree, and fir the female, in many European and Asian traditions.

Medicinal Uses

Constituents: *L. laricina* bark: vanillic acid glucosides, 4-hydroxybenzoic acid glucoside, vitexin, laricinan (beta-1,3-glucan), syringetin-3-glucosides, paracoumaric glucosides, arabinogalactans and leucoanthocyanins, 13-epitorulosol, 13-epicupressic acid, lariciresinol-3-acetate, lariciresinol-coumarate, rhapontigenin, piceatannol, taxifolin (dihydroquercetin), rhaponticin, labdane type diterpenes, including cis-19-hydroxyabienol, 8-alpha-hydroxy-12Z, 12-labdadien-19-al, 19-acetoxy-13S-hydroxy8(17), 14-labdadiene, the stilbene 3-methoxy-3,3f,5f-trihydroxystilbene, 23-oxo-3alpha-hydroxy-cycloart-24-en -26-oic acid, and 13-epitorulosol.

Heartwood: taxifolin, aromadendrin, quercetin, esters of ferulic, phthalic and long-chain fatty acids, beta-sitosterol, eicosanol and nonan-2-ol, D-galactose, and L-arabinose.

Needles: beta-glucosides of vanillic acid and p-coumaric acid, alpha-glucoside of p-hydroxybenzoic acid.

L. occidentalis: bark: lignans; inner bark: arabinogalactans (3,000–100,000 Da).

L. gmelinii bark: taxifolin (dihydroquercetin).

L. sibirica bark: suberin, phenolic acid esters, particularly alkyl ferulates, methyl pimarate, methyl abietate, and phenolic acids like ferulic, coumaric, and caffeic. Unsaponifiables are docosanol, tetraconsanol, and beta-sitosterol.

Knot wood: dihydroquercetin, and lignans (-)-secoisolariciresinol and (+)-isolariciresinol.

L. decidua bark: oleoresins (50–65%) larixinic acid (maltol), and alpha- and beta-laricinolic acid; lignans including lariciresinol, liovil, and secoisolariciresinol; labdane type diterpene resins, acids such as labdanolic acid, larixol, larixyl acetate, arabinogalactans, d-glucaric acid.

needles: melezitose.

L. kaempferi cones: eight abietane diterpenes.

Larch needles: flavanones (naringenin, hesperitin, hesperidin), flavones (apigenin, vitexin), and flavonols (kaempferols, quercetins, isorhamnetins, myricetins, syringetins).

The inner bark of Tamarack is decocted to help bleeding of the lungs or throat and to soothe bleeding hemorrhoids. It will reduce excessive menstruation and is good for the liver and spleen when enlarged and hardened, combining well with red root. The cooled, strained decoction is used in an eyecup for inflamed eyes, or to relieve earache.

The decoction wash will resolve gangrene or old skin ulcers, while a decoction of wood ashes is better for healing burns and scalds. Fresh inner bark, containing galactic acid, is a healing poultice for wounds and frostbite. In cases of constipation, add licorice and calamus roots to the inner bark and simmer slowly, 1 teaspoon of each to 1 pint of water for 20 minutes. Drink 4 ounces as needed.

The Eclectic physician John King recommended tamarack bark decoctions for their laxative, tonic, diuretic, and alterative properties in obstructions of the liver, rheumatism, jaundice, and various skin diseases. A famous prescription called Dr. Bone's Bitters contained larch bark, prickly ash, tansy, and aloe as a stimulating cholagogue and alterative. Cook (1869) suggested that "*Apocynum* (dogbane) might profitably replace the aloes; and if horseradish were added, the compound would meet some cases of dropsy." Combine tamarack with spearmint, horseradish, and juniper berries for dropsy and other water-retention issues.

The *United States Dispensatory* of 1916 mentions tamarack bark tincture for treating bronchitis and chronic inflammation of the urinary tract. Chronic nonresponding urogenital infections will be helped by either bark tincture or decoction. Think of tamarack bark when children have chronically over-used antibiotics for respiratory and bladder infection and no longer respond effectively to the drugs. Tamarack bark decoction, with equal parts by weight of hops infused after removal from heat, makes an acceptable cough syrup with addition of honey. Decoction of the needles has been used for hemorrhoids, menorrhagia, diarrhea, and externally as a cool wash for skin disease, ulcers, and burns.

Tamarack cambium and bark has been found to possess high antioxidant activity, and may possess antidiabetic activity (Fraser et al. 2007). Further work by Shang et al. (2012) identified several compounds with antidiabetic activity. Rhapontigenin, previously identified, showed glitazone-like insulin-sensitizing activity. A unique compound 23-oxo-3alpha-hydroxycycloart-24-en-26-oic acid showed strong adipogenesis activity at EC_{50} of 7.7 μM. Another compound 13-epitorulosol potentiated adipogenesis EC_{50} of 8.2 μM. This suggests benefit in prevention or treatment of obesity. Like metformin and rosiglitazone, tamarack bark increases glucose uptake and adipogenesis, activates AMPK, uncouples mitochondrial function, and improves ATP synthesis (Harbilas et al. 2012). Work by Smiley et al. (2012) looked at in vitro effects of rhaponticin on metabolism of the antidiabetic drug gliclazide. Rhaponticin and the aglycone did not show significant effects on repaglinide or gliclazide inhibition. The algycone rhapontigenin showed effect on various

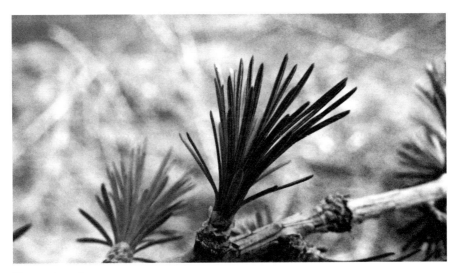

Tamarack needles

liver enzyme metabolic pathways, suggesting potential in vitro drug interactions (Cieniak et al. 2013). Rhaponticin inhibits fatty acid synthase and down-regulates its expression in human breast cancer MCF-7 cells (Peng Li et al. 2014). Rhaponticin is found in fenugreek seed and roots of various rhubarb species.

Larch and tamarack resin help relieve muscle cramps. The resin soothes and strengthens the respiratory tract, helping dissolve old mucus in cases of chronic sinus congestion and upper respiratory tract infections. Chronic sinusitis is often associated with food allergies, and this possibility should be fully explored. A small piece of resin, chewed like gum, increases or brings on menstrual flow, so caution is advised. McCutcheon et al. (1992) found branches of western larch active against nine of eleven bacteria tested. Arabinogalactans are plentiful in nature and are found in small amounts in carrots, radish, wheat, and tomatoes. They are also present in some immune-enhancing herbs like *echinacea*, *Thuja*, and *Angelica* species and the medicinal mushroom *reishi (Ganoderma lucidum)*.

Larch arabinogalactans are composed of galactose and arbinose units in a 6:1 ratio with a trace of uronic acid. The bark is extracted to produce light cream-colored powder with a slight pine odor and sweet taste. It is 100% water soluble, with low viscosity, and is a 3,6-beta-D-galactan–type compound. The polysaccharides encourage natural killer (NK) cell and macrophage activation, helping strengthen the immune system's effectiveness. Specific cytokines are increased, including interferon-gamma, TNF-alpha, interleukin-1-beta, and interleukin-6 (Hauer and Anderer 1993). L. S. Kim et al. (2002) looked at the effect of low-dose arabinogalactan and two *echinacea* species on 48 females in a randomized double-blind placebo-controlled study. At 1.5 grams per day, complement properdin increased 18% with a combination of two extracts. Properdin deficiency is linked to susceptibility to fulminant meningococcal disease. Causey et al. (1999) looked at 20 subjects taking 30 grams of arabinogalactan powder daily and found white blood cell, monocyte, neutrophil, and lymphocyte counts increased. Udani et al. (2010) found an extract increased IgG and IgE antibody response to pneumonia vaccine in a randomized double-blind placebo-controlled pilot study of 45 healthy volunteers.

The absence of response following influenza vaccination suggests involvement of T cells, and a role for arabinogalactan in cold infections (Dion et al. 2016). It is speculated it may have a direct effect on the immune system via gut-associated lymphoid tissue. It has properties that make it an ideal carrier to deliver agents to hepatocytes via the asialoglycoprotein receptors. Its activity is stronger than *echinacea*, with no allergenic or insulin response. Larch arabinogalactans are an excellent source of dietary fiber and have been shown to increase the production of short-chain fatty acids, particularly propionate and butyrate, necessary to nourish colonic cells and prevent diarrhea, constipation, and bowel cancer. They act as a prebiotic fiber to promote the growth of healthy intestinal *Bifidobacterium* and *Lactobacillus* and reduce the amount of ammonia produced in the colon. Reductions of *E. coli* and *Salmonella* bacteria have been found. Healthy production of good bowel bacteria has been shown to reduce serum cholesterol and inhibit the overgrowth of yeast. It works like modified citrus pectin by inhibiting the attachment of cancer cells and competitively binding to liver lectin (hepatic galatose receptor).

Arabinogalactans can decrease both incidence and severity of childhood otitis media, especially associated with gram-negative bacteria. Consider combining this sugar complex with xylitol from birch for increased synergy. Arabinogalactans alleviate dry eyes and may help heal corneal wounds (Burgalassi et al. 2007). Larch arabinogalactans also enhance vascular permeability. Species of larch in Japan show inhibitory effects from the bark pro-anthocyanidins on dental caries. Mitsunaga et al. (1997) found inhibition of glucosyltrans-ferase derived from *Streptococcus sobrinus*, associated with the development of dental caries. This suggests potential for creation of new dental care products.

The green tissue contains myricetin, a compound that exhibits strong antigonadotro-phic activity. Arabinogalactan has properties that make it suitable as a carrier for delivering diagnostic or therapeutic agents to hepatocytes. Work by Prescott et al. (1995) has looked into this possible application. Work in Germany has shown that cytotoxicity in arabinoga-lactan interacts like the action of mistletoe (*Viscum album*). Owen and Johns (1999) found tamarack extracts inhibit xanthine oxidase at 86.33%. This is a measure of possible suc-cess in treating gout. Phenolic and tannin contents are believed responsible for the activity. Tamarack showed the greatest inhibition among the 26 species from 18 families evaluated. The compound cis-19-hydroxyabienol is active against colon carcinoma cell lines DLD-1 (Pichette et al. 2006).

European larch bark tincture is used to treat bladder and urinary infections such as cystitis and urethritis. It is useful for respiratory troubles such as pharyngitis, bronchitis, and tracheitis, and more serious bleeding associated with purpura hemorrhagia as well as passive hemorrhage. The bark, collected in spring, was official in the *British Pharmacopoeia* of 1885.

The tree resin is applied to wounds to both protect and counter infections. Bark decoc-tions are used as a wash for eczema and psoriasis conditions. The resin has been used as an antidote to phosphorus poisoning, while turpentine has traditionally been used for cya-nide and opium poisoning, as well as a disinfectant in gangrene. Maltol gives a burnt-sugar aroma and is used to impart a "freshly baked" odor to breads and cakes. It is present in roasted malt and chicory roots. D-glucaric acid helps remove harmful chemicals from the body and inhibits tumors of the colon, breast, liver, lung, skin, and bladder in mice and rat studies. This compound is present in apples, oranges, and *Brassica* species.

The needles, in summer, exude a sugar known traditionally as Briançon manna. The needles of European larch inhibit various human cancer cell lines, albeit in laboratory set-ting (Frédérich et al. 2009). Siberian Larch has been investigated and found to contain prostaglandin E (1 and 2) similar to that found in animals (Levin et al. 1983). Diquercetin, an industrial bioflavonoid derived from larch, increases the antiradical activity of vitamin C up to 20% when combined in 1:3 up to 1:10 ratios. Larch bark contains 3-arabinosides of dihydroquercetin, with antioxidant, anti-inflammatory, diuretic, hypolipemic, and hepatic protective properties.

A new product, ResistAid, combined arabinogalactans with flavonoids from larch bark such as taxifolin and quercetin, increasing antioxidant capacity benefitting the immune system. A double-blind randomized placebo-controlled trial of 199 healthy volunteers was conducted for three months. The control group suffered far more cases of the common cold than the arabinogalactan group (Riede et al. 2013). Another product containing dihydro-quercetin and vitamin C, called LarchVita, is on the market. Taxifolin (dihydroquercetin) is nearly five times more effective as a capillary protector than the well-known bioflavonoid quercetin. This compound is antiviral and shows activity against Coxsackie B4 virus in vitro. It is most active in early stages of viral reproduction.

It would combine well with astragalus root (*A. membranaceus*) in treating mycocardial infections as well as pancreatitis (Galochkina et al. 2016). Taxifolin, from the bark, called Lavitol, has been widely studied and is recognized as GRAS by the European Union as a food additive. This compound and larch lignans enhance properties of brain neurons and reduces inhibition of activated astrocytes in vitro. This suggests benefit in the treatment of acute and chronic neurological disease (Loers et al. 2014). Labdane-type diterpenes in *Larix* species are TRPC6-selective inhibitors that mediate pathophysiological response within heart and kidney disease (Urban et al. 2016). It also acts via pathways in reducing produc-tion of beta-amyloid, associated with Alzheimer's disease (Junfeng Wang et al. 2015).

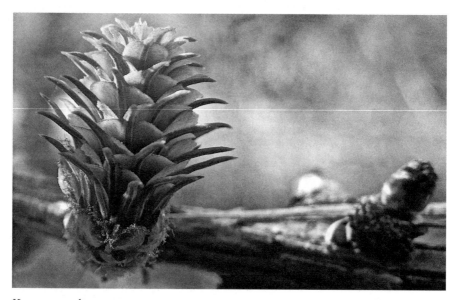

Young tamarack cone

Homeopathy

Vinton McCabe (2007, 92–93) wrote an amazing book in which he compared the Bach flower essences to homeopathic remedies:

In terms of homeopathic remedies, it is easy to find the parallel to Larch. The remedy Lyco-podium [Clubmoss] most closely resembles Larch's psychological situation. Like Larch, Lycopodium feels inferior and is beset with issues of self-confidence. Lycopodium patients may also collapse into an inert state, convinced that whatever they attempt is doomed to fail. But they are more likely to use their inferior state and their feelings of overcom-pensation to fuel their way to success. With each success, Lycopodium patients can, for a moment, forget their feelings of inferiority, only to have them return soon. Like Larch, Lycopodium's life is a balancing act between the desired result and the tendency to quit when times get tough. Both have deep feelings of inadequacy, and both use these feelings to color and control their experience of life.

Homeopathic Terebinthina Laricina (tamarack turpentine) is indicated for anxiety about the future, fear of accidents, confusion of mind, and dullness, as if enveloped in fog. Everything seems unreal, as if in a dream. The patient cannot weep, even though sad. There is dryness of eyes, lips, and throat. Offensive sweat, with underarm perspiration and bad odor, looking like raw meat. There is a desire for warmth. Feeling of bubbles in head, racing up through nose and middle cortex. The patient can hear them. Ringing in ears on waking, tingling soles of feet, heavy upper limbs.

Dose: 12th C potency. Proving by David Riley with 14 females and three males in 1995.

Essential Oils

Tamarack produces oil from both the twigs (0.8–1.2%) and needles (0.2–0.3%). The twig oil is composed mainly of alpha-pinene (up to 38%) and 3-carene (up to 28%), with lesser amounts of camphene, bornyl acetate, beta-pinene, mycrene, terpinen-4-ol, longifolene, caryophyllene, cadinene, and germacrene. The needle oil is mainly camphene and bornyl ace-tate (18.5%) as well as alpha-pinene (17.9%) and lesser amounts of the constituents above. Of note is the content of germacrene D (11.7%) in twigs that is not present in needle oil.

Needle oil from *L. laricina* in Saskatchewan contains thujone and isothujone, not pres-ent in either Alberta or British Columbia oils. In fact, it is usually only found in higher amounts in *Thuja* species. Hmm. Due to the content of alpha-pinene and 3-carene, the oil oxidizes quickly and should be stored in a dark, cold, air-tight container. This is a fantastic oil for treating respiratory conditions through inhalation. I particularly enjoy its fragrance in our aromatic steam, particularly when I feel run-down, either physically or mentally. It also makes an excellent rub when diluted to 5% in a good vegetable or nut oil for lumbago, neuralgia, and sciatic pain.

Western larch yields an essential oil averaging 0.86% from the twigs and 0.28% from needles. The needles are composed mainly of alpha- and beta-pinene and lesser amounts of car-3-ene, camphene, bornyl acetate, and humulene.

Twig oil varies a great deal depending on the site. The most variable terpenes are car-3-ene, sabinene, alpha-terpineol and its acetate, citronellol, cadinene, nerolidol, farnesol isomers, and manool. The oil, like the needle, is mainly alpha- and beta-pinene (50%). Alpine larch twig oil yields a very substantial 2.78%, composed mainly of monoterpenes, alpha- (39%) and beta-pinene (14%), car-3-ene (6.7%), sabinene (7.48%), and lesser amounts of mycrene, beta-phellandrene, camphene, borneol, bornyl acetate, gamma-terpinene, terpinen-4-ol, citronellol, sesquiterpenes like nerolidol, cadinene and cadinol isomers, germacrene-D, carophyllene, longifoline, and beta-elemene. Sabinol and myrtenal are absent in alpine larch. In general, the twig oils are easy to gather and have higher yields and similar profiles to the leaf oils.

European larch needles yield an important essential oil composed mainly of monoterpenes such as alpha-pinene (70%), beta-pinene (6.5%) and limonene; alpha-terpineol, bornyl acetate, delta-3-carene (10%), beta-pyrones (3%), and cadinols (sesquiterpene

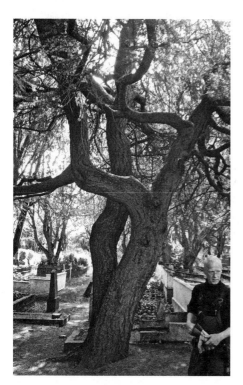

alcohols). The oil is used medicinally for its antiseptic and anti-infective action, particularly against *Pneumococcus*. It is therefore indicated in various bronchitis and pneumonia conditions. The oil is a neurotonic, helping induce states of relaxation. This can be useful in cases of nervous fatigue, exhaustion, and stress-related disease of the nerves and muscles. It will find good application in cases of muscular dystrophy and related myalgias as well as other hardening or contraction of muscles.

The resin of tamarack or larch is known as Venetian turpentine. The oil is obtained from the resin by distillation. Larch turpentine, as it is also known, is barely pourable at room temperature. It is light amber to pale yellow and has a soft, balsamic terpene-like odor. It is composed mainly of 70% alpha-pinene, 10% delta-3-carene, beta-pinene, beta-pyrene, traces of limonene and borneol,

European larch in a Reykjavik, Iceland, cemetery

and neutral labdane compounds such as epimanol, larixol, and larixyl acetate. It has been used in Europe as a low cost amber-like fixative in some industrial perfumes, and to adulterate balsam fir essential oil. The oil is anthelmintic, emmenagogue, and vulnerary. However, it must be used in very small amounts, as it is extremely irritating. It is used in veterinary medicine for hoof disease and skin wounds.

Laurie and I had the great honor to study and spend time with Daniel Pénoël, a well-renowned French aromatherapist. In 1992, we invited Daniel and his wife, Rosemarie to present a four-day medical aromatherapy workshop in Edmonton. He brought up a personal case study using turpentine oil for an extremely difficult health crisis. A middle-aged woman was brought to his clinic with severe lymphangitis, one leg swollen to three times its normal size. He put one drop of turpentine oil onto the inner groin on that side and waited. The oil created the opportunity for lymphatic drainage, and within twenty-four hours her body drained over twenty-six pounds of retained water.

Suggested dosage for tapeworms is five drops morning and evening in dispersed water for four days, no longer. Use the same dose twice daily for bloody diarrhea. It must be used with dispersant to avoid irritating mucous membranes. The oleoresin is used externally to treat ringworm and to ripen boils. Apply neat for no more than thirty minutes. If it irritates, dilute in vegetable oil.

The balsam of *L. decidua* is obtained by drilling into the trunks. The balsam obtained has up to 20% essential oils. Trees yield 8–9 pounds of turpentine annually for up to fifty years. At the end of this time, the wood is useless as timber and is used for firewood. The balsams are used in 10–20% concentration in various ointments, gels, and oils for rheumatism, coughs, bronchitis, fevers, colds, and tendency to infections.

In Russia, the resin from the trunks burned by forest fires is gathered and traded under the name *orengurg gum*. Maltol has that burnt-sugar caramel-like odor. It is found in roasted malt, chicory, pine needles, and wood tars. Larixol and labdanolic acid from the resin is used as a starting point for ambergris-like fragrances.

Hydrosol

The needle hydrosol is also useful. It has a very pleasant minty-balsamic note and taste that is much different than other conifer waters. The pH is 3.5, indicating good stability. Suzanne Catty (2001) suggests using it internally and externally for the lymphatic system. It is less astringent than juniper berry and is a good diuretic when there are no acute symptoms. Rudolph Balz suggests using the hydrosol as an eyewash for infection. Darcy Williamson, friend and noted herbalist, suggests it is an effective stimulant of the circulatory system, without changing blood pressure. Use one dropper daily in water. It cleanses and stimulates the lymphatic system. Use 20–30 drops to increase or quicken menstruation. Use with caution. Catty (2001) recommends the hydrosol for cleaning crystals, energy clearing, and healing in general.

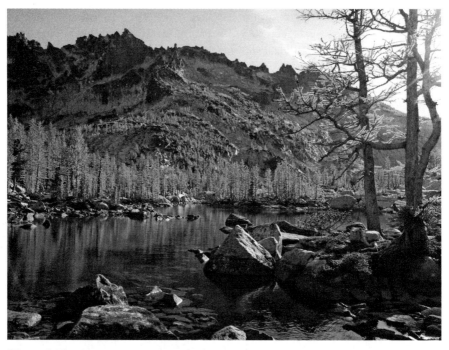

Western larch

Flower Essences

Laurie spent time in the midst of three tamarack in a journey to connect with their essence, which is found in the Prairie Deva flower essence line. Three tamarack mark the magical entrance to a special plant kingdom. The flower essence may help promote a feeling of safety and protection. It provides a safe place to rest and reroute one's life. Tamarack may help one relax through release. Through it, one may become more comfortable and confident, allowing a letting-go of old patterns and tensions. It is a ground essence that helps connect people to life in an earthy, solid manner. This is especially important for dreamers who need a safe place to land and reorient. Tamarack essence reflects stability, strength, and peace. It is an essence of abundance. Edward Bach developed the flower essence for the European larch.

Larch relates to the soul quality of self-confidence. In the negative state, the Larch person feels inferior. It is not a matter of doubting one's abilities but a conviction of inferiority. They expect to fail. The foundation is often rooted in childhood and becomes an automatic response. Richardson-Boedler (1998) expands on this idea:

> One may feel intimidated, depressed, hesitant and irresolute, and unmotivated. Mixed feelings of envy, respect, and shyness in regard to those in charge of themselves and their

work. Sense of inferiority may be defended against by exaggerated, overly ambitious attempts to achieve or "show off" and prove one's worth.... Suggested use of Larch in psychosomatic illness: Gastric and duodenal ulcers—overambitious patients or dependent patients. Hyperventilation syndrome. Migraines. Skin diseases (urticaria and atopic dermatitis—adolescence and adulthood).

Spiritual Properties

Chase and Pawlik (1991) looked at European larch and its spiritual properties. European larch is one of the confidence builders, broadening your vision of who you can be. For example, if you are a trim carpenter and are attracted to European Larch, perhaps you are being told it is time to expand your creative potential. Larch heightens your enthusiasm for new possibilities. Starting your own business may suddenly seem appealing and distinctly possible to execute. European larch aids you in dissolving a narrowness of vision, fear, or self-doubt, so that you can bring your dreams into reality with confidence and excitement.

Beresford-Kroeger (2010) offered this insight into tamarack:

A tree commonly called the tamarack or larch is the water baby of the conifers. This tree sits like a rebel in a pool of water and snubs its nose at its eight remaining rustic sisters worldwide. The tamarack has learned how to survive in bogs and fens, muskegs and marshy woods. These are places where no self-respecting conifer should be found.

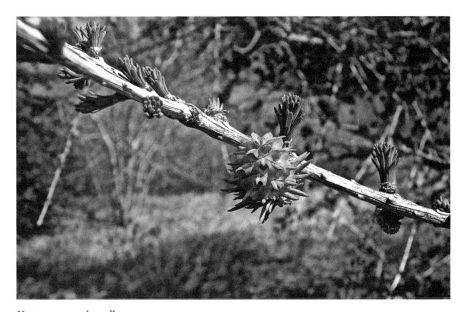

Young cones and needles

Myths and Legends

Related by Turner (2014, 263–64), from the Okanagan comes a legend, "Tamarack, the People Eater," of how tamarack (western larch, *Larix occidentalis*) came to be used for medicine.

Fox traveled along, but he hadn't gone far when he met again with Coyote, and told him about a long, tall tree, growing high up in the mountains, which was a people eater. This tree was Tamarack. Tamarack killed people by grabbing them when they got too close—around the base of each of these tall trees were the bones of many victims.

Coyote went over to the place where Tamarack could be found. He took with him a large club, so that he could smack the tree when it bent down to grab him. He got close to Tamarack. The tree began to bend down, but before he could hit it, Tamarack smashed him and threw him a long way. Coyote died. As usual, Fox knew that Coyote had been killed—he came over to the spot where Coyote lay, and stepped over him, bringing him back to life. Coyote scolded his partner, "Why did you bother me? I was just lying down to rest."

"No," said Fox. "You were killed by Tamarack, that people eater. I'll help you—I'll give you a weapon, tipped with black flint. When Tamarack tries to grab you, hit him with this, and he'll bother you no more."

So Coyote went back to Tamarack with his new weapon. Tamarack bent down to grab him, but Coyote yelled out, "Don't kill me yet! I have something to say to you." When Tamarack hesitated, Coyote whacked the top of the tree. Coyote then passed judgment: "Henceforth, when the transformed people come to this land, you will not be a people-eater. You will be used as medicine. Today, the tops of the tallest Tamarack, high up in the mountains, are all bent; this is because Coyote made it that way."

RECIPES

Decoction: Dried bark (1:32) 2–4 ounces, up to 4 times daily.

Tinctures: The bark is stripped in late spring and dried. The bark tincture is prepared at 1:5 ratio and 40% alcohol. 5–30 drops 3 times daily. Resins are tapped in autumn, not spring.

Tamarack bread: Scrape off the soft wood and inner bark of tamarack, mix with water, and ferment into a dough to be mixed with rye meal and buried under the snow for a day. Fermentation begins, and the dough can then be cooked as camp bread or dumplings, the sweet wood pulp acting as a sugar for the yeast in the rye.

Larix: One to two 00 capsules up to 3 times daily as needed.

Powdered bark: 1 tablespoon 4 times daily in cold water.

Salve: Cover 1 part by weight of inner bark with 5 parts by volume of coconut oil and heat in low-temperature crock pot for 4 hours. Strain. Use for skin conditions such as eczema, psoriasis, and skin ulcers.

Caution: Do not use arabinogalactans in active tuberculosis, according to some authors. Clifford Cardinal, noted Cree healer, suggests tamarack bark should not be used in combination with antibiotics (Young et al. 2015).

7

Egg-Hatching Moon Herbal Allies

Red Osier Dogwood and Bunchberry

Red Osier Dogwood • Moose Wood—*Cornus sericea* ssp. *sericea* L. • *C. stolonifera* Michx. • *C. sericea ssp. stolonifera* (Michx.) Fosberg

Pagoda Dogwood • Green Osier—*Cornus alternifolia* L. f.

Dwarf Cornel—*Cornus suecica* L.

Bunchberry • Chicken Berry—*Cornus canadensis* L.

> *When the dogwood flowers appear*
> *Frost will not again be here.*
>
> —Old saying

> *After all, I don't see why I am always asking for private, individual, selfish miracles when*
> *every year there are miracles like white dogwood.*
>
> —Anne Morrow Lindbergh

> *Outside of a dog, a book is a man's best friend. Inside of a dog it's too dark to read.*
>
> —Groucho Marx

Cornus derives from the Latin *corneolus*, meaning "of horn," in reference to the hardness of the wood. It may come from the Latin *corna*, the brilliant red drupes of the *cornus* or cornelian cherry tree, or more obscurely from the Greek *kranon*.

The Romans prized the hard wood of cornelian cherry for javelins, spears, and sword handles. In early England, skewers to roast kebabs on an open fire were called "prickes" as the stems pricked the meat. The shrub offering these strong sticks, without leaves or flavor, was known as a pricke timber tree.

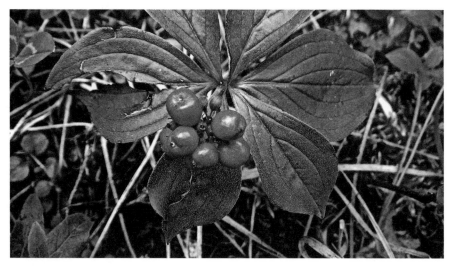

Bunchberry

The common name *dogwood* is derived from the Norman *dague*, the name of a pointed steel weapon. This became later the English *dagg*, meaning "stab," and eventually *dagger*. In the English manor, skewers for roasting meats were made from this bush, which became known as dagge wood and later doggewood.

Other suggestions for the origin of *dogwood* include the use of leaves and bark as decoction for washing mangy dogs, that dogs like chewing on it, that the fresh-cut wood smells like dog poop, or the inferiority of the berries, not even fit for a dog. All of these suggestions are less likely. Dogwood does not resemble a dog but was a contemptuous term for the poor wood in days when dogs were not valued a friend of man. It meant the fruit was only good for dogs, and various English phrases refer to a dog's life, dog-drunk, and dog latin, meaning a coarse or illiterate form of the language. Different than pig latin!

In fact, the Cree use the term *dog* as part of conventional animal metaphors for people; *atim* or "dog" means a worthless person. Other examples are *maskwa*, meaning "bear," or an adolescent girl, *omidāhcis*, meaning "wolverine" or "thief," and *wāpiscānis*, "marten" or "attractive woman."

The beaver is the national animal of Canada and there are way too many jokes relating our national animal to the female pubic region. The name for beaver in Cree is *amisk* and has been transposed into meaning both the animal and an incestuous human. This relates to the ongoing tension in Cree society, related to sexual encounters and marriage with close relatives, and the Roman Catholic Church's disapproval of such unions.

Stolonifera means "bearing root suckers," or the ability of the stolons to take root. *Sericea* means "silky." Many authors suggest this refers to the texture of the leaves, but the juice of the mature white berry is very silky. *Alternifolia* means "alternate leaves." *Suecia* is the Latin name for Sweden. *Osier* is from the Old French *osiere* or *auseria*, a Gallic-Roman word from the Gaul *auesa*, meaning "bed of a river," which is the plant's natural habitat. Other authors believe *osier* is from the Latin *oscaria*, meaning "bed of willows." Osiers are canes used for basket-making, traditionally from willow, but *Cornus* genus stems were also widely used. Red originates from the bright red stems observed on many but not all trees. The anthocyanins in bark are believed to improve photosynthesis and give protection from the sun, depending on whether the plant is fully exposed or has partial shade. The bright red stems against white snow are a beautiful winter scene. In the language of flowers, dogwood symbolizes love in adversity.

It may not appear at first glance that dogwood and bunchberry are related, but look closely at the white flower, or rather what appears to be white petals, which are actually the bracts; the true flower is a small yellow-green cluster in the center. Bunchberry has four leaves before it is mature enough to flower, and six leaves in the years after. Bunchberry flowers open in less than 0.5 milliseconds, one of the fastest movements yet observed in nature. Dogwood and bunchberry leaves contain latex that holds gently broken leaves together.

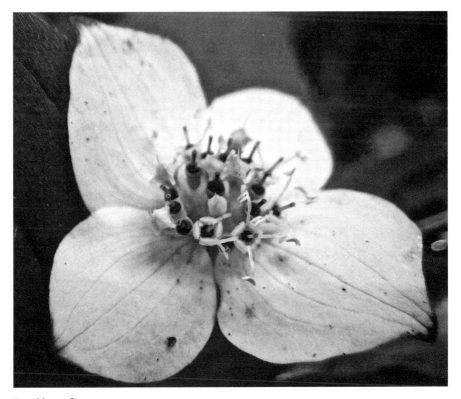

Bunchberry flower

Traditional Uses

Bunchberry is known as *kawiscowimi* or "itchy skin berry" to the Wood Cree who nibbled on the fresh fruit (drupe). It is also known as *pihew menis*, meaning grouse berry, and *githukistomina*, itchy beard berry. The berries (drupes), when rubbed on the skin or face, feel itchy. Bunchberry is known as *jikonaze* to the Dene or Chipewyan people of northeastern Alberta. They also call the fruit marten berries, a name sometimes attached to northern comandra (*Geocaulon lividum*). The name Chipewyan is derived from the Cree word for "pointed shirt," a traditional clothing style. They call themselves Dene, meaning "the people." The Dena'ina, of Alaska, name for bunchberry and dwarf cornel is *ch'enlq'ena*, meaning "crunchy" or "hard to chew."

The Eastern or Swamp Cree call the plant *saguninan*. They boil the whole plant together with creeping wintergreen (*Gaultheria hispidula*) for colds. The Iroquois used decoctions of the whole bunchberry, including roots for coughs, fevers, cancer, and tuberculosis. This is due to the ability of the leaves to stimulate endorphins, elevate mood, and improve the immune system. Iroquois and Ojibwe decocted the roots to treat colic in children. The Ojibwe refer to the plant as *caca' go min* or *ode'iminijiibik*. The name of the Iroquois Confederacy is derived from the Algonquian word meaning "real snakes." The name Haudenosaunee is now considered more appropriate, as is Kanansionni, meaning "people of the longhouse."

The Mik'maq or L'nu'k of Eastern Canada added the berries in combination decoctions for epilepsy and used the leaf tea for bed-wetting. The Anishinaabe (original people) or Algonquin used the root decoction for colic in babies and a lighter infusion for coughs and fevers. *Algonquian* is the native word for "puckered," referring to the moccasin style. *Algonquin* is a French corruption of either the Maliseet word *elehgomoqik*, "our allies," or the Mi'kmaq place name *algomaking*, "fish-spearing place."

The Montagnais steeped the plant to treat those with paralysis. The Forest Potawatomi call it popcorn weed. The Potawatomi now prefer the name Bode'wadmi, the traditional religious role of "fire-keepers." The Nlaka'pamux along the Fraser River in British Columbia used the powdered leaf or its burned ash to sprinkle on sores, while the root tea was reserved for infant colic. It is known as Three Leaves, which makes little sense, as the plant leaves are in fours and sixes; it is also known as Cluster-on-the-Ground Dogwood.

The red bunchberries were not considered edible, but chewed for "insanity" as well as a source of orange-red dye for baskets. They are not that tasty, but rather insipid and dry. The Yakutat Tlingit heated the leaves on a stove and applied them to cuts, burns, and cataracts. The leaves were applied to a mother's breast for sore nipples or to stimulate milk flow.

The Gitksan of northern British Columbia used bunchberries as a thickener when boiling berries, helping the dried berry rolls stick together. Rolling long flats of cooked berries laid out on skunk cabbage leaves and then turning them over was tricky work. The cracks were often filled with bunchberries to ensure the rolls stuck together. Other indigenous groups chewed the berries and applied them to burns. Steeped in hot water, the leaf tea was used to treat paralysis or combined with bearberry leaves for bee stings, poison ivy rash, and other skin problems.

Bunchberry has a most unusual method of pollination. There is no scent, no nectar, but when an insect touches a stick from one of the closed petals, they pop up, releasing the stamens, which send a cloud of pollen into the air. The stamens accelerate with a force of 99,000 feet per second, faster than a rocket.

The Laplanders of Scandinavia use *C. suecia* to make a pudding of whey and crushed berries. The berries are rich in pectin and make good extenders or thickeners for low-pectin fruit. A natural hybrid occurs between this plant and bunchberry in parts of Alaska. In Gaelic, *C. suecia* is called *lus-a-chraois,* meaning "plant of gluttony," based on its reputation to stimulate appetite. Dwarf cornel is a creeping or alpine perennial with red berries that seldom grows taller than six inches. The berries were eaten by the indigenous people of North America and in parts of Europe as a tonic for appetite.

The Cree used red osier dogwood, or *mihkwapimakwahtik,* in the same manner the Iroquois made use of bunchberry. Other variations are *mikwapanuk, mehkwa, pemakwa, mikobimaka,* and *mikwapimakwa,* meaning "red willow," *mikwa piskaw,* for "red wood," and *mehkwapemak,* "red stem." Russell Willier, noted Cree healer from Sucker Creek First

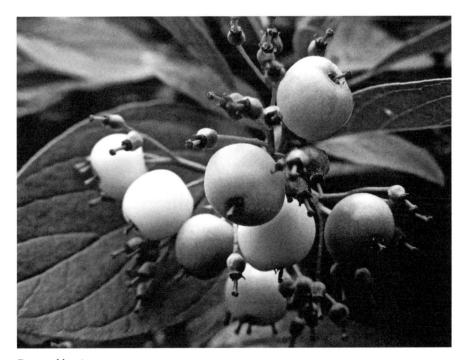

Dogwood berries

Nation, boils the top four inches of new growth for energy and as a blood tonic. He uses the berries to break a love charm, and the inner bark for smoking mixtures (Young et al. 2015). The white berries (drupes) were made into a wash for snow blindness, while the pith of the branches was used for cataracts.

Brenda Holder, a former student, passed on from her Cree medicine grandmother the use of the ripe white berries as a superior hair conditioner. The juice may be frozen as ice cubes for use anytime. Birds love the fermented berries, and will eat them to excess, spitting out the seeds, and getting drunk from the adventure.

Stem tea was used for chest troubles, coughs, fevers, and the ripe fruit for tuberculosis. The leaf tea was consumed for dysuria, the inability to urinate. Dogwood inner bark is sedative and useful for insomnia, as a decoction, or in smoking mixtures, called kinnikinnick. The outer bark can be removed with a vegetable peeler and then the inner bark collected and dried. Or you can feather the whole stem and dry it by a fire. The inner bits are then removed and give a somewhat sweet addition to smoking mixtures.

The Eastern Cree of Hudson's Bay know it as *milawapamule* and used warm bark decoctions as an emetic in coughs and fevers. A red dye can be obtained by decocting the rootlets. Millspaugh (1887) considered it similar to *C. florida* in action, although more astringent and less bitter. It appears stronger on the heart and causes more cerebral congestion than its famous cousin. The Gitksan used Red Osier root bark for fractures and an analgesic by pounding and applying it to affected area as a poultice. The inner bark was decocted and applied to sores and to help relieve pain. The tree is known as *khlaahl*.

The Dene (Chipewyan) call the shrub *k'ai k' oze*, meaning "willow that is red." The Dene Tha (Slavey) of Greater Slave Lake boiled the ripe white drupes for half an hour as a tea to treat tuberculosis. Sophie Thomas, a Saik'uz elder and herbalist, calls it red willow, or *k'endulk'un*. The bark shavings are soaked in hot water, and when it turns yellow, applied as a fomentation to swellings. The branches are chewed to relieve headache (Young and Hawley 2004). The Dena'ina of Alaska call it boreal owl's berry or great horned owl's berry. Fruit not considered edible for humans was often attached with an animal name. The white berry relates to the color of snow owls. The Wet'suwet'en (Hwotsotenne) decocted the inner bark and used the cool wash to treat psoriasis. The same tea was used internally for postpartum hemorrhage. Some tribes combined the edible but hardly tasty white berry with saskatoon berries, calling them "sweet and sour." I have picked the two together when ripe and definitely appreciate the sweet-sour combination. Sometimes the stones were separated from the drupes and eaten later as a snack.

The Cree dried the inner bark as part of a smoking mixture, what today is widely known as kinnikinnick. Some people apply this as a common name to the plant bearberry (*Arctostaphylos uva-ursi*); the dried leaves are also used in many smoking combinations. The Alberta Elders' Cree Dictionary calls kinnikinnick *mihkwapemakwa ka pihtwat-amihk.* This is known as red willow or *muskomina*. A branch with the bitter outer red bark was cut into, and the inner bark curled back for six or eight inches in clusters. The sharp end of branch was then stuck in the ground near a fire and roasted until dry. The dried inner bark was then ready to smoke. Some native healers suggest the bark is best when harvested from a dormant plant in winter. It is interesting to note that three of the main herbs used in smoking mixtures are associated with the color red, representing blood, or the essence of life. Red osier dogwood bark is obvious; the red-berried bearberry is another example, and so are the leaves of sumac, which turn brilliant red in fall. The Nimipu (Nez Perce) tell a legend of how red osier dogwood received its color from the red blood of a girl shot by her brother. He hid the bloody arrow in the shrub, and ever since it has been red.

Midwives of this community used a strong bark decoction to stimulate uterine contractions and bring on childbirth. The fine scrapings of the inner bark were used to cure coughs and fevers, or induce vomiting as necessary. Finely ground and powdered bark was used as a styptic on bleeding and wounds that refused to heal.

The leaves were dried and used in smoking ceremonies. Early French settlers called it *bois de calumet*, meaning "pipe wood." They would push the soft pith from the center of the hard stems and use them for pipe stems. The Cree and other native peoples let nature do the work. They would find a patch of goldenrod and look for a round gall halfway up the stem. This is the winter home of the Goldenrod gallfly (*Eurosta solidaginis*). It lives there an entire year, producing a type of antifreeze substance to protect it through the cold winter.

It is said the height on stem at which this insect makes its winter home portends the height of snow that winter. This has never been my observation. The live, white larvae was inserted into one end of a dogwood stem and sealed in. The insect had no choice but to

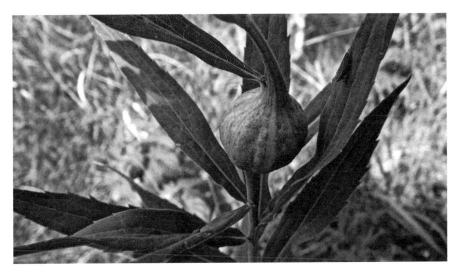

Goldenrod gall

transit the entire length to exit, thus creating a perfect pipe stem for those with time to wait. The pipe bowl was carved from large wild rose (*Rosa acicularis*) roots, or from red pipestone found in various waterways.

The sacred pipe stem and bowl are carried separately. A hush will be heard as the pipe keeper purifies and joins them together. After filling with smoking mixture and being lit, the pipe is passed sun-wise, and each participant takes four puffs. The hollow bowl and stem symbolize the female. "The hole for receiving the stem symbolizes the vagina, which is symbolically (and linguistically in some languages) equated with Earth. The most awesome part of pipe ceremonies is when the two parts of the pipe are joined, when the male stem is inserted into the female bowl, at which time ritually significant pipes become potent (Paper 2007, 154).

Various ethnobotanists through the centuries have mistaken the true use of smoking mixtures by indigenous peoples. In some cases, extremely derogatory remarks were written in journals, alluding to those poor natives running out of tobacco and having to smoke twigs, bark, and leaves. Nothing could be further from the truth. In the southern plains of Canada, various tobacco societies would trade for seeds farther south and then plant and carefully tend their crop. By fall, the plants were barely a foot tall, with no flowers and containing very little if any nicotine. But the plants did contain harmine, harmane, and other alkaloids, also found in buffalo berry. These monoamine oxidase (MAO) inhibitors were combined with various other ingredients for a specific purpose. In the case of red osier dogwood, the analgesic and anti-inflammatory activity was increased and extended by combination. In other cases the MAO inhibitor was combined in smoking mixtures to bring about spiritual journeys, séances, and entheogenic adventures. The mixtures were not random.

Dream catchers are often made from this genus, due to its connection with lucid dreams and charms:

> Native Americans have long associated spiderwebs with protective and healing powers. Orb webs were placed directly on top of a puncture wound to stop the flow of blood. A web painted on a shield was thought to be protective, like an actual spider's web, whose sticky strands and long radiating support lines cannot easily be destroyed by arrows or bullets, which pass through, leaving only tiny holes. Similarly, protective web designs are sewn and painted on baby hoods and cradles to stop bad dreams from penetrating a baby's open fontanel. And throughout North America today small nets known as "dream catchers" are made by cutting the supple willow or red dogwood branch, bending it into a circle, and weaving plant materials or sinew into a spiraling orb within the circle (Tedlock 2005, 116)

The Secwepemc (Shuswap) of British Columbia made a tea for children who wet the bed from red osier inner bark. The Wisconsin Potawatomi used the root bark of red-stemmed bush (*C. stolonifera*) as their most efficient remedy for diarrhea. The Abenaki used infusions of this bark, as well as willow and hazelnut, to treat eye problems.

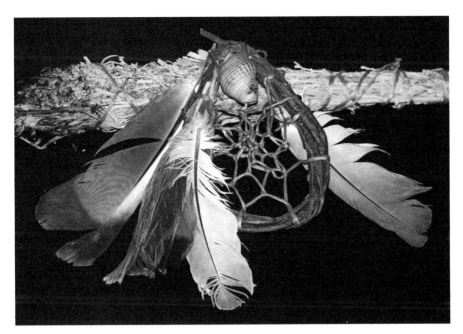

Dream catcher

The Nlaka'pamux (Thompson) called the white fruit bitter tail or bitter gray and ate them with dried snowberries for intestinal worms. The wood, bark, and leaves of little red stick or little red wood was decocted and given to women after childbirth. The fresh inner bark was poulticed on painful sore nipples from babies biting with first teeth during breastfeeding. For vomiting and diarrhea, the bark was combined with wild rose and chokecherry branches.

Natives of Haida Gwaii used the branches to make animal-skin drying frames and sweat lodges. It is known as *sqiisqi* or a similar variation of the spelling. Gary Raven, a traditional healer from Manitoba, mentioned combining the inner bark of red osier dogwood and tamarack as a special tea for pregnant women. It was given for one week before childbirth and one week after for purification.

The wood was used for tipi stakes, forks, arrow shafts, baskets, and fishnets. Dogwood hole-pins were used in boats built on the south shore of Nova Scotia. The Basque of northern Spain used it for divining rods, replacing hazel in that part of the world. The Blackfoot covered split beaver teeth with bark to make gambling wheels. They call the shrub *mekotsi-pis* or *mis kwabi mic*. The bark was used for dyeing and tanning of hides.

Moose love the tops as a winter food. It is often called "moose candy" and is consumed in amounts of up to sixty-five pounds per day by a mature animal. Moose is from the Algonquin *mus*, meaning "to tear away." In laboratory studies the plant will survive temperatures as low as −320°F, or 83 Kelvin, by freezing the water in an extracellular manner.

Alternate-leaved, or pagoda, dogwood is rare on the Canadian prairies and restricted to the southeast region. It has bluish-black fruit and pinkish red stalks. Natives of the region used the root of this tree as an attractant or charm on muskrat traps. The leaves are alternate, unlike other dogwood leaves, which are opposite. The Chippewa (Ojibwe) used it for utility and medicine and called it moose plant, or *muj'omij'*. The Potawatomi used bark infusions of moose wood as an eyewash. Various *Cornus* species produce mild antiseptic compounds that may help keep fresh water fish farms healthy and avoid the overuse of antibiotics.

Medicinal Uses

Constituents: *C. canadensis* plant and drupe-cornin (verbenalin), cornic acid, cyanin, quercetin, phenylethylamine, tannins, campesterol, stigmasterol, beta-sitosterol, alpha-amyrin, beta-amyrin, pelargonidin-3-robinobiosides, and cyanidin-3-robinobiosides. Some endorphin-like substance has not yet been identified.

fruit: cyanin, pelargonin, stigmasterol.

C. stolonifera stem bark: anthocyanins, cornic acid, cornin (verbenalin), cornuside, halleridone, tannins, hyperin, quercetin, kaempferol, gallic acid and various fatty acids, C24:C26 alkanes, fumaric acid, hyperoside.

Leaves: contain 13.44% crude protein.

Drupe: calcium, copper, cornus tannin, gallic acid, iron, magnesium, malic acid, potassium, tartaric acid, ursolic acid, zinc.

C. alternifolia berries: anthocyanins.

Leaves: iridolactone, alternosides A–C, cornalternoside, kaempferol(-3-)-beta-glucopyranoside.

All dogwoods appear to have similar medicinal properties, although *C. florida* and *C. circinata* have been studied in greater depth. The root bark of red osier dogwood is tonic, astringent, and mildly stimulating. In many ways it possesses similar action to cinchona or Peruvian bark. It disperses intermittent fevers and invigorates the body's vital forces without stimulating circulation.

Cornin acts as a weak parasympathetic stimulant and has both smooth-muscle relaxing and laxative properties. Cornic acid is similar but weaker than acetylsalicylic acid, according to my herbal friend and colleague Terry Willard. A major difference is that cornin can be used by individuals sensitive to salicylic acid. This is important not only for some individuals but for the veterinary treatment of cats, who are very sensitive to salicylic acid.

Cornin induces angiogenesis, meaning that it may promote cancer tumor growth by increasing blood vessels (Kang et al. 2013). Angiogenesis is part of the wound healing process, but cornin may be an ill-advised supplement in cancer patients with blood vessel–fed tumors. Maybe. Other studies show cornin exhibits growth inhibition against colon, breast, lung, central nervous system, and stomach human cancer cell lines (Vareed et al. 2007). At the same time, cornin may protect against cerebral ischemia, due in part to antioxidant properties (Jiang et al. 2010). Recent work by Xu et al. (2016) identified an increase in expression of phospho-CREB and phospho-Akt by cornin helps exert cardiac protective action in myocardial injury. Earlier work by same research team found cornin significantly improved functional recovery after stroke.

Work by McCune and Johns (2002) found methanol extracts of red osier dogwood similar to green tea in antioxidant activity. Verbenalin, quercetin, and betulinic acid combine to give a great treatment for fevers and coughs and colds. The glycoside verbenalin affects serotonin pathways associated with smooth-muscle relaxation, calming and relaxing the mind, and remaining open to dreams and meditative practice. This compound is found in vervain and blue vervain (*Verbena* species). Verbenalin showed good therapeutic effect on a prostatitis mouse model (Miao et al. 2016).

Infusions are valuable for checking vomiting, especially in pregnancy, as well as lower back pain and uterine problems, including prolapse. Menstrual pain, especially during the first day, is relieved. The dried bark is best decocted at very low temperatures or as a cold infusion gently warmed for hot dry conditions such as fevers, headaches, and hot dry lungs. It makes a good gargle for sore throat and mouth ulcers.

The dried bark tincture is a good analgesic, with benefit in dysmenorrhea, asthma, and other spasmodic and neuralgic irritations. It combines well with crampbark in these situations. The bark:

> will relieve cramps on the base of the foot even when the reason for the cramps is unknown. It also will strengthen the interior walls of the lower intestine. A decoction of the bark is good for elders or younger people who have a weakness in their intestines. It will increase the circulation and clean out any pockets of festering material trapped in the intestines that give a person constant gas or a grumbling stomach. (Geniusz 2015, 150)

The dried inner bark makes a good tincture for headaches, fever, and liver disorders. The fresh bark decoction is a good laxative. The powdered inner bark is a suitable dentifrice that strengthens soft gums. The bark is best collected in early spring before leaves appear. I find the easiest way to harvest inner bark is to cut long strips and lay outer bark down on a table in the spring sun. Wait for a few hours, and the inner and outer bark begin to separate, and you can pull it out more easily. This tip can save you hours and hours of scraping.

Roots can be harvested and dried for relief of diarrhea, while the fresh bark is more laxative. Infusions of the white sepals can be used as a substitute for *C. florida* in the treatment of colds, flu, and colic. The flowers can be gathered, dried, and infused for a calming and relaxing tea. Ethanol extracts of the flower clusters and leaves exhibit activity against

Staphylococcus aureus (Borchardt et al. 2008). Earlier work by McCutcheon et al. (1994) found moderate antifungal activity. Cook (1869) writes:

> *The bark is similar to that of* Cornus florida, *but partakes more of the characters of a pure astringent and less of those of a tonic. It is also more stimulating than the other dogwoods. It expends a considerable influence upon the uterus and is of service in atonic conditions of that organ. Combined with* Caulophyllum *[blue cohosh], it promotes parturition in cases where the system is lax and the pains inefficient; with* Convallaria *and* Mitchella *is good for prolapsus, degenerate leucorrhea, and chronic menorrhagia; and with an excess of* Dioscorea, *will often benefit the sympathetic vomiting of pregnancy.*

Fumaric acid is an antitumor and antioxidant and a protectant against liver cancer. Hyperin is anti-inflammatory, antitussive, antiviral, and induces capillary formation. Hyperoside and hyperin are both present in more significant amounts in St. John's wort. Cornuside is immune-modulating and inhibits inflammatory response in sepsis. Halleridone is cytotoxic. Anthocyanins from *C. alternifolia* fruit display growth inhibition against colon, breast, lung, central nervous system, and stomach human cancer cell lines (Vareed et al. 2006).

The leaves contain kaempferol-3-O-beta-glucopyranoside, which exhibits potent agonistic activity on peroxisome proliferator–activated receptors PPAR-alpha and PPAR-gamma,

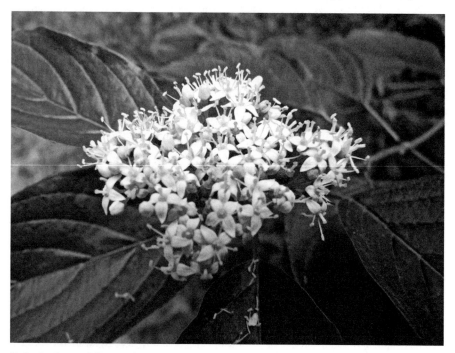

Red osier dogwood flowers

as well as liver X receptors (He et al. 2012). PPAR agonists affect weight loss and blood sugar dysregulation and related conditions such as diabetic retinopathy.

Bunchberry leaf contains cornin that has a mild aspirin-like effect that decreases inflammation, pain, and fever—with no stomach irritation. It can be used safely by those allergic to salicylates in plants such as poplar and willow as well as aspirin.

Cornin is also known as verbenalin, a relaxing component of vervain (*Verbena officinalis*). The leaf tea works wells for fevers that cause chills and shivering with clammy headaches. There may be nausea with damp neck and back. Pulse is usually weak. Tinnitus, dizziness, and deafness may be present. Use the hot leaf tea for colds and flu, or strain and cool for an effective eyewash in a sterile eyecup. Both leaf and root can be infused for kidney issues, taken internally at body temperature. It can also be used for irritability of the intestine; it soothes ulcerative colitis, diarrhea, and chronic gastritis.

Verbenalin shows benefit in mice models of prostatitis (Miao et al. 2016). The orange-red berries can be crushed and the pectin applied to burns like a poultice. Even more effective is decocting a cupful of the berries in ½ cup of tannin-rich water (i.e. uva ursi) for poison ivy, bee stings, and other skin problems. Diane Beresford-Kroeger (2010, 117) writes:

> The [orange] color of the berry sends a hidden message to the avian eye.... This color is made up of two very closely related molecules with very different abilities. One, pelargonin, has the capacity to transcend the old problem of mixing oil with water.... The other, cyanin, affects the avian eye and improves its vision to see at night. The cyanin bonds with different sugars to make this night vision more powerful.

The whole plant, including fruit, is used for bed-wetting in children, urinary frequency due to cold deficient conditions, and degenerative kidney conditions such as glomerulonephritis and chronic nephritis.

Mors Kochanski calls bunchberry the happy plant. A coffee cup full of the fresh leaves can be decocted or eaten to give a strong cappuccino effect, or eat one leaf at a time. He also says the dried leaves in a ratio of 1 part to 7 parts water can be boiled for a tea that helps one mellow out and helps increase endorphins. Fresh leaves are stimulating, and dried leaves are sedating. Interesting! Mors also found that when he ate the fall leaves that turn red-purple, it created a ravenous hunger. The chemistry involved is unknown but worthy of investigation. Some authors believe the fresh red fruit is best for stimulating appetite.

The whole plant is used for headaches, pain, paralysis, and seizures. The root can be decocted and cooled as tea for infant colic. Anthocyanin derivatives of pelargonin and cyanin have some potential as natural red food coloring. McCutcheon et al. (1992) found aerial parts active against 9 of 11 bacteria tested, as well as significant inhibition of *Pseudomonas aeruginosa* K99. Pelargonin is hydrotrophic, helping water and oil mix together. Cyanin improves night vision.

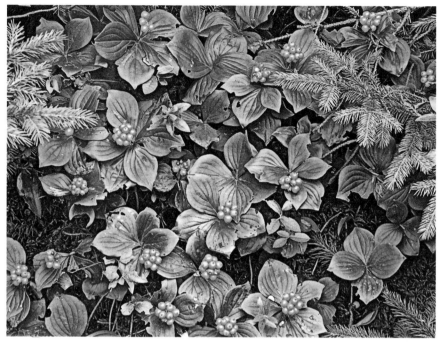

Bunchberry patch

Homeopathy

Various species have been investigated for homeopathic applications. Round-leaved dog-wood *(C. circinata)* is indicated in homeopathic form when there is a burning in the mouth, throat, or stomach. Loose windy stools immediately after eating may be present, with burning of the anus and dark bilious diarrhea. Vesicular eczema in breast-feeding infants is relieved. The mind may be confused and forgetful of familiar matters. There is an inability to fix the mind on any subject. The client may read without appreciating the ideas of the subject. A depression of spirits, great drowsiness, and aversion to household duties may be noted. Coffee helps headache, but rather than causing sleeplessness, makes one sleep better. There is a desire for sour drinks, and general debility from summer heat.

Dose: 1st to 12th potency. First proving by Marcy with one female and seven males at 1st, 3rd, and 12th dilutions in 1855.

Swamp walnut *(C. alternifolia)* is for the weak and tired, with disturbed sleep, fever, and restlessness. The skin may be cracked and the chest can feel cold like it is full of ice. There is no ambition to do anything for any length of time. An uneasy feeling may come toward night, as if something terrible will happen. They suffer restless and sleepless nights and hear every little noise and sound. Pressing frontal headache may exist. There is sensation as if something is lodged in the throat. Coughing and feeling of something heavy on the chest and throat may be present, as well as a dull pain in left shoulder. Dreams may include spending summer in countryside, fires, dead rats, and sex.

Dose: Tincture to the 30th potency. The first proving was by Lutz in 1896 and another male with tincture and 30th potency.

Flowering dogwood (*C. florida*) is for heartburn, with general debility, night sweats, and loss of fluids. There may be neuralgic pains in the arms, chest, and trunk as if broken in two. Intermittent fevers with chill proceeded by drowsiness may be present. The patient feels cold but is warm to touch.

Doses: Tincture to the 30th potency. Proving by Bute potentized to 30th potency in pure snow water in 1838. Proving by Macfarlan in 1890s.

Dwarf Cornel (*Cornus sericea*) shows anxiety with eruptions of the lower limbs, white vesicles with red borders.

Doses: Tincture to the 30th potency.

Flower Essences

Many years ago I worked with the small flowers of bunchberry, preparing a flower essence one summer day. The flowers are so small that a lot of attention was required. It is one of the Prairie Deva Flower Essences. Bunchberry flower essence is for bringing to awareness the qualities of deception—including self-deception. For deeper insight into situations and individuals where there is "more than meets the eye," this flower essence helps unveil and give a more objective, dispassionate observation. Bunchberry helps uncover and explore the

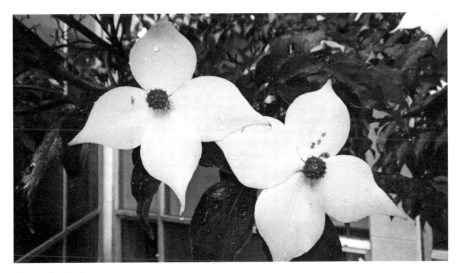

Cornus florida *flower*

various levels or layers of reality that can coexist at one time. According to modern string theory, associated with quantum physics, there are at least eleven space dimensions and one time dimension.

Bunchberry is the essence for exploration of myths and their impact on issues involving life and death and questions of wonder. It is the essence for exploring the subtle levels of our own consciousness and appreciating the gifts we receive daily that remind us of our connection. It can help to filter out some of the static associated with modern lifestyles, including traffic noise, pollution, and electromagnetic influence from cell phones, microwaves, televisions, and computers. It combines well with Toadflax flower essence and Wood Ear mushroom essence for issues surrounding hearing and listening.

Darcy Williamson (2011) has looked at dogwood as a flower essence. She found it "tempers awkward and painful awareness of the body, emotional trauma stored deep within the body while promoting grace-filled movement and physical harmony."

Myths and Legends

Nancy Turner and Barbara Efrat (1982, 64) recorded the following:

A native myth of the Hesquiat tells of an unhappy wife who was driven to the top of a tree for punishment by her husband. As she climbed the tree she was bleeding from menstruation, and where the blood fell, a bunchberry grew. Her brother came to find her when he heard her singing. The wife died as a result of the ordeal, and her brother disguised himself as his sister and sought for the husband in a nearby village. He was found out by mallard duck sisters, because he did not harvest bracken fern like a woman.

Guillet (1962) collected and preserved this legend:

Long ago a monster thunderbird swept down from the north and tore the young tobacco plants to shreds with his cruel wings. Then he caused a deluge of water that carried the uprooted plants away. The Indians managed to rescue a few plants and carried them to Nanibozo to ask him what to do with them.

Nanibozo was a god who liked to destroy things too, but he hated thunderbirds. At times he was kindly and told the people to dry the tobacco leaves, also sumac leaves and the inner bark of dogwood. When they had done this, he told them to mix and powder the leaves and then fill their pipes. He bade them smoke first to the north, then to the south, then to the east, and lastly to the west. Finally, they must smoke to the great god Nanibozo in gratitude for his advice. Thus originated the favorite smoking mixture of the Indians—the kinnikinnick.

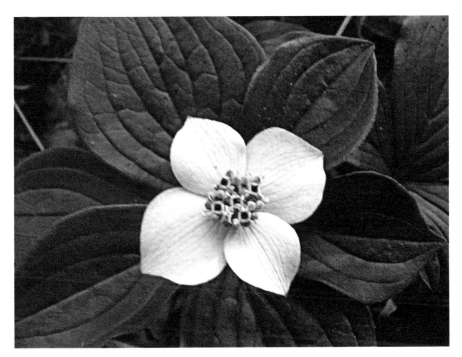

Bunchberry flower

John Hellson (1974, 49) writes:

According to a certain myth, there was a time when the bark of this bush (C. stolonifera) was white and not red. Naapi saw some gophers playing in the warm ashes of a campfire. They would bury each other in the ashes, and when it got too hot, they would cry out and the other would uncover them. Naapi joined the game and persuaded them all to get in the ashes.

Only a pregnant gopher resisted, and Naapi let her go, saying that she was necessary to propagate the species. Then he roasted the gophers and made a frame of C. stolonifera, which he used as a plate while he ate them. That was how the bark turned red, and to this day the grease from the gophers drips from the branches when they are heated.

Annora Brown (1970, 222) recorded this legend:

When held over a flame, the red-stemmed dogwood oozes grease which spreads along the stem. This characteristic is explained by the story that Old Man, after roasting his meat in the coals, usually spread it to cool on the stems of the red dogwood. The stems absorbed the fat that dripped over them, and they kept it there in their fibers, only to become visible when melted near a fire.

RECIPES

Infusion: Steep 1 ounce of dried bunchberry leaves in 1 pint of boiled water. Drink cool, 1–2 ounces up to 3 times daily.

Tincture: 20–60 drops 3 times daily. Dried inner bark is tinctured at 1:5 and 40% alcohol. Fresh leaves of dogwood or bunchberry are tinctured at 1:4 and 60%. You must grind the leaves well to get this ratio.

Decoction: ½ teaspoon of inner bark to 8 ounces of water for 15 minutes. Then steep for 30 minutes more. Take 4 ounces 3–4 times daily.

Syrup: Take 4 cups of bunchberries, 2 cups water, and 1 cup honey. Mix and boil until it is a thick sauce. It is a very different taste, but great on pancakes.

Bunchberry burn ointment: Mash fresh berries in glass pan and set in the sun for 24 hours. Scrape the partially dried pulp into a jar and cover with an equal part jojoba oil and ¼ part balsam bud oil. Set in a warm area for three weeks, or use a low-temperature crock pot. Add beeswax to the desired consistency (Williamson 2011).

Fireweed

Fireweed • Willow Herb—*Epilobium angustifolium* L. • *Chamerion angustifolium* (L.) Holub.

Each spike [of fireweed] produces its own bunch of flowers, a head composed of a quantity of loose-jointed watery little flowers dangling flabbily by their necks from the main stem: insignificant, rickety, ill-nourished looking flowers, cold pink in color and without smell. The head of the fireweed spike ends in a weakly green point. You would not expect anything so rank of growth to be sensitive, but fireweed is exceedingly touchy and flops in a wilt at any provocation.

—Emily Carr

And only where the forest fires have sped,
Scorching relentlessly the cool north lands,
A sweet wild flower lifts its purple head,
And, like some gentle spirit sorrow-fed,
It hides the scars with almost human hands.

—Tekahionwake (Pauline Johnson)

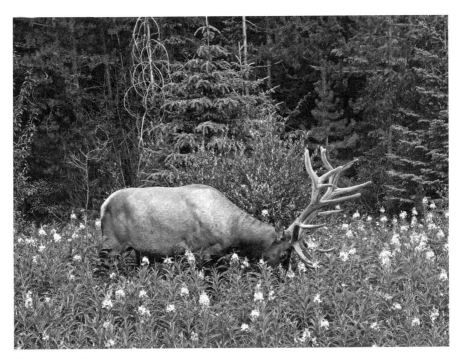

Elk grazing on fireweed

Epilobium is derived from *epi*, meaning "upon," and *lobium*, for "pod" or "capsule." It refers to new flowers being superior, above or on top of the seedpods. *Boisduvalia* is named in honor of Jean Baptiste Boisduval, a nineteenth-century French naturalist and author of a floral book of France. *Angustifolium* means "narrow-leaved." *Chamerion* is derived from the Greek *chamai*, meaning "dwarf," and *nerion*, for "oleander," due to its similar leaf shape.

Fireweed is perhaps derived from the German *feuerkraut*, the name given by Gesner in 1561 for a plant that flourishes on ground cleared by fire. In England, the common name bombweed was given for the quick restoration of bombsites. It was the first colonizer of Mount St. Helens after it erupted. In the first year, 81 percent of the new seedlings on the devastated land were fireweed.

Traditional Uses

The Cree call it *ihkapaskwa* and noted it flowered when the moose were fattening and mating. Other Cree names include *askapask*, *athkapask*, and *akapuskwah*. The root was macerated and applied to boils or infections. The leaves were plastered on bruises. The raw roots were a popular native food source. Even the summer stem was split open with the thumbnail or between the teeth to extract the inner edible pith. It tastes a bit like cucumber but is very sweet and can give a sugar buzz when needed. It was used later in the season to sweeten buffalo berry whip, also known as Indian ice cream.

The Kamtschadalis of eastern Russia boiled the plant with fish and used the leaves as tea. The stem pith was scraped out with shells, tied in bundles, and sun-dried. Known as *kipri*, it was boiled into a thick, sweet wort and used to make *quaffe*, a fermented drink of malted rye, flour, and wild mint. Six pounds of *kipri* was mixed with one pound of cow parsnip stalks and fermented into vinegar.

Fireweed is a popular food of moose, with one study showing more than 70 percent of the rumen content from July to October consisting of fireweed, birch twigs, and blueberry leaves. In winter, red osier dogwood is the staple. The Woods Cree of Saskatchewan made a tea of the whole plant for intestinal parasites. The root is crushed and applied to boils or abscesses, or to draw out infection from open wounds. The root is used by the Cree of Wabasca, Alberta, as part of a decoction to reveal whether or not a woman is pregnant. If the decoction, when drunk, causes a violent nosebleed, she's pregnant. Otherwise, menstruation will soon begin.

A Métis healer from Sucker Creek, Alberta suggested eating the young tops to "get the blood up if the blood is weak." This reminds me of the approach to blood in Southern states articulated by noted herbalist Phyllis Light. This condition suggests low blood, meaning either low in nutrition, low in blood pressure, or lower-down problems in the body. The Métis of northwestern Canada call it *bouquets rouge*, or *eñ narbaazh di feu*. They infuse the leaves for a tea to calm the nerves. The Blackfoot rubbed fireweed flowers on their mittens and rawhide thongs as waterproofing. The inner pith from the stems was dried, powdered, and rubbed on the hands and face as protective talc from winter's icy grip. The Ojibwe call it *zhoshkidjeebik* or *oja'cidji'bik*, meaning "slippery root" or "soap root." They would moisten and pound the root until it lathered up and then apply it as a poultice to bruises, boils, furuncles, and sores. An alternate name is *kêgi'nano'kûk*, meaning "sharp pointed weed."

The northern Dene (Chipewyan) call fireweed *gon dhi'ele*, meaning fire new branch. Natives of Nunavut ate the tops of *paunnait* as summer food. The young stems are full of sweet water and can be sucked out. Sophie Thomas, a Saik'uz elder and herbalist, suggested drying the root and then boiling it to treat asthma. Many native groups, including the Gitxsan clan of British Columbia, used fireweed syrup as a type of glue to keep their berry rolls stuck together. When not available, they would use bunchberries as glue. To the Gitxsan, fireweed is called *haast*. The *k'ilhaast*, or single fireweed, was considered the first totem pole, and *gisk'aast* is the name of one of the four *pdeek*, or clans, of the Gitxsan. One totem pole of Kitsequecia shows the flower as a crest, and fireweed was used as the name of one clan, or society, within the tribe. This is somewhat unusual, as traditionally a clan would be named in honor of a mammal, bird, or fish. One account records *k'ilhaast* planted in front

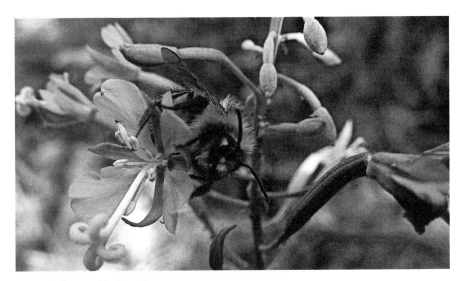

Fireweed flowers visited by a bee

of a house and overnight it grew so tall that it pierced the sky (Johnson 1997, 140). The term *totem* is a variation of the Anishinaabe word *dodem*. Jordan Paper (2007, 17) writes:

> *It is first found in the work written in 1791 by John Long, an English trader traveling north of the Great Lakes:* Voyages and Travels of an Indian Interpreter and Trader. *In his slim book, Long somewhat accurately describes a personal* dodem *as a "favorite spirit … that never kills, hunts, or eats the animal whose form they think this totem bears.*

The modern Western concept of totem animal is derived from the Greek concept of daemon, which later underwent Christian conversion to demon. A *dodem* pole represents a clan symbol or personal *manido* (derived from Manitou) or spiritual being.

The fireweed was first chewed and crushed to remove all the sour juice. The ground fireweed was mixed with seal blood and then oil to make *aluk*. Various tribes rubbed the fresh leaves on bowstrings to help preserve them. The Nlaka'pamux used the small twisted roots as good luck charms. The Haida peeled the young shoots and ate them to purify their blood, make them handsome, or to "move stuff around one's insides," referring to its tonic and laxative effect.

The Dena'ina of Alaska place the raw stem on cuts or boils to draw the pus and prevent infection. A decoction of the aerial parts was used in parts of Alaska and throughout the Arctic to initiate breast milk secretion (Birket-Smith 1931). Newcombe (1897) noted cordage is made from the stem fibers: "From the fibrous skin or bark after the outer layer had been got rid of by prolonged immersion in water, a string used to be spun, which was afterwards made into nets." It is not as strong as fiber derived from stinging nettle or dogbane. It worked well enough to use for thread, and then three could be braided into larger diameters. The outer stem fibers are very tough and can be twisted into snare cordage, usable but inferior to dogbane. It should be peeled off the stem and dried in June or July, before the plant flowers and the stems become too hard. Later, the dried strips are soaked in water and twisted or spun into twine for nets or to make pack straps. Six or more strands require braiding to possess any great strength. The roots were used medicinally by the Haida in an unspecified manner. According to Swanton (1905), a game called "woman's pubic bones" used fireweed stalks as an item of wager. Sounds like an interesting game!

Fireweed is a healer of burns, including those of mother earth. Wherever forest fires have devastated, the beautiful magenta blooms begin the healing process and prepare the soil for willow and poplar to follow. Fireweed is indifferent to soil pH and is adaptable to both acidic and alkaline soils. Fireweed starts flowering from the bottom up, each blossom lasting only two days. On the first, it produces sticky turquoise-colored pollen, and on the second no pollen, but it is receptive to fertilization and gives off a strong fragrance from its nectar. Older blossoms contain more nectar, giving bees a drink first before they climb up to scrape pollen out of the younger flowers. The stickiness of the turquoise pollen is due to a lipoid coating, pollenkitt, and viscin threads. This helps ensure cross-pollination, with each plant capable of producing up to forty-five thousand seeds.

Early French settlers called the young shoots *asperge* and steamed them as an early green. The unopened buds can be added to salads or pickled like capers for winter. Fireweed was introduced back to Europe, where today it remains a popular vegetable. Fireweed contains ninety times the vitamin A and four times the vitamin C of oranges. I harvest the new

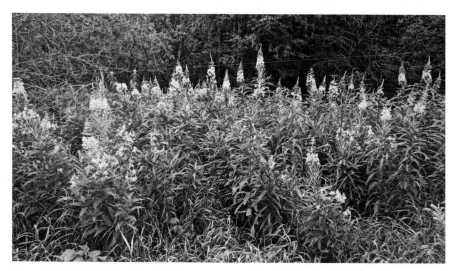

A patch of fireweed

shoots when they are from six to ten inches tall and are very flexible. Although some people steam them, I prefer to oven-roast them on a cast-iron pan to let the sugars come out and caramelize the tasty shoots.

In Greenland, the leaves are combined with seal blubber for a spicy treat. Research in Sweden found the roots make an acceptable survival food if soaked in ash water for several hours. The Inuit have been reported to eat the roots after boiling. Further south, the Algonquin grated the fresh root as a poultice to treat furuncles.

The fluff from ripened pods is used as tinder to start fires, and when carbonized is extremely susceptible to the smallest spark or heat friction. "Wick up" refers to the use of rolled fluff as a wilderness candlewick inserted in tallow or other fat. If the fluff is rolled up and inserted into a fat, it will produce light without carbonizing and burning up, ensuring nighttime illumination. Or at least until your squirrel fat is used up. The insulating and water resistant quality of fireweed fluff was utilized. The natives of Puget Sound wove the fluff together with mountain-goat hair, and later dog hair, to make waterproof blankets. Other tribes used duck feather cattail–fireweed combinations. Down feathers and fireweed fluff make excellent comforters. Balsam poplar fluff can be substituted when necessary.

It also makes an excellent wilderness bandage combined with balsam pitch. The Cheyenne of Montana call it red medicine. A tea from the root and leaves was taken for rectal hemorrhage. The natives of Kamchatka brewed a stupefying ale that combined fireweed aerial parts, cow parsnip stems, unripe bog blueberries (*Vaccinium uliginosum*), and dried *Amanita muscaria* mushroom into a fermented drink. I was invited to the Telluride Mushroom Festival in 2013 and presented a formula for Kamchatka Ale, created with the help

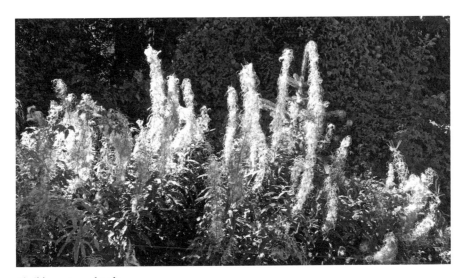

Fluff from ripened pods

191

from my brewing buddy, Patrick Tackaberry. The ratios are all-important. For all of these ingredients to be available at the same time, late summer would be the ideal time to prepare this potent preparation.

Dried Fireweed leaf tea is relaxing and calmative, reminiscent of green tea but caffeine-free. An oven-roasted leaf tea from Russia is called Kurilski chai, kapoorie, or Kurile tea. The fresh-leaf tea is sour and not particularly pleasant to me. Some people really enjoy it, so try it for yourself. In Siberia, the leaves are first fermented and used for tea. It is called John's tea or Ivan chai. The roots may be roasted and prepared as a coffee substitute.

Fireweed honey is an important commercial bee product, with a distinctive buttery caramel taste. Sugar yields from individual flowers range from 0.66 mg per flower per day to over 4.0, with yields increasing with temperature up to 75°F and decreasing thereafter. Flower life is 5–6 days at 57°F. Work in Russia reported honey production as high as 9,000 pounds per acre, an unbelievable (and probably greatly exaggerated) yield. I believe they missed a decimal point. Fireweed honey is highly prized by confectionary chefs due to its unique aromatics and texture. The honey possesses activity against *Streptococcus pneumoniae, S. pyogenes*, and both regular *Staphylococcus aureus* and MRSA (Huttunen et al. 2013).

Fireweed is the floral emblem of Yukon and the national flower of Russia. White-flowered variations are probably the result of mutation from radiation near uranium deposits, and in the wild, may well help geologists find this mineral. When additional nitrogen is made available to fireweed, a noted increase in asparagine and glutamine content is found. One unusual experiment, carried out in Russia in 1972, was the injection of a water extract from fireweed racemes into the stem of a barley variety. This produced earlier maturation, resistance to lodging, and higher protein content in the grain. I don't believe it made it to commercialization. In Quebec, the flowering of fireweed signals the optimal time to pick the ripe mature cones of white spruce to sell to tree nurseries.

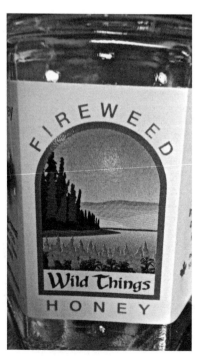

Fireweed honey from Yukon

Hall's willow herb is a rare relative found around Lesser Slave Lake. The flower is white, often fading to pink, with distinct fireweed leaves, and it is found on moist ground or in the wet boreal forest. I thought I had discovered a new species and became quite excited; but alas, it was named long ago. The related, but smaller, river beauty (*E. latifolium*) inner stems were a choice edible of the Bella Coola people. The Inuit of Baffin Island call it broad-leaved willow herb, dwarf fireweed, or *paunnat*. The leaves are eaten raw or mixed with fat, while the flowers are mixed with crowberries, blood, and oil. In Greenland the plant is known as *niviaqsiaq*, meaning "little girl." It is considered by many to be the country's national flower. In the U.S. Southwest, *Epilobium glandulosum* root was used for leg pain. The Navaho-Kayenta traditionally used plant infusions as a lotion and the roots as a poultice for muscular cramps. The Potawatomi use root infusions to stop diarrhea. Their name is *wisigi-bag*, bitter weed.

Medicinal Uses

Constituents: *C. angustifolium*: mucilage, ellagitannins (up to 20%), including oenothein B (14–23%), chaermenericm, olenolic and maslinic acids, ursolic and 2-hydroyursolic acids, sugars, starches, pectin, ascorbic acid, calcium salts, beta-sitosterol caproate, sitosterol glucoside, and sitosterol 6g-acetylglucoside; various sitosteryl esters, including propionate, caproate, caprylate, caprate, and palmitate; and flavonoids, including myricetin-3-O-beta-D-glucuronide; quercetin (0.42%), quercetin-3-O-glucuronide, myricetin (0.32%), kaempferol (0.37%), sexangularetin, and various sterol acetates comprising beta-sitosterol (66.8%) kaempesterol (1.2%), and stigmasterol (0.4%). Total sterol content is 0.1221/100g. Various acids, such as ferulic, gallic, protocatechuic, ursolic, maslinic, cinnamic, caffeic, gentisic, and chlorogenic are also present. Flavonoids include flavonol aglycones and flavonoid glycosides, including afzelin, juglalin, avicularin, hyperoside, isoquercetin, and miquelianin. The leaves, buds, and stem tips contain 28–31% protein and cellulose of 9–10%. In 58 g of young fireweed leaves there are 8 mg calcium, 1 mg iron, 332 RE vitamin A, 0.49 mg riboflavin, and 57 mg vitamin C.

Flowers: sexangularetin, chanerol, chanerozan.

Pollen: linoleic, linolenic, lauric, margaric, capric, myristic, myristoleic, nonadecanoic, oleic, pentadecanoic, stearic, and palmitic acids.

E. latifolium: beta-sitosterol and various flavonoids including quercitrin, myricitrin, and isoquercitrin.

Fireweed leaves and flowers are useful for a multitude of skin problems, including psoriasis, eczema, acne, burns, and wounds. The leaf is both cool and drying. Fytokem, a former biotech company located in Saskatoon, Saskatchewan, produced a patented Canadian Willowherb Extract with clinically proven anti-inflammatory properties. Studies using 5% extract were tested against 1% cortisone cream and control over a 24-hour period on irritated skin. The extract showed improvement in redness and irritation of 35.5% within 1 hour and 40.5% in 24 hours. Cortisone cream had a 10.75% improvement in 1 hour and 25.75% over 24 hours. The company was purchased by Lucas Meyer (Unipex) in 2009.

Whole quarter-sections (160 acres) of fireweed are grown as a commercial crop to supply the growing demand. The highest content of flavonoids and highest radical scavenging activity is found in full blooms. Glucuronic acid is a growth factor and has been used in the past in abdominal surgery as a detoxifying agent and in therapeutics for arthritis and rheumatism. The flowers can be infused and gargled for sore throat, pharyngitis, and laryngitis, and combined with the leaf as a tea for insomnia and relief of headaches caused by nervousness. The flower juice is very antiseptic and can simply be squeezed from the fresh petals. I like to juice the flowers and then preserve in ice cube form for use year round.

Cool decoctions of the whole plant are used in hiccups, whooping cough, and asthma, slowly sipped until the spasms subside. Leaf tea is mild but helpful in cases of persistent slow hemorrhage conditions from the lungs, nose, bladder, or uterus. It is mild, like bugleweed, and may be combined with cranesbill root, shepherd's purse, or fleabane for more severe cases of internal bleeding. Fireweed leaf decoctions soothe stomach problems like ulcers, gastritis, and colitis, and serious conditions such as gastric tumors, whether of a malignant nature or not. Leaf decoctions are demulcent with mild astringency and can be useful in subacute stages of diarrhea and dysentery. Watery diarrhea due to a change of drinking water is relieved. Poultices of fresh leaves and flowers are applied to inflammations of the ears, throat, and nose. In arthritis and rheumatism, it plays a key role with its anti-inflammatory and kidney-cleansing properties.

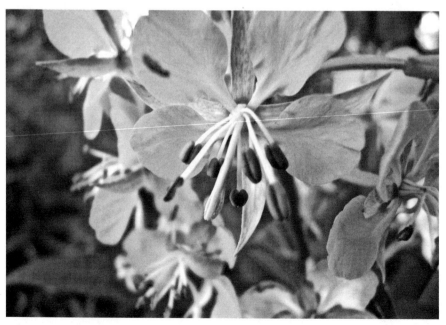

Fireweed flower close-up

Fireweed (*E. angustifolium*) leaf and flowering tops show strong activity against *Staphylococcus aureus* and *Candida albicans*, and moderate activity against *E. coli* and *Pseudomonas aeruginosa* (Borchardt et al. 2008). Fireweed also shows inhibition of the bacterium *Klebsiella pneumoniae* (Battinelli et al. 2001). Recent work found activity against various bacteria, including *S. aureus*, *Micrococcus luteus*, *E. coli*, and *Pseudomonas aeruginosa* in a manner more effective than vancomycin or tetracycline (Bartfay et al. 2012). Ethanol extracts of the root show activity against *C. albicans* (Jones et al. 2000).

Extracts are effective in treating tinea capitis and fungal skin conditions. The ellagitannins are antifungal and may act as an ileocecal valve tonic in chronic candidiasis. Colic and other irritated conditions, including chronic diarrhea, are relieved. Although the author is not a biochemist, I would suggest some of the caprylate compounds may be responsible in part for the antifungal activity. McCutcheon (1994) found aerial parts and root active against all nine fungal species tested. It completely eliminated elastase activity, suggesting skin healing and support. Inhibiting elastase is the basic mechanism of many skin antiwrinkle products that only temporarily create smooth skin.

The rhizomes contain fewer tannins and no mucilage but contain flavonoids useful for anti-inflammatory processes involved with prostatitis and enlarged prostate. Michael Moore (1993, 138), the late, great Southwest herbalist wrote:

The single specific indication for fireweed is chronic, pasty diarrhea, without heat and fever, and green or yellow in color. This is a common complaint in the spring in the north country due to changing from a meat-and-potatoes winter diet to one of green and red spring plants. Some prescription drugs for ulcers, colitis, and arthritis can induce a lingering low-level swelling and dryness in the descending colon, and in men, a low-grade prostate heaviness; two or three cups of tea a day for a week will help, and fireweed has no contraindications with drugs.

It is most useful in subacute and chronic diarrhea when the bowel is tender and the watery discharge needs astringency. Darcy Williamson (2011) writes:

Certain forms of cholera infantum, especially with greenish discharges of undigested aliment, have been controlled by fireweed tea or tincture where the ordinary remedies prescribed by physicians failed to have any beneficial effect. Use 2 teaspoons of the dried leaves per cup of boiling hot water and take as needed. Use 1 to 2 teaspoons of tincture in boiling hot water in more severe cases.

Traditional Eclectic indications are a red, dry, and contracted tongue with pinched, emaciated, and nearly effaced papillae. The skin also looks dry and contracted with a pinched or emaciated look in the face. Studies confirm the anti-inflammatory and prostaglandin inhibition properties. It appears to reduce chronic inflammation through modulation of the arachidonic acid pathway. This is due in large part to the myricetin

3-O-beta-D-glucuronide that inhibits release of prostaglandins PGI2, PGE2, and PGD2. It is at optimal levels during and just after flowering.

Lesuisse et al. (1996) found the tannin oenothein B, from various fireweeds, to be the active compound inhibiting 5-alpha-reductase in the human prostate. This same compound possesses antiviral and antitumor activity. Extracts of the herb, administered with testosterone, increased estrogen receptor alpha activity by 9% and decreased ER-beta by 36% in a rat model. Fireweed may be useful in polycystic ovary syndrome, menorrhagia, vaginal weakness, chronic cystitis, and acute prostatitis. Oenothein B is found in all species of *Epilobium*.

Hevesi et al. (2009) found the compound to possess antioxidant activity equal to Trolox and vitamin C. Fireweed exhibits significant antioxidant activity (Fraser et al. 2007). Ducrey et al. (1997), found oenothein A and B inhibit 5-alpha-reductase and aromatase. Aromatase inhibitors are a class of drugs used for male and female hormone–sensitive cancers. Kiss et al. (2006) found oenothein B extracted from *E. angustifolium* inhibits proliferation of cell lines with high neutral endopeptidase expression (NEP). This suggests use in disturbed metabolism of signaling peptides by an unbalanced NEP activity. Oenothein B from this species exhibits immune modulation both in vitro and in vivo (Schepetkin et al. 2009). Maslinic acid in vitro inhibits serine proteases, key enzymes necessary for the spread of HIV in the body. It shows antiproliferative effects on various cancer lines, including human prostate cancer (Park et al. 2013). Other studies show activity against adenocarcinoma, lung, melanoma, colon, breast, and gall bladder cancer cells.

It may also have benefit in cerebral ischemic injury by promoting the clearance of glutamate via NF-kappa-B–mediated GLT-1 up-regulation (Guan et al. 2011). Maslinic acid is found in olive skin wax. Afzelin (kaempferol-3-O-rhamnoside) is antibacterial and possesses antioxidant, anti-inflammatory, and anticomplement activity. It also inhibits ACE, suggestive of benefit in cardiovascular conditions (Schepetkin et al. 2016). Hyperoside, also present in St. John's wort, suppresses vascular inflammation and relieves the pain of thrombosis. Isoquercetin and quercetin inhibit alpha-glucosidase, suggesting benefit in blood sugar dysregulation, but preventing uptake of sugar in the small intestine (Liu et al. 2016).

Miquelianin (quercetin-3-O-glucuronide) is the major flavonoid glycoside in fireweed. It stimulates depressed immune function and is anti-inflammatory. It ameliorates insulin resistance in skeletal muscles that are inflamed and suppresses plasmin-mediated mechanisms of cancer cell migration (Liu et al. 2016). Pharmacology studies comparing *E. angustifolium* and *E. parviflorum* show remarkable similarity with flavonoid content of the former at 6.6% and the latter at 5.9%. Triterpene and sterols were 4.2% and 4.7%, respectively (Nowak and Krzaczek 1998). Water extracts of the former show five times greater inflammatory power (Hiermann et al. 1986).

Several authors identify the leaves as possessing the highest antioxidant levels. The leaf infusion can be used as a wash for infant skin problems, including cradle cap. Work by Battinelli et al. (2001) found *E. angustifolium* active against human prostatic epithelial cells and to be strongly analgesic in nature. The leaf contains an unknown substance that, like grapefruit juice, enhances the action of drugs four to seven times, according to Mors Korchanski. Liver involvement is unknown.

A phase II, randomized, double-blind, placebo-controlled trial by Coulson et al. (2013) showed benefit for benign prostatic hypertrophy. Just as exciting is a finding by Stolarczyk et al. (2013) that fireweed induces apoptosis in prostate cancer cells. River beauty tops contain steroid compounds that act as gastrointestinal astringents to soothe the digestive tract.

Infused and Essential Oils

An excellent sun-infused oil can be produced from young flower heads and buds of fireweed. Use a 1:5 ratio, weight to volume. Set for 2 weeks, shaking daily in coconut oil. If weather is cool and cloudy, consider a low-temperature setting on a crock pot to avoid spoilage. A 12-hour wilt of flowers and buds will remove excess moisture and produce a better product. This can later be strained and used for highly effective rectal suppositories for hemorrhoids, anal fissures, and prostate inflammation as well as childhood eczema.

Fireweed yields low levels of essential oil. In dried plant material, the steam-distilled volatiles were 16–56% trans-2-hexenal, and 2.6–46.2% trans-anethole. When fresh plant material was used, cis-3-hexenol (17.5–68%) was found. Alpha- and beta-caryophyllenes accounted for 2.4–52% of all volatiles, both fresh and dried. The yield is extremely low, but the hydrosol is very useful.

Hydrosol

Fireweed hydrosol has a most subtle and peculiar fragrance. It has literally no taste so can be taken orally by all ages. Much research needs to be done on the water, but external spritzing on skin conditions such as burns, sunburn, and other inflamed states would be worthy of trials.

Members of the Alberta Natural Health Agricultural Network, including Heather Kehr, steam distilled fireweed. They took the hydrosol to an aromatherapy conference in California and found great interest in the product. The hydrosol shows antimicrobial effect against a number of bacteria, including *Propionibacterium acnes*, associated with acne.

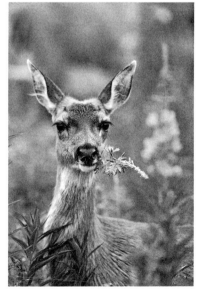

Deer munching on fireweed

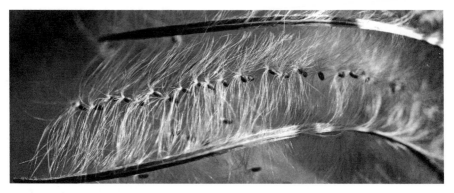

Fireweed seeds and fluff close-up

Spiritual Properties

Hilarion (1982) offered the following insight:

> Fireweed has the ability to connect the soul with higher levels. It isn't of much use to the
> majority of souls now on earth, but for seekers and those whose spiritual vibrations are
> already heightened. A tea made from the whole blooming flowers will produce energies in
> the lower bodies, which open the soul to input from the higher realms.

Flower Essence

Jim Steele was a former student in the 1990s. I invited the class to explore flower essence
preparation and observation for themselves. Here is a report on his experience with
fireweed:

> Just wanted to let you know that I did some follow-up on the course of study for fireweed.
> I prepared a flower essence using the described procedures in August 1997 on a beautiful
> sunny day.
>
> I did not follow up with the other preparations as I had been "corrupted" along
> the way by the repeated references I came across for this herb in a number of texts
> while trying to maintain some forward momentum in the learning sphere. What I
> did determine, at least for myself, was the psychological impact of the flower essence.
> About four days after I prepared it, I took 4 drops of the mother tincture under the
> tongue and had an immediate and strong physical reaction. I felt as if someone was
> pushing on the base of my breastbone accompanied with an overwhelming feeling

of sadness. Along with this powerful emotional response was the strong direction of acceptance.

It was as if whatever stored up over a lifetime was brought right back to the surface. The impression I was left with was that the essence of fireweed offers acceptance of undeniable and unpleasant truth.

This is an incredible gift, as many of us tend not to bring ourselves to accept those things that for whatever reason we can't change or control. My feeling is that this essence may be of value for those recovering from the loss of friends or family, recovering from marital breakup, or accepting terminal disease in oneself or in a loved one. The opportunity for growth flourishes after acceptance of mortal tragedy.

All of these realizations came in less time than it has taken to type this. I've also spent a great deal of time reflecting on my impressions, and they haven't changed in over a year. I did not proceed with journeying with the essence as I find the experience so incredibly intense in a manner that I'm not completely comfortable with that it's very much like dragging the proverbial horse to water. I've never had a bad experience in journeying, although there have been some harrowing contacts in the past, and what I feel is a sort of fear about entering that level of consciousness. Maybe I'm a little afraid about what I'll learn about myself.

Personality Traits

Pam Montgomery (2008) offers her experience with fireweed:

She introduced herself as Fiona, a spirit of fireweed. She had an incredible mix of passionate, powerful energy combined with softness and kindness. She held these two energies in complementary balance. She explained that before one comes to passion, they must first experience compassion.

Myths and Legends

Annora Brown (1970, 230) preserved this native legend:

One legend of the fireweed tells of an Indian maiden. To rescue her lover from an enemy tribe that was preparing to torture him, she set fire to the forest about their camp. While they fled before the flames, she lifted the wounded man and carried him off through the woods.

Some of the tribe, unfortunately, saw what she was doing and followed her. With her heavy burden she could not travel fast enough to escape, but wherever she touched her moccasined feet to the black ashes of the forest floor a flame sprang up in her wake and drove the enemy backward. When at last they gave up the chase, flames continued to leap about her, but they took the form of a brilliant flower that blazed through the blackened skeleton of the forest long after she had passed.

Courtney Milne (1998) was an amazing photographer from Saskatchewan. He preserved and recorded this legend:

The First Woman of the Tlinget people, Asintmah, initially appeared near the Athabasca River in northern Saskatchewan, Canada. As Earth Mother, she walked over the land, collecting fallen branches to make her loom. Asintmah wove a blanket from the fibers of fireweed, the willow herb loved by Earth. Then she gathered the sacred cover and walked in all four directions, spreading it over Earth's body.... Finally, Asintmah wove threads of music and sang as Earth heaved and birthed her children, bringing Mouse, Rabbit, Cougar, Caribou, and all the other animals onto the land.

RECIPES

Infusion: Take 2–4 ounces of steeped dried leaf tea 5–6 times daily. The flowers are difficult to dry and preserve, easily turning to fluff. Use a ratio of 1 part plant by weight to 20 parts water by volume.

Tincture: 10–20 drops up to 3 times daily. Make the whole aerial plant tincture including root at 1:4 and 60% alcohol.

Caution: Fireweed extracts decrease the effectiveness of ciprofloxacin against *E. coli* by four times. Do not use concurrently.

Decoction: 1 ounce of whole plant, including root, to 1 pint of water. Simmer slowly for 20 minutes. Take 1 tablespoon every 5 minutes.

Fresh flowers: Juice and pour into ice cube trays. Freeze and then pop out, bag, label, and return to the freezer.

Oil: The carrier oil can be made into salves and ointments for burns, cuts, childhood eczema, and ulcerous sores. For hemorrhoid suppositories, you can use coconut oil or harden other oils with beeswax.

Lilac

Common Lilac—*Syringa vulgaris* L.

> *Still grows the vivacious lilac a generation after the door and lintel and the sill are gone, unfolding its sweet-scented flowers each spring, to be plucked by the musing traveler.*

—Henry David Thoreau

> *April is the cruelest month, breeding*
> *Lilacs out of the dead land, mixing*
> *Memory and desire, stirring*
> *Dull roots with spring rain.*

—T. S. Eliot

Syringa is from the Greek *surigx* or *syrinx*, "pipe" or "trumpet," probably in reference to the hollow stems that were at one time used to make pipes. In Greek mythology, the god Pan was chasing a young maiden, Syrinx. She escaped briefly but was turned into a reed that Pan then turned into his musical pipes. A 1759 painting by François Boucher titled *Pan and Syrinx* portrays the story. Lilac symbolizes the youth and acceptance, or first emotions of love in the West, while in China, it represents friction and strife. Lilac is associated with May 13. In Scotland, it is considered unlucky to bring blossoms into the home, while in Germany, lilac blooms are said to make people tired and indolent. *Lilac* is derived from the

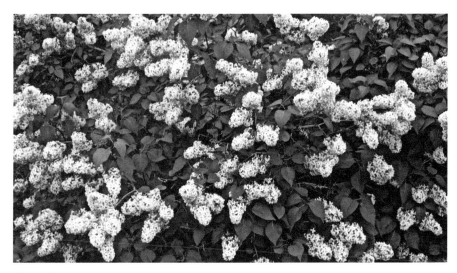

Lilac bush

Persian *lilag* or *lilac*, meaning "bluish flower." This is believed in turn to originate from *nilak*, "bluish," from *nil*, an indigo-blue dye of Arabia. The Persian name Lila, given to a young girl, means "evening." *Lilith*, meaning "night," may be from same origin.

Lilac is the flower of welcome to summer. Our previous home in Edmonton was surrounded with seventeen different lilac cultivars, different in color, shape, and scent. It is said that bees don't like lilac, and I have never seen many bees on these flowers—maybe one or two. In Wales, the blossoms indicate changes of weather. If flowers keep closed longer than usual, this is an indication of fine weather; if they quickly droop, it means a warm summer; and late flowering indicates rain. The blossoms are quicker to open in the morning when rain is on the way, and slower when the air is dry. Finding a five-petal blossom is considered good luck.

Traditional Uses

The best flowers grow in the coldest and most difficult climates, hence the great interest by gardeners in northern Canada. The original lilac is a small flowering shrub native to the Carpathian Mountains of western Romania. It was brought to the New World in the 1600s. Purple lilac is the state flower of New Hampshire because it is "symbolic of that hardy character of the men and women of the Granite State." Early Canadian settlers were given free lilacs by the government, hence their proliferation across the prairies on deserted homesteads.

If anyone can be called the founder of the modern lilac, it would be Victor Lemoine and his sons, working at their nursery in Nancy, France. A small plant with double flowers that he discovered and moved to his garden thirty years previously was finally hand-pollinated in 1870. From one hundred pollinations, just seven seeds were collected, and the next year only thirty. From these beginnings, two hundred and fourteen cultivars were developed over seventy-one years and are sold today as French hybrids.

There is also a Canadian connection. Isabella Preston, working at the Central Experimental Farm in Ottawa in the 1920s, produced over fifty crosses and introduced forty-seven varieties. The Royal Botanical Gardens in Hamilton, Ontario, is the international center for the registration of lilac varieties. Harvard's Arnold Arboretum grows the world's largest collection of lilacs, with five hundred named varieties, some over three hundred years old.

The Cree did not use the introduced plant medicinally, as far as I know. They named it *nipisisa ka watihkwaniwiw*. The Iroquois chewed the bark or leaves for sore mouths. Its gentle action made it effective and useful for children as well. The petals are often employed in candy novelties like flavored marzipan. They can be added to ice cream or yogurt, adding a lemony, pungent, and floral scent and taste.

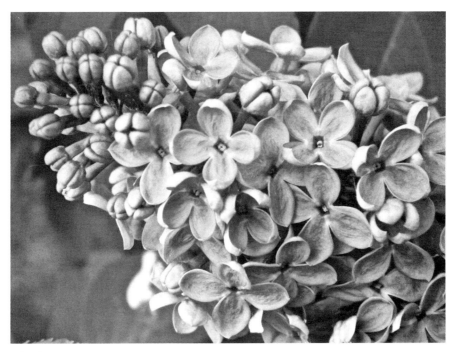

Lilac flowers

The purple lilac is associated with the first emotions of love, or an awakening love. The white lilac represents youthful innocence but is also linked to death. Some people refuse them entrance into their homes. My mother loved the scent of lilacs, and when I smell them it reminds me of her love. In Victorian times a lilac sprig was sent to the fiancé when asking that an engagement be broken. An old proverb declared that she who wears lilac would never wear a wedding ring. Walt Whitman used purple lilac to symbolize the cycle of grief and optimism experienced by those who remain after a death.

In magic, the lilac is planted to drive away evil from the property. It is associated with Venus and the water element. Fresh flowers are placed in haunted houses to clear the vibrations. The Ainu of Japan used lilac poles as "fetish" or protection from evil. Poles were placed on the eastern side of new lodges, during death ceremonies, or alongside a bear feast (Batchelor 1892). In China, the flowers, *sung lo cha*, of small-leaved lilac (*S. microphylla*) are used as a tea substitute. In Russia, the flowers are used to make a special liniment for rheumatism. The hollow stems were used for pipe manufacture in Europe, where tobacco was introduced about the same time as lilacs. And the dried wood, when burned, contains the sweet fragrance of the flower.

Medicinal Uses

Constituents: *S. vulgaris*: bark and leaves: a bitter glycoside variously called lilacin, syringing, and ligustrin; lignans (+)-lariciresinol, 4-beta-D-gluco-pyranoside, and (-)-olivil-4-beta-D-glucopyranoside; verbascoside; various iridoids and secoiridoid glycosides, including oleuropein, ligustroside, nuzhenide, epikingiside, syringalactones A-B, and demethyloleuropein; sugar esters acteoside (verbascoside) and neoacteoside; phenylpropanoids such as syringin, syringopicroside, syringoxide, verbascoside, coniferin, acetoside, lilacoside, fliederoside, and forsythiaside; the coumarin esculetin; kaempferol-3-O-rutinoside; astragalin, a flavonoid; D-mannite; mannitol; and tyrosol.

Flowers: acteoside (2.48%), neoaceteoside, echinacoside (0.75%), oleuropein (0.95%).

Green fruit: syringin, oleuropein (1.09%), nuzhenide (0.42%).

Leaf: various sugars, including mannitol.

Lilacs are not considered a medicinal herb by many people, even a majority of herbalists. But it is very a very useful herbal ally if you look more closely. The fruit (seed) of lilac is a good tonic and febrifuge when extracted. The fruit and leaves are bitter and subacrid, but the isolated glycoside is odorless and tasteless.

The flowers can be steeped in boiling water and drunk cool for acid indigestion. Lilac blossoms, eyebright, lady's mantle, avens, and valerian root can be mixed and steeped in cold water overnight. Gently bring to a boil in the morning and infuse for three minutes. A piece of linen soaked in the cool infusion, and applied to closed eyes several times daily for a period of time, will remedy weeping eyes.

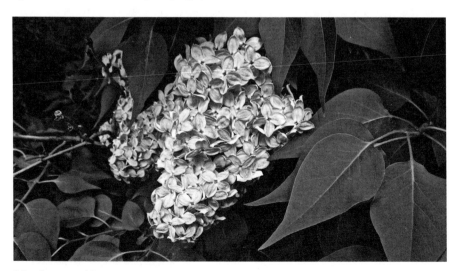

Lilac flowers and leaves

Syringin, from the leaf and bark of lilac, has neuroprotective, tonic, adaptogenic, and immune-modulating properties. Syringin has been found to enhance secretion of beta-endorphin from the adrenal medulla, resulting in lowered blood sugar levels in type 2 diabetic rats (Niu et al. 2008). Syringin modulates the immune function of abnormal cells and the balance of cytokines in an arthritis study in rats (Song et al. 2010). The leaf extracts appear to reduce inflammation associated with induced ulcerative colitis (Liu and Wang 2011). Syringin appears to decrease neuronal cell death, suggestive of use in dementia conditions (Yang et al. 2010). It increases acetylcholine release from nerve terminals and enhances insulin secretion from the pancreas (Ko-Yu Liu et al. 2008). Syringin is a compound found in the root and rhizome of *Eleutherococcus senticosus*, formerly misnamed Siberian ginseng. Lilac leaves show antimicrobial activity against *Staphylococcus aureus*, *Proteus vulgaris*, and *Aspergillus niger*. Kaempferol-3-O-rutoside, a flavonoid extracted from the fresh flowers and leaves, shows a hypotensive effect in laboratory studies. This effect was not inhibited by antihistamine nor antimuscarinic agents (Ahmad et al. 1993). It also exhibits antiglycation activity (Lal Shyaula et al. 2012). Syringin, derived from the bark, lowered blood pressure but had no effect on the pressor effect induced by norepinephrine or carotid occlusion (Ahmad and Aftab 1995).

Acteoside, also known as verbascoside, isolated from violet lilac flowers, exhibits hypotensive activity, with a decrease in systolic, diastolic, and mean arterial blood pressure (Ahmad et al. 1995). Verbascoside shows significant wound healing and anti-inflammatory activity (Korkina et al. 2007). Verbascoside derived from lilac may be useful in reducing inflammation associated with periodontitis (Paola et al. 2011). Verbascoside exhibits anti-oxidant protection, and in a study on human keratinocytes and tumor cells, it exhibited photoprotection of human skin (Kostyuk et al. 2008). See "Mullein" in Chapter 9 for more properties of verbascoside.

Forsythiaside, found in bark and leaves, is also present in the TCM herb *Forsythia suspensa*. Mouse studies have found the compounds protect against cigarette-induced lung injury by activating the anti-inflammatory cytokine Nrf-2 and inhibiting the NF-kappa-B signaling pathway (Cheng et al. 2015).

The bark and stems can be decocted and given warm to children for fevers accompanying measles, mumps, or chickenpox. By helping move the infective state to the exterior, the condition is more quickly resolved, helping prevent possible complications. This decocted tea is good for rheumatism and gout, again drunk at body temperature.

The leaves and bark contains oleuropein, also found in olive leaves and a few other plants. In laboratory in vitro studies, it is highly active against *Mycoplasma* species, *E. coli*, *Klebsiella pneumoniae*, *Pseudomonas aeruginosa*, *P. fluorescens*, *Enterococcus faecalis*, *Listeria monocytogenes*, and *S. aureus*. A rabbit study involving acute pyelonephritis initiated by drug resistant *P. aeruginosa* found increased survival rates, and when oleuropein was combined with a relatively ineffective antibiotic, amikacin, the survival rates nearly doubled.

The oleuropein group showed levels of IL-6 and TNF-alpha, and bacterial counts were all reduced. Stephen Buhner (2013, 185) contributes:

> *Besides its antibacterial actions, oleuropein is strongly protective of cells from bacterial membrane constituents. It protects endothelial tissues from inflammation, stops angiogenesis, reduces monocytoid cell adhesion to cytokine-stimulated endothelial cells, inhibits VCAM-1, and inhibits NF-kappa-B.... Oleuropein inhibits nitric oxide, IL-1beta, IL-6, TNF-alpha, iNOS, COX-2, and MMP-9.*
>
> *Interestingly, oleuropein stops the development of morphine antinociceptive tolerance. Over time, as people take opiates for pain, even with years between doses, the receptors in the brain that react to morphine stop doing so. The more you take, even if it is for a week for back pain and then five years later for a broken bone, and so on, the less responsive the brain receptors become. Then, later, if you get cancer, the morphine does nothing. Oleuropein stops this process.*

In fact, oleuropein may be a useful therapeutic agent in the treatment of neuroblastoma (Secme et al. 2016).

The leaf compound improves insulin sensitivity in a randomized placebo-controlled crossover trial by De Bock et al. (2013). Forty-six middle aged men were given an extract containing 51.1 mg of oleuropein and 9.7 mg hydroxy-tyrosol or placebo for 12 weeks, crossing over to the other treatment after a 6-week washout. A 15% improvement in insulin sensitivity was found compared to the placebo as well as the 28% improvement in pancreatic beta cell responsiveness.

A compress of the fresh flowers may be placed over the pancreas (belly button) to assist with addressing blood sugar imbalance and to regulate the function of the gland. The leaves have been shown to reduce inflammation in mouse models of ulcerative colitis (Liu and Wang 2011). The leaves contain syringopicroside and related metabolites that exhibit significant activity against MRSA in a mouse peritonitis model (Zhou et al. 2016). Oleuropein is active against *Staphylococcus aureus* and shows synergistic effect with ampicillin, suggesting herbal-drug increased efficacy.

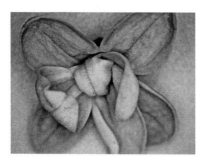

Close-up of lilac petals

The fruit (seeds) contain nuzhenide, a compound in seeds of the European ash (*Fraxinus excelsior*). Montó et al. (2014) found nuzhenide and another secoiridoid may be useful in the prevention of metabolic syndrome, which exhibits obesity, insulin resistance, glucose intolerance, high levels of triglycerides, and high blood pressure. Nuzhenide may also be useful for the prevention and treatment of osteoporosis (Chen et al. 2013). The flowers contain echinacoside, found in various *echinacea* species. Acteoside and echinacoside may be useful in the treatment of liver fibrosis (You et al. 2016).

Gemmotherapy

Gemmotherapy is a novel preservation of flower, root, or leaf buds with alcohol and glycerin. Lilac buds act specifically on the arteries of the heart. It is an effective antispasmodic, which assures better nutrition of the myocardium through vasodilation, and is therefore indicated in cases of angina pectoris and other heart irregularities. It should be prescribed with caution in the elderly patients who are on blood thinners. This is because the senile myocardium may initially have difficulty adapting to the increasing heart irrigation.

Dose: 15–20 drops 2–3 times daily.

A 1:10 ratio infusion of the swollen buds has been used traditionally in southeastern Russia for diabetes (Moskalenko 1987).

Essential and Sun-Infused Oil

As mentioned above, the lilac is a much sought-after fragrance. The lilac will not give up its heady scent to steam distillation, and solvent extraction (done very rarely) will not capture the true quality. In 1971 the constituents of lilac oil were published in Japan. It is, therefore, commonly sold as synthetic fragrance oil, and next to rose and jasmine, is the perfume most frequently created from synthetic and natural materials. In schools that specialize in training noses for the perfume industry, creation of lilac and lily of the valley scents are often the assigned exam. A product from France called Butaflor Lilac comes close, but most of the absolutes do not approach the true scent.

The ordinary lilac has an odor characterized by hydroxycitronellal and a rose odor against a rather heliotropin background and a slight suggestion of hawthorn (anisaldehyde). The purple lilac has a darker color and a warmer, more pronounced hawthorn odor. All have a distinct but mild green odor. Extracting flowers with petroleum ether to produce concretes results in a "green" odor reminiscent of basil but more unpleasant. The yield is about 0.377%, but there is no market for it. However, the discovery of carbon dioxide extraction has led to a fragrant oil used in high-quality perfumes such as Chamade, Soir de Paris, Florissa, and Tweed. It is known as Syringa in the fragrance industry.

Ordinary, everyday lilac gives a rose-heliotrope scent with a slight suggestion of hawthorn. Purple lilacs provide a reddish-purple oil with more color and a warmer, more pronounced hawthorn odor. Persian lilac is more suggestive of hyacinth, while the white versions tend more to the jasmine-like odor.

Headspace vacuum concentration of lilac fragrance shows the presence of E. ocimene (37%), Z 3-hexenol (9.5%), benzyl, eugenol and isoeugenol methyl ethers, and anisaldehyde in the purple lilac. The red lilac contains only small amounts of ocimene, and the white higher concentrations of indole.

A reasonable perfume is produced by covering fresh lilac flowers with 96% alcohol for six hours. Remove the flowers and store the alcohol in the fridge. The next day, add more flowers without any green stems or leaves. Repeat for a few weeks.

A sun-infused oil that is close and acceptable can be made with canola oil. The flowers, placed in a mesh bag, are wrung out and changed every day for up to three weeks in the sun. Use a ratio of about 1 part by weight to 5 parts of oil by volume. Those with laboratory equipment could attempt to do a pure ethanol extraction from the resulting concrete, but it would probably best be done under vacuum. My wife, Laurie, and I have done this, and we were very happy with the oil obtained. The scent is not authentic to fresh lilac blooms but adds a wonderful fragrance to bath oils.

Flower Essence

My beautiful wife, Laurie, journeyed with lilac flower essence she prepared and discovered the following (this essence is from the Prairie Deva Flower Essence line): lilac flower essence helps heighten the imagination and sense of play and fantasy of the user. It is an essence preferred by the inner child who wishes to play and express without constraints. Lilac can help us view our past with compassion, finding within it times of joy and meaning. It helps us merge our present, past, and future selves in insightful ways. This can aid us in shamanic journeying, meditation, and dream work, or anytime we need to locate some insight and inner wisdom. In the same way, it is useful for doing intuitive work such as tarot reading or astrology analysis.

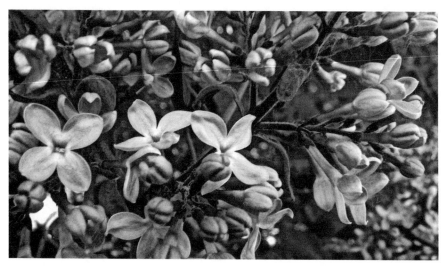

Lilac blossoms

This essence is wonderful for nurturing. It helps us see beauty and joy in little things. It reminds us of the fragility and beauty of each moment. It brings the poetry of our souls into every-day life. This essence brings out a sense of sweetness and femininity in individuals. It is an essence that provides receptivity and kindness. It can also enhance feelings of security and appreciation.

Spiritual Properties

Aversano (2002) contributes this image of lilac:

In calling on the spirit of the plant, a beautiful young woman of innocence, dressed in shim-mering white, appears to me. With her arms dancing with subtle movements of grace, she moves her feet in harmony to the gentle sounds of the wind. She saunters around the lilac bush, enchantingly picking its flowers.

Call on the spirit of this wonderful plant when one is transitioning through life. Lilac is symbolic of transition. It assists a woman energetically as she transitions through menopause.

Myths and Legends

Guillet (1962) collected and shared this lovely legend from Persia:

The Persians tell of an avaricious merchant who never had enough. One day he saw a poor old man in a little garden tending his plants with loving care. "Which one do you value the most?" asked the merchant. The man pointed to a small lilac shrub. "You must sell it to me," the merchant said.

The old man hesitated, but he did not dare offend the rich and powerful man. The merchant named a pittance, and sorrowfully the old man dug up his cherished plant.

"Plant it where it is cool and sunny, and give it many drinks of water," he begged.

"I'll plant it were I choose," scornfully replied the merchant. The old man could not forget the plant.

In a few days he stole into the merchant's garden and there stood the great man surveying the wilted and dying lilac shrub. He turned angrily on the old man. "You have deceived and cheated me," he stormed. "Give me back my money and take your wretched plant." The old man tenderly uprooted the little shrub, and when he reached his garden, he planted it in the choicest spot.

Day after day he nursed it back to health. In the spring the shrub put forth heart shaped leaves and later there came great plume-like clusters of lilac flowers. Amazed, the old man wept with joy and cried.

"Thou art lovelier than my dreams of thee."

The shy plant replied, "My flowers are perfumed by the sweetness of your thoughts for me, my roots are cool with the water that you have given me; my heart shaped leaves are a tribute to your generous heart."

Batchelor (1892, 93) wrote:

The chief inao should be made, so far as the stem of it is concerned, of lilac, because this is said to be a hard kind of wood, and does not quickly rot even if stuck in the damp ground out of doors. Upon questioning an Ainu on this subject, he said: "It is not considered wise to use any wood other than the lilac for making the stem of this kind of fetich, for in ancient times a certain man made one of Cercidiphyllum, the end of which rotted after a short time, so that it fell over." Not many months elapsed before the owner himself became weak and died. This was owing to the influence of the fetich being withdrawn. For this reason it is now known that the stem should be made of lilac only, that being the most durable wood of all."

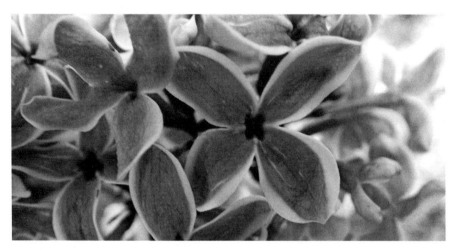

Lilac flower close-up

RECIPES

Decoction: 1 tablespoon of dried bark to 1 pint of water. Simmer for 10 minutes. Syringin is highest in the bark in May, and then again in September, averaging 2.7%.

Infusion: 1 ounce of fresh leaves to 1 pint of water. Infuse for 20 minutes. Take 1 cup as needed. Infusion can also be made from the flowers and seeds, although they are more bitter.

Tincture: The fresh bark, leaf, and flower is tinctured at 1:4 and 60% alcohol. The dried bark is prepared at 1:5 and 40% alcohol. A pleasant flower tincture is produced by using 40% alcohol for up to 6 hours, no more.

Bath: Take a large handful of lilac flower heads and put into a muslin bag. Tie the bag to the bath tap and run a hot bath. Squeeze the bag periodically during your bath.

Labrador Tea

Common Labrador Tea—*Rhododendron groenlandicum* (Oeder) Kron & Judd ✦ *Ledum groenlandicum* Oeder ✦ *L. palustre* var. *latifolium* (Jacq.) Michx. ✦ *L. latifolium* ✦ *L. palustre* ssp. *groenlandicum* (Oeder) Hulten

Northern Labrador Tea ✦ Narrow-Leaf Labrador Tea—*Rhododendron tomentosum* Harmaja. ✦ *Ledum palustre* L. ✦ *R. tomentosum* ssp. *subarcticum* (Harmaja) G. Wallace ✦ *L. tomentosum* Stokes. ✦ *R. subarcticum* Harmaja ✦ *R. decumbens* ✦ *L. decumbens* (Aiton) Lodd. ex. Steud ✦ *L. palustre* ssp. *decumbens* (Aiton) Hulten

Glandular Labrador Tea ✦ Western Labrador Tea ✦ Trappers' Tea—*Rhododendron neoglandulosum* Harmaja ✦ *R. columbianum* (Piper) Harmaja ✦ *Ledum glandulosum* Nutt.

> *Not being able to find any* tripe de roche, *we drank an infusion of Labrador tea and ate a few morsels of burnt leather for supper.*
>
> —John Franklin

I first became acquainted with northern Labrador tea while living on the south shore of Lesser Slave Lake. I was told the leaves made a good herbal tea, so I gathered a few leaves, dried them, and steeped a hot beverage. It was okay. The next week, I visited a Cree neighbor

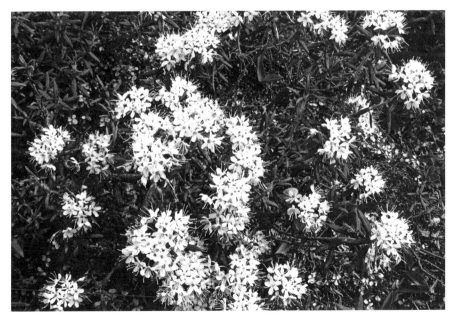

Labrador tea patch

and sampled some marsh tea slowly decocting on the back of his woodstove. There was quite a difference in both the flavor and potency.

At the time, my good friend Terry Anderson and I had started a herb tea company called Home Grown Products. We dried some Labrador tea leaves and tried to market the packaged product at the local farmer's market. We were both working for the Company of Young Canadians at the time, similar to the Peace Corps in the United States. One of our initiatives was to plan and implement a farmer's market in High Prairie, which I believe is running to this day, some forty years later. The Labrador tea was a hard sell, particularly as the local people could go into their backyards and pick it for themselves. Wild mint (*Mentha canadensis*) was also readily available, but the dried leaf tea sold well for us.

Ledum is derived from the Greek *ledos,* meaning "woolly robe," in reference to the under-leaf; or from *ledon,* which was the Greek word for *Cistus* or rock rose. It may derive from the Latin *laedere,* meaning "hurt," in reference to its intense scent, causing headaches. This is less likely. *Palustre* means "of the marshes." The name Labrador may originate from the 1500s, when the Portuguese are said to have touched down in eastern Canada and loaded a ship with enslaved Inuit people. *Lavradores* means "worker" or "slave." An early Italian map of Newfoundland is named Terre del Laboratore, or Land of the Worker. João Fernandes Lavrador explored the area after explorer John Cabot in 1498.

My great-great-great grandfather spent two years on an English ship cod fishing off the Grand Banks of Newfoundland. After this time of servitude he was given a small piece of land on which to build a house in the now deserted outport of Grole. Maybe that explains why I enjoy cod so much. Early Acadians heard "Labrador" as *la bras d'or,* meaning "golden arm." This was attached to the beautiful Bras d'Or Lake of Cape Breton.

In 1996, the *American Horticultural Association* folded *Ledum* into the genus *Rhododendron.* This is based in part on similar-looking leaves and other taxonomic similarities. Labrador tea or muskeg tea, as it is known to northerners, makes a pleasant camp tea. Its strong flavor makes it a good substitute, like sweet gale, for bay leaves in soups and stews. The Arctic explorer John Franklin wrote in 1823 that the leaf tea smelled to him like rhubarb. When you have tired of the taste of muskeg tea, simply add a pinch of salt. This will give it a chicken soup-like flavor. Of course, if you are in the bush any length of time, you can make your own salt from sweet coltsfoot leaf ash. The dried leaves add a spicy flavor to meat, soups, sauces and other dishes.

The sweet, camphor-like, and yet narcotic scent of the flowers is never quite forgotten. It is said that falling asleep in a patch of blooming Labrador tea, will induce drowsiness and produce an intense headache in many people. I cannot imagine this happening. Generally speaking, the areas most loved by this plant are hillocks in coniferous swamps, very wet and full of mosquitoes. The plant emits volatile oils, including ledol, palustrol, and ledene that are absorbed by neighboring birch leaves, and then released to deter herbivores that would eat them.

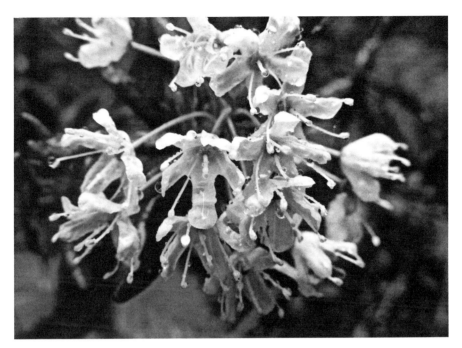

Labrador tea flowers after a rain shower

Traditional Uses

In Finland, ale containing the herb is given to the groom on the eve of his wedding, causing him to fall asleep. The bride then takes advantage to crawl between his legs, in an apparent means of ensuring an easy childbirth when the time comes. It sounds very much like a transference ritual that passes the pain of labor onto the father.

The Sami of northern Finland and Norway used the plant as a salt substitute and leaves as a beverage for cough and colds, including whooping cough. For rheumatic pain, the leaves were poulticed with chickweed and aspen poplar inner bark. Three-day-old decoctions were taken internally for joints swollen from frostbite. The tea was ingested for various conditions including high blood pressure, bladder catarrh, and diphtheria. The leaves were sometimes chewed as a breath freshener and boiled and steamed for snow-blindness.

The Russians believe the smell of the flowers can cause psychosis, with a sense of impending doom. Siberian shaman smoldered the plant and breathed in the strong-smelling narcotic smoke to induce trance-like states. The flowering tops were added to traditional beer recipes to enhance the stupefying effects. Korean herbalists use the leaves for female disorders. The drying of the plant should not be done in a confined space, as the fumes affect the heart of those who are sensitive.

Thoreau (1906, 492) described the fragrance "between turpentine and strawberries," especially the flowers in full narcotic bloom. This aggressive scent can be used to protect woolens, can be added to grain and rice bins to discourage rodents, and can even be added to mosquito repellents. Strong decoctions will kill head lice. Like juniper, a sprig of Labrador tea was hung in homes and closets to repel ghosts and ill health.

The northern Cree call it *maskihkohpakwa*, "plant of the muskeg," and made use of the dried leaves, even gathering it from beneath the snow. This is the Cree name used by noted healer Russell Willier, who uses the leaves for kidney problems and as a diuretic. It is used in combinations by Russell as an herbal ally for bad blood and stressed liver, and to help lower blood sugar levels. The Wood Cree of Saskatchewan and closer to Hudson's Bay call it *kakikipak*, referring to the fact the leaves stay on the plant a long time. It is known to Métis as *timaskik* or *maskekopakwati*, meaning muskeg leaf tea, and even *muskakopukwu*, meaning medicine tea. The Métis of northern Canada also call it *ti maskik* or *muskego*. The leaves were crushed and combined with animal fats to treat burns externally. The leaves and flowers were infused for colds, and with calamus root for more severe conditions like whooping cough.

Lawrence Millman, noted ethnobotanist and author, shared the Labrador Cree name as "plant that never dies" due to its availability for medicine when harvested under the winter snow. Eastern Cree call it *wesukipukosu*, meaning "bitter herbs," while the Potawatomi

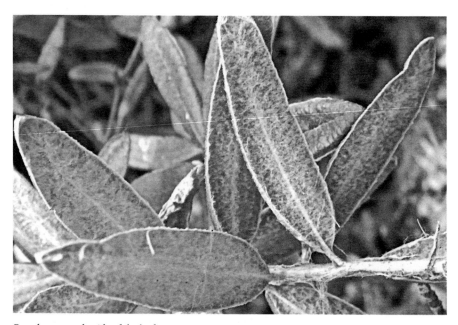

Rust-brown underside of the leaf

name is *wesawabaguk*, "yellow leaf." The Potawatomi are also known as Boodewadamii, from *boodawe*, meaning "those who build a fire." They are the Keepers of the Sacred Fire of those who call themselves Anishinaabeg. The Anishinaabe name for this swamp tea is *mashkiigobag*. Other names include *mamiji'bagûk*, meaning "hairy leaf," and *mamîzhi'bagûk*, "woolly leaf." I have also heard swamp-growing tea, swamp tea leaves, yellow leaf, hairy leaf, and woolly leaf. Lots of choices!

The Hudson's Bay Company imported the leaves into England as a beverage under the name Weesukapuka. Samuel Hearne wrote that the tea was "much used by the lower class of the Company's servants as tea, and by some is thought very pleasant. But the flower is by far the most delicate, and if gathered at the proper time, and carefully dried in the shade, will retain its flavor for many years and make a far more pleasant beverage than the leaves" (Hearne 2010). I find the flower tea is very pleasant and one of my favorites.

The Dene (Chipewyan) call it muskeg tea in English, and *nagodhi* in their own language. The Gitksan of northern British Columbia call it *sk'an dax do'oxwhl*. The K'ómoks (Comox) of northern Vancouver Island steamed the leaves in a shallow pit, alternating with licorice fern roots, until the leaves were dark brown. These leaves were pulled up, dried, and then stored in a cedar box until needed for a tea. Infusions of the flowering tops were used for fevers, chest colds, insect stings, rheumatism, and to quiet the nerves. The powdered leaves were applied to wet eczema to lessen the irritation and pain or sprinkled on baby rashes. The Blackfoot powdered the leaves and made an ointment with bear grease for burns and scalds. They boiled and drank the leaves as a strong emetic. Women of various indigenous tribes drank leaf decoctions three times daily before giving birth.

The Chippewa (Ojibwe) call it *muckig' obug*, swamp leaf, and apply dry powdered roots of Labrador tea and chokecherry bark to skin ulcers. When the powder becomes damp, the area is washed and more powder is applied. The Dene boiled the roots of Northern Labrador Tea to cure sharp chest pains and combined fireweed and Labrador tea leaves in a decoction to help bring on labor. The Roman Catholic brother Marie-Victorin Kirouac (1935) wrote, "It is apparently a mild narcotic; Indian women of certain tribes took some of it three times daily just before giving birth, and the powdered leaves are taken for a headache." The Inuit used the leaves to moisten very dry hands. It is known as *qijuktaaqpait*, meaning "a large amount of fuel for a fire." It is used to treat toothache and eye disorders as well as heal canker sores of the mouth. The stems and leaves are boiled as tea and gargled for sore throat.

The leaves of *R. tomentosum* vary a great deal in phenolic content based on the time of picking, including daylight hours (Black et al. 2011). Natives of the Kodiak Islands of Alaska drink Labrador tea for lung problems, including tuberculosis, as well as upset stomachs. The Dena'ina of Alaska call the narrow-leaf subspecies *k'eluq'ey*, meaning "forked branches," and the larger wide-leaved *L. groenlandicum* is called *quchukda*, "their grandmother," a term of endearment. Both were used as a spice for meat by throwing leaves into the same boiling pot. The leaves are used for hangover, as a laxative, and for dizziness, arthritis, stomach problems, and heartburn in the form of a strong tea. The Haida call it *xaaydaa tiiga*, meaning literally Haida tea, and the Skidegate Haida call the plant *k'usinga xilga*, "tuberculosis-leaves" or "tuberculosis medicine." They generally pick the leaves before the plant flowers for tea and again with the flowers for medicine. An alternate name used by the Massett Haida is *xil qagann*, meaning "cold medicine." The peeled root is used to treat colds, or in large amounts, it acts as an emetic. The Gwich'in of the Mackenzie Delta prefer *maskig*, or *L. palustre*, over the taller, big-leaved *L. groenlandicum* for taste. Both can be used for medicine, however, including the root for an even more concentrated tea.

Matthew Wood (2009) mentions the use of leaf tea as a strengthening tonic after sweat lodge. "It is also used in the fall to stop excessive sweating, in preparation for winter, and is one of the most important Anishinaabe Ojibwe cold and flu remedies in northern Minnesota. It is traditionally used for excessive urination and diabetes mellitus." Today, the Germans and Scandinavians use *Ledum* leaves to make strong beer and ale. It potentiates the beer in a manner similar to the sedative and muscle-relaxing effect of elephant head (*Pedicularis* species). The flowers bloom at around the same time as the mating of bears, suggesting extra caution in the woods. The elector Georg III of Lower Saxony prohibited its use for brewing in 1723 due to the intoxicating effects. At least one author suggests this is the beverage responsible for the often-mentioned frenzy of the Berserkers. This is very doubtful. If anything, the fly agaric (*Amanita muscaria*) mushroom may be a more suitable guess. See "Fireweed," earlier in Chapter 7, for a beer recipe.

Siberian shamans began each engagement by rubbing their knee with heated leaves of Labrador tea. Shamans of Giljak and other Amur residents laid dried leaves on glowing coals and bent over the thick-scented smoke as part of a healing ritual. They would sometimes chew the root as well as inhale the smoke. Ainu shamans of northern Japan use Labrador tea to treat menstrual and colic cramps. Labrador tea, stinging nettle, and devil's club root tinctures combine for an excellent muscle rub. Russian homeopaths boiled the flowers in butter as an ointment for rheumatism, bruises, and skin diseases.

The flowers are used in various cosmetic products, including hand creams, antiwrinkle face creams, and body oils. The antifungal and toning effects of the plant extract find application in hair and shower products as well as foot-care applications. Saunas and steams are greatly enhanced by splashing the leaves on hot rocks, at least before they burn. The twigs, with leaves attached, are soaked in water and used as sauna whips in parts of Scandinavia. Today in Russia, *Ledum* leaves are still used for tanning leather due to the high tannin content (6.4–8.88% of dry weight).

Northern Labrador tea (*L. palustre* ssp. *decumbens*) is, of course, circumpolar and is used in China to treat asthma and coughs as well as lower blood pressure, and is prized for its antifungal activity. It is known as *tu xian*. Labrador Tea can survive the harsh, cold, and drying winters thanks to its own sugary natural anti-freeze and leaves that minimize moisture loss like desert plants. Sustainable harvests of old leaves are possible, but when all the leaves are removed, up to two-thirds of plants die off (Tendland et al. 2012).

Glandular Labrador Tea has a paler underleaf surface with dense resin glands and short, white scales. It is more common to the subalpine regions. This species is poisonous to livestock, especially sheep. It is not recommended for humans. The Secwepemc name for this variety translates as "dogs wash nose," referring to washing the nose of hunting dogs with tea to sharpen their sense of smell.

Medicinal Uses

Constituents: *R. groenlandicum* aerial parts: andromedotoxin, ericolin, ericinol, leditannic acid, palustroside, fraxin and esculin (coumarin glycosides), stearophen, valeric acid, ledol, 5-hydroxy-7,4f-dimethoxy-6-methyl-flavone, vitispirane, perillyl alcohol and aldehyde, iso-pinocamphone, two monoterpenes (lepalone and myrcene), palustrol, alloaromadenllrene, cyclocolorenone (sesquiterpene lactone), citric, tartaric, and malic acids, and essential oils.

Vitamin C content is 98 mg/100 g, and iron 184 mg/100 g in the leaves.

R. tomentosum aerial parts: coumarins including fraxin, esculin, and palustroside, esculetin (6-O-beta-D-[6f-(3-hydroxy-3-methylglutaryl)] glucoside), umbelliferone, scopoletin, flavonoid glycosides such as quercetin 3-beta-D-(6-p-coumaroyl) galactoside, and 3-beta-D-(6-p-hydroxy-benzoyl) galactoside, triterpenoids such as taxerol, uvaol, ursolic acid, as well as beta-sitosterol and oxybenzoic acid. Chlorogenic acid, p-coumaric acid, and three caffeic acids are present, as well as procyanidins and (+)-catechin, hyperin, avicularin, and quercitrin.

Flowers: flavonoids, hydroxycinnamic acids.

Labrador tea is a respiratory tonic, useful in small amounts for coughs and irritations of the lungs and pleural membranes. It combines well with butterwort and sundew in cases of whooping cough. It is believed the essential oils and ledol provide the expectorant and antitussive effect. Other plants with some ledol content are hyssop, chaste tree, hops, eucalyptus, peppermint, and valerian. The plant also contains uvaol, a compound that reduces allergic response in pleurisy and asthma models (Agra et al. 2016). Uvaol and ursolic acid are found in black cherries (*P. serotina*) and produce vasodilation by increasing nitric oxide and hydrogen sulfide production.

Darcy Williamson (2011) suggests a decoction or tincture for prostatitis, combining well with fireweed. She finds a hot cup of tea settles a nervous stomach or relieves nervous tension and mild stress. There is mild yet persistent diuretic effect that tones the kidneys due to its overall drying nature. Decoctions of the leaves are very useful for itch and other skin disorders, especially when fever and skin eruptions are present. The tea can be used internally and externally. An ointment of flowers and leaves is useful for skin and scalp conditions.

The aerial parts inhibit xanthine oxidase associated with gout (Owen and Johns 1999). This may be due in part to the content of esculin and fraxin, which enhance uric acid excretion in mouse studies and benefit kidney dysfunction (Li et al. 2011). Honey syrups can be used for coughs and hoarseness of the throat. These are best prepared with fresh leaves and honey in a 1 to 4 ratio in the top of a double boiler. Use adequate ventilation in the kitchen while slowly simmering the mixture for at least one hour. Labrador tea has a vitamin C content second only to rosehips in the northern forest. It possesses higher antioxidant properties than plantain, sage, chamomile, or uva ursi (Bol'shakova et al. 1998).

Injections of angelica root and Labrador tea before irradiation showed protection of lab animals from injury to the gastrointestinal and blood systems. These experiments by Narimanov (1991) raise interesting questions regarding Labrador tea as a radiation protectant for humans. Labrador tea is used in a new medication for drug addiction in China. It is supposed to remarkably relieve symptoms of withdrawal as well as eliminate the psychological need for drugs and increase immunity (Yan 2010).

Studies by Fokina et al. (1991) confirm increased resistance to tick-borne encephalitis (TBE) virus in lab mice as well as increased survival rates and longevity. Swedish studies suggest it has greater efficacy against nymphs of the tick *Ixodes ricinus* than wormwood (*Artemisia absinthium*) or *Myrica gale* essential oils or extracts. Another study in Sweden found extracts of Labrador tea, *Myrica gale*, and yarrow significantly reduced *Aedes* species mosquito biting. See the "Essential Oil" section below.

Infusions of *L. palustre* enhance activity of several antituberculosis drugs (Guseinova et al. 1992). McCutcheon et al. (1992) found branches of Labrador tea active against *E. coli*, *Bacillus subtilis*, and MRSA. Borchardt et al. (2008) found ethanol leaf extracts active against *S. aureus*. Jin et al. (1999) identified flavonoid glycosides from *L. palustre* active against various fungi and KB cancer cell lines. The latter were originally thought derived from an epidermal carcinoma of the mouth, but were later determined to be contaminated by HeLa cervical adenocarcinoma cells. Many cancer cell lines used

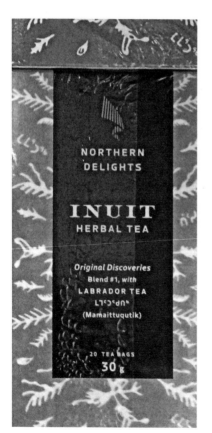

Labrador tea commercial product

for biomedical research are contaminated with more aggressive cancer cells. The problem is widespread. Plant extracts show anti-thrombin and anticancer activity (Goun et al. 2002).

Labrador Tea leafy shoots, in 40% ethanol extracts, exhibit anti-inflammatory activity. This property is present in the fresh leaf and still present in the fresh oilcake after steam distillation. Research in Quebec led by Dufour et al. (2007) found methanol extracts of the leaf possess anti-inflammatory and antioxidant properties. The twigs are active against DLD-1 colon carcinoma and A-549 lung carcinoma cells, with ursolic acid identified as partly responsible for this cytotoxic effect.

Spoor et al. (2006) found Labrador tea (*R. groenlandicum*) extracts appear to possess insulinomimetic and glitazone-like activity. This may explain in part the use of Labrador tea by the northern Cree as a favored beverage. Type 2 diabetes is prevalent among many First Nations people, with over 50 percent incidence in populations over age thirty-five. Epidemic or economic-social genocide is the politically incorrect, but proper word for it. Further studies suggest Labrador tea prevents the absorption of sugar in the small intestine due to alpha-glucosidase inhibition. It appears to help in type 2 diabetes through prior ingestion or when taken with the meal, making this one possible approach to this health epidemic (Baldea et al. 2010). Rapinski et al. (2015) found the shrub reduced adipogenic activity, suggesting its use for obesity. High blood sugar, high cholesterol, and high blood pressure are part of the pattern associated with diabesity. Shilin Li et al. (2016) found Labrador tea improved renal function in mice fed a high fat diet for eight weeks.

Older texts suggested the herb contains arbutin and a toxic diterpene, acetyl andromedol. Not true.

Homeopathy

The plant has long been prized in homeopathy. *Ledum palustre* is particularly valuable for puncture wounds where there is redness, swelling, and throbbing pain, and when the wounds feels cold to touch but is relieved by cold. It should be considered for black eyes or any severe bruising where there is numbness and cold. As a rule, rheumatic pain that starts in the feet and moves upward calls for *Ledum*. The soles of the feet are painful but feel better from exposure to cold.

Lung congestion and other breathing difficulties, such as double inspiration and sobbing, also calls for *Ledum*. Some homeopaths use it for acne, gout, rheumatism, and intercostal neuralgia, all provided that symptoms are relieved by cold. Skin eruptions may be symmetric. Desire for wine is noted. It is good for cystic acne with lesions on the forehead. *Ledum* is said to be an antidote to spider poisons.

Dose: 3rd to 30th potency. Dr. Nash says that for a black eye, the 200th potency has no equal.

The mother tincture is made from dried young shoots reduced to powder, and 1 part by weight is added to 20 parts, by volume, of alcohol. Let it sit for 8 days, and decant the clear liquor. First proving was by Hahnemann with seven male provers. Lembke self-experimented with the tincture in 1848 and 1865. Lippe looked at side effects of 2C given for rheumatic pain in feet.

A homeopathic gel containing *Ledum*, nettle, *echinacea*, and witch hazel extract reduce erythema from mosquito bites (Hill et al. 1996). Following is a delightful poem about homeopathic *Ledum*.

Materia Poetica

Whenever there's a bite
A wound that goes in deep
Ledum comes to mind
A useful remedy
Punctures aren't the only thing
For which he does apply
Rheumatism, alcoholism
A puffy, bloated guy
All this booze he's drinking
Is bound to cause some gout
Broken down by alcohol
Living life alone
He's absolutely chilly
But so prefers the cold
I guess it helps his achy limb
Helps the surly state he's in
Arthritic, chilly, cranky guy
Ledum's life, no cherry pie.

—*Sylvia Chatroux (1998)*

Essential Oil

Constituents: *R. tomentosum (L. palustre)*: aerial parts: monoterpenes, including pinene, sabinene, limonene, and terpinene; sesquiterpenes (selinene, ledene and selinadiene); ledol, borneol, and palustrol; lepalox, lepaxonebutyric acetate, cyclocolorenone, myrtenal aldehyde, vitispirane, perillaldehyde, isopinocamphone, and germacrone. Flowering tops yield about 1.2%, nonflowering 0.35%.

Shoots: palustrol (16–53%), ledol (12–18%), gamma-terpineol (0.0–32%), p-cymene (0.1–14%), lepalone (0.7–6.5%), lepalol (1.0–6.5%), and cyclocolorenone (1.0–6.4%). Different chemotypes are present.

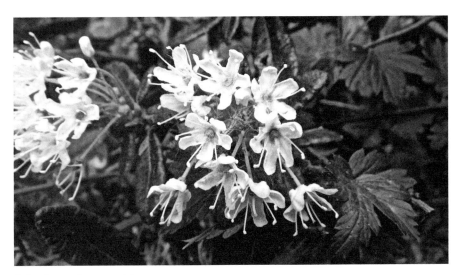

Labrador tea flowers and leaves

Yields are from 0.14–0.87%.

R. groenlandicum: leaves: sabinene (15.7%), terpinen-4-ol (7.6%), beta-selinene (5.7%), myrtenal (3.5%), bornyl acetate (3.3%), gamma-elemene (3.1%), and minor amounts of gamma-terpinene, beta-pinene, pinocarvone, alpha-caryophyllene, alpha-pinene, alpha-selinene, cuminaldehyde, camphene, (Z)-carveol, alpha-terpinene, p-cymene, and (+)-limonene.

High germacrone levels (62%) before buds open, high sabinene levels (22%) during flowering, and high limonene levels (24%) with the flowers only.

Steam-distilled essential oil (yield 0.3–2.5%) is very valuable, both to the herbal practitioner and the producer. The young shoots give three to four times the amount of precious oil and larger amounts of terpenoids than older plants. Palustrol levels are higher in aged than younger leaves. Wide variation in oil content is observed from different regions, in different seasons, and under various weather conditions. The highest levels of ledol are found in flowering plants. *Ledum* essential oil has a bitter and yet pleasant coriander-like fragrance, with hints of mint and a persistent green note. At present, the oil commands over $1,000 per pound, but it is worth every penny.

The reddish-yellow oil is used for kidney disorders and has been found clinically effective for patients awaiting kidney transplant. I have successfully used the oil for pending kidney failure, combined with cool infusions of goldenrod and stinging nettle seed tea. Nephritis and glomerulonephritis may be treated using this two-pronged protocol.

Vegan diet and watermelon-seed tea are also beneficial. The essential oil relieves the pain and inflammation that accompanies prostate enlargement, even with infection present. It plays a smaller role in liver sluggishness and viral hepatitis.

In Russia, the cough medicine Ledin is based on the essential oil. It is an expectorant, an antitussive, and an antispasmodic. The tablets contain 50 mg of ledol and are used for acute and chronic bronchitis, pneumonia, asthma, pulmonary tuberculosis, cystic fibrosis, and frequent, dry cough. For inflammation of the adenoids, tonsils, and other lymphatic congestion, it can be used internally and externally. The oilcake left over from steam distillation can be made into a tincture product, as mentioned above. Nervous energy, spasms of the solar plexus and hyperthyroid conditions are calmed. Insomnia and heart palpitations that accompany these conditions are also relieved. It may balance low thyroid condition as well. Black spruce oil is a useful adjunct for thyroid issues.

Wagner et al. (1986) found *Ledum* leaf oil has a great inhibitory effect on prostaglandin and is therefore useful in inflammatory and rheumatic conditions. Work by Baananou et al. (2015) found hydro-distilled oil significantly reduced edema in a manner similar to the drugs piroxicam and ketoprofen. Kurt Schnaubelt recommends the oil for liver and kidney detoxification, especially after an acute illness. He also uses the oil to counteract insomnia and allergies. A few drops in a diffuser will help sensitive individuals by creating a safer-feeling home environment.

Labrador tea essential oil can be used in mosquito and tick repellants to good advantage (Kiss et al. 2012; Jaenson et al. 2005). It is superior to wormwood and sweet gale for antitick activity, as mentioned above. Sweet gale, Labrador tea, and yarrow significantly reduced mosquito biting in a study conducted in southern Sweden. Germacrone was the constituent shown in studies to be the main reason Labrador tea is not browsed by rabbits. Ledol is a central nervous system stimulant that can result in convulsions and paralysis in high amounts. Mice studies found the oil demonstrated a dose-dependent reduction in motor activity and ability to maintain balance as well as increased sleep time when given with a barbiturate or alcohol.

Dose: 2 drops daily in water.

The seed oil contains palustrol (38.3%) and ledol (27%) as well as smaller amounts of beta-pinene oxide, isomenthyl acetate, nerolidyl acetate, cadalene, and guaiazulene. The picking of seeds is a tedious task.

Sun-Infused Oil

One Sunday morning I was drawn to a huge swath of flowering Labrador tea in a tamarack forest. Initially I was going to take the flowers home and dry them for a winter tea. They are vastly superior to the leaves for fragrance and flavor. Things intervened, so instead of letting them sweat and decompose, I covered one part of flowers by weight with five parts by volume of organic olive oil. I sat the jar outside in the sun, and covered the top with cheesecloth.

I shook the glass container every day for two weeks and then opened it. It possessed a remarkably fruity scent, reminiscent of raspberry fruit. It was a really pleasant surprise.

My wife later created an all-natural perfume from various essential oils and carriers oils, extracted from twenty-two plants native to Alberta. Laurie found the Labrador tea oil an important constituent for helping create an out-of-doors effect. The perfume was called Prairie Essence. We poured the precious blend into a seven-milliliter rose-colored perfume bottle, shaped like a wild rose, Alberta's provincial flower. It quickly sold out in our store.

The flower oil can used externally for muscle pain, spasms, and inflamed, swollen conditions, according to Williamson (2011). The flower oil combines well with mullein flower oil for inflamed swollen glands, lymph node enlargement, and ear inflammation. Sun-infused leaf oil can be made before or after flowering and is valuable for insect repellent mixtures. It really keeps mosquitoes away.

Hydrosol

Labrador Tea hydrosol is very complex and potent, with a somewhat hot and spicy scent reminiscent of bay rum with a cinnamon stick thrown in. The taste, however, is more camphorous and penetrating. It is very close to the scent of the fresh leaves, but not the flowers. It has a pH of 3.8 to 4.0, and although it is clear, it has small icicle-like spikes in the water that settle with time.

The hydrosol, like the oil, is very potent and should be used with caution, with half the recommended dosage of other distilled waters. *Ledum* water left over from the steam distillation can be used for facial cleansing like rose water, or drunk for an enlarged or inflamed prostate. The water is a liver detoxifier and appears to strengthen the immune system, with particular use after surgery and for convalesce.

Suzanne Catty (2001) suggests its use with yarrow hydrosol to ease withdrawal from addictions such as tobacco and alcohol. I would recommend calamus root and licorice root waters as well. She suggests trying ½ teaspoon in water just before bedtime for insomnia. Veterinarians and complementary and alternative medicine (CAM) practitioners have used the hydrosol successfully for Lyme disease in animals and humans. Williamson (2011) suggests one dropper of hydrosol in one liter of water drunk throughout the day. She notes to take it for ten days, then take five days off, and repeat until symptoms have ceased.

Caution: Avoid use in young children, during pregnancy, and in epileptics, following the same contraindications as the medicinal herb.

Flower Essence

One day I produced a flower essence from Labrador tea. It is a research essence of the Prairie Deva flower essence line. *Ledum* flower essence is related to the cold element. Some individuals have a general lack of body heat, and yet ironically the warmth of bed at night causes discomfort. With this body sensation may be irritability and depression as well as delusional thinking. The flower essence helps calm the nervous system and allows energy to move more evenly throughout the body. It combines well with bearberry flower essence to release and move kundalini energy up the spine.

I have yet to see data suggesting grayanotoxin is present in North American Labrador tea species. This is a common toxin in *Rhododendron* species honey in other parts of the world. In northern Alberta, the commercial bee industry places few if any hives in the Labrador tea environment, so I am not sure about the validity of these studies. Mad honey (grayanotoxin) poisoning is rare. An article by Dampc and Luczkiewicz (2015) examined North American Labrador tea and toxicity of ledol; no grayanotoxin was found. Mad honey is produced chiefly from the nectar of *Rhododendron ponticum*, which grows in Japan, Nepal, Brazil, parts of North America, Europe, and Turkey. It is purchased for its reputed benefit in sexual performance, but this misadventure often ends in dizziness, hypotension, and bradycardia. Atropine will antidote the myocardial irregularities.

RECIPES

Infusion: Take 1 heaping tablespoon of leaves and flowers (dried or fresh) to 1 pint of boiling water and steep 20 minutes.

Cold extract: As above, in 4 ounces of cold water for 10 hours. Take ½ cup daily.

Decoction: As above, but simmered.

Tincture: Up to 20 drops 2 times daily for pertussis and respiratory inflammation with spitting of blood. The tincture is prepared in full flower, with leaves, at 1:4 and 50% alcohol. Some authors advise against use of fresh plant tincture. This is probably due to lack of practical experience with the plant.

Homeopathy: 10 drops every 15 minutes in the acute stage; 3 times daily only in chronic cases.

Essential oil: 2–5 drops in water up to 4 times daily. Externally, a 5% dilution to the affected area. Do not use during pregnancy.

Ledum **ale:** Mash malt with water at 150°F for 90 minutes. Boil total of 5 gallons of water, 1 pound of brown sugar, and sparge mash. Boil with 2 ounces of fresh flowering tops of Labrador tea. Let cool to 70°F, place in the fermenter, and add yeast. Place 2 more ounces of flowering tops in a muslin bag with a rock and lower into the container. Ferment until complete. Prime bottles with ½ teaspoon sugar, fill, and cap. It is ready in 2 weeks. You can also take your favorite beer recipe and for the final fermentation add fresh Labrador tea and yarrow aerial parts. This results in an interesting, somewhat mood-altering beverage that is quite pleasant.

Caution: Labrador tea is a uterine stimulant and should not be used during pregnancy or lactation. Some authors cite the content of ledol and restrict drinking to 1 cup of tea per day.

The timing of harvest can influence anti-inflammatory and antioxidant activity (Black et al. 2011).

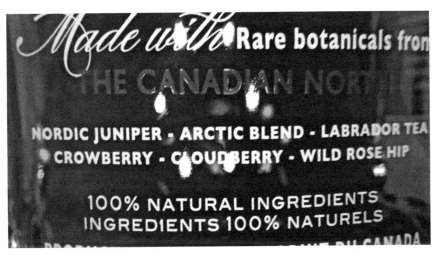

Quebec produced gin containing Labrador tea and other northern medicinal plants.

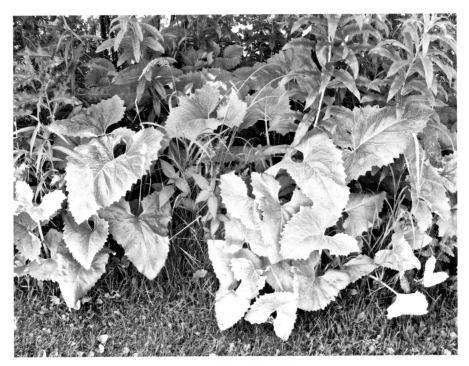

Sweet Coltsfoot (P. frigidus)

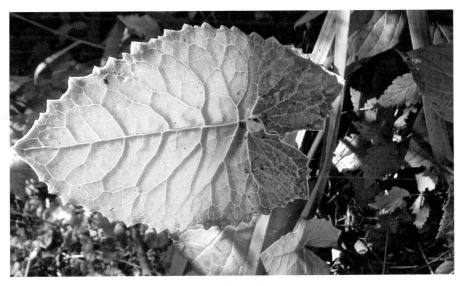

Coltsfoot leaf

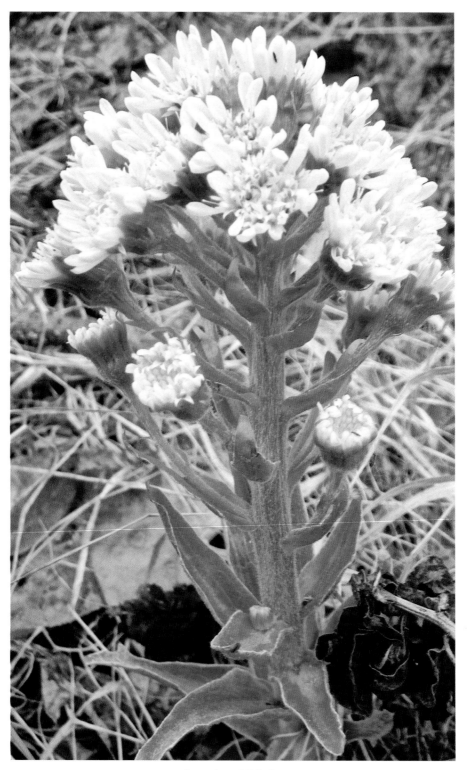

Arrow-leaved Coltsfoot

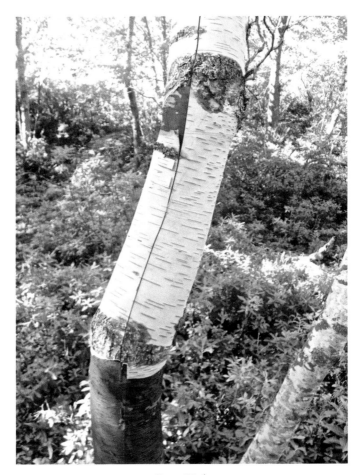

Paper Birch

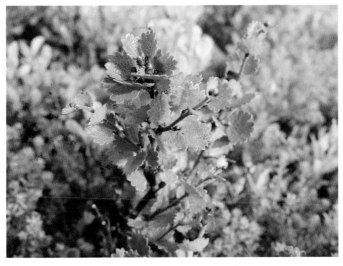

Bog Birch (Betula glandulosa)

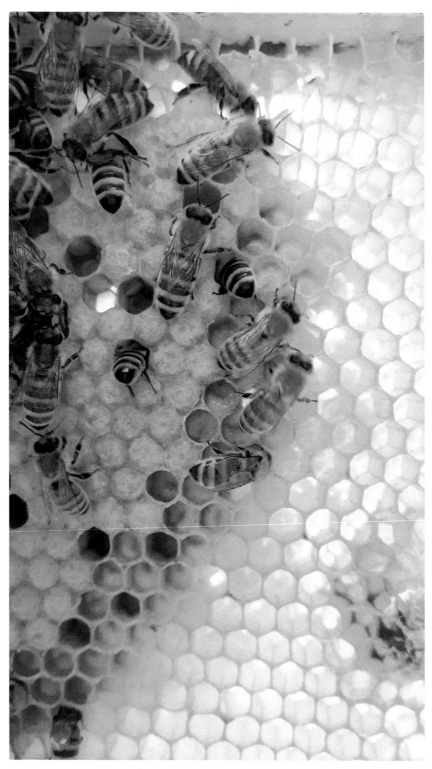

Female worker bees and larvae

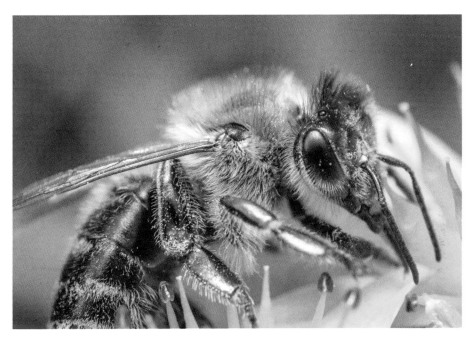

Close up of bee covered in pollen

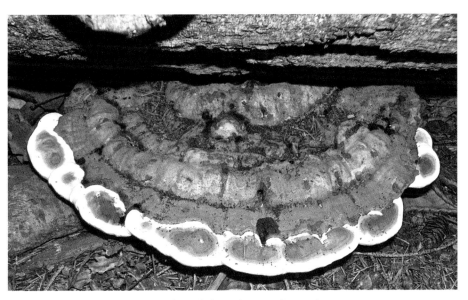

Artist's Conk (Ganoderma applanatum)

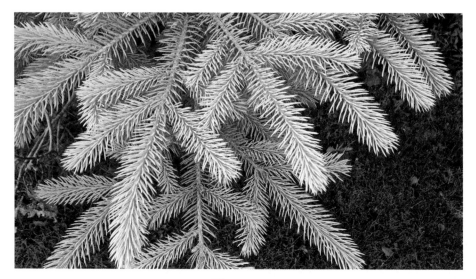

Blue spruce

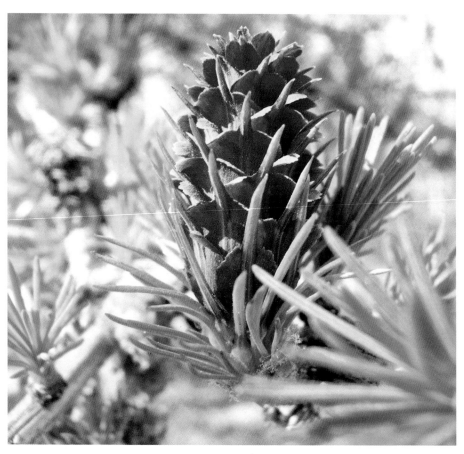

Young tamarack cone

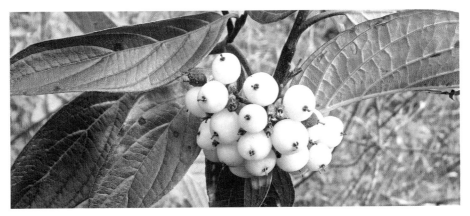

Red Osier Dogwood berries

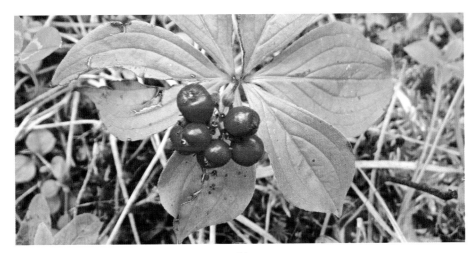

Bunchberry

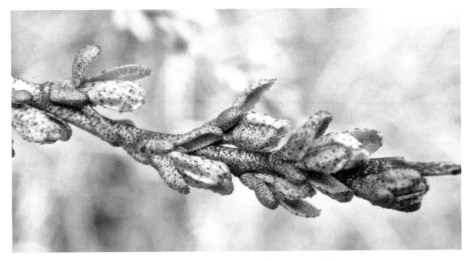

Buffalo Berry stems and leaves—note distinct spotted appearance

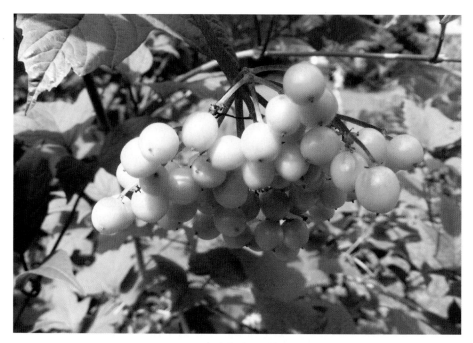

Unripe high bush cranberries

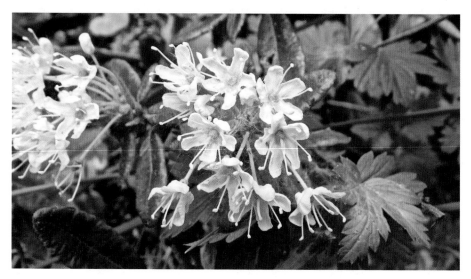

Labrador Tea

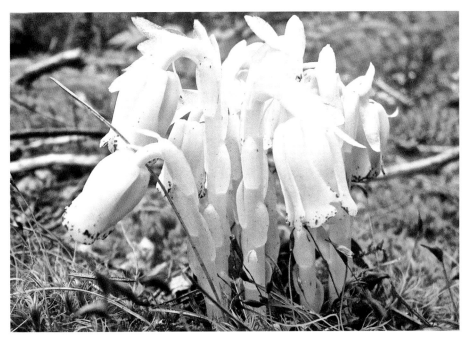

Ghost pipe

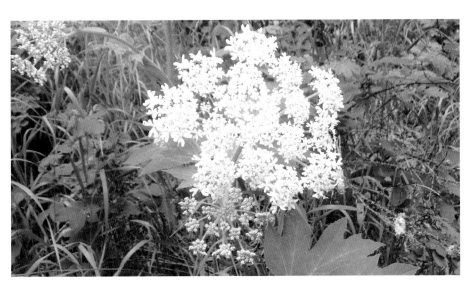

Cow Parsnip flowers

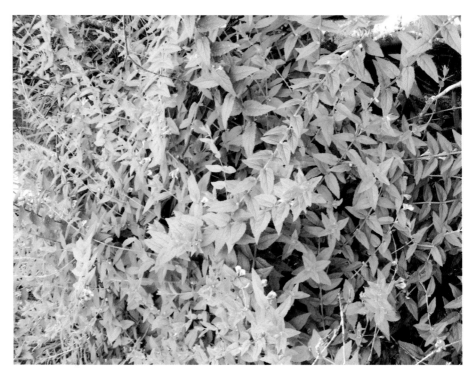

Wild Blue Scullcap (S. lateriflora)

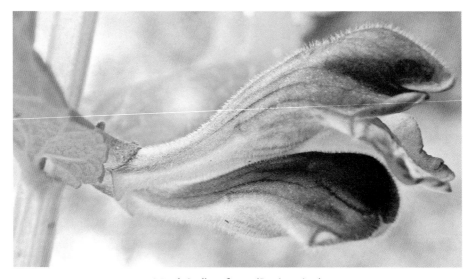

Marsh Scullcap flower (S. galericulata)

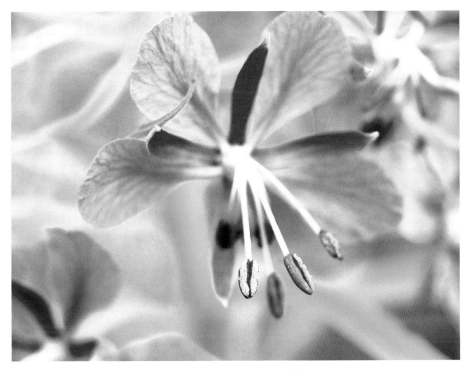

Fireweed—note turquoise pollen

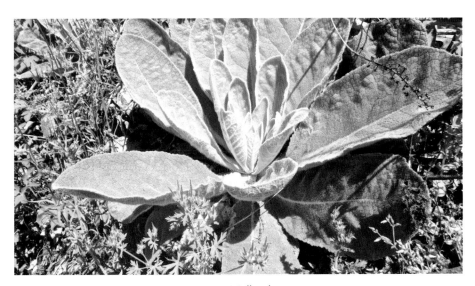

First year Mullein leaves

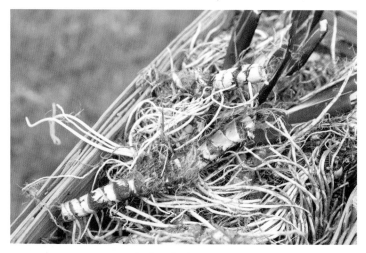

Basket of calamus root

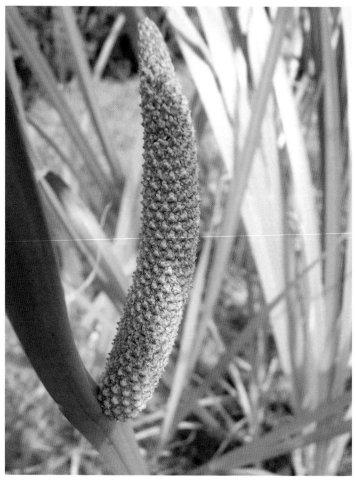

Ripe, fertile seed head of Acorus americanus.

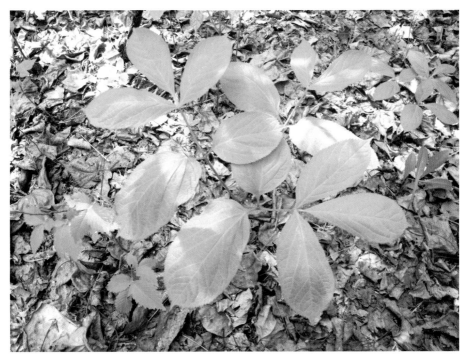

Wild sarsaparilla (Aralia nudicaulis) *in shaded forest*

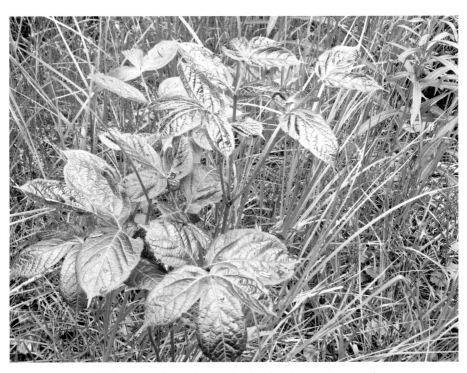

Wild sarsaparilla turning purple when forest canopy is removed

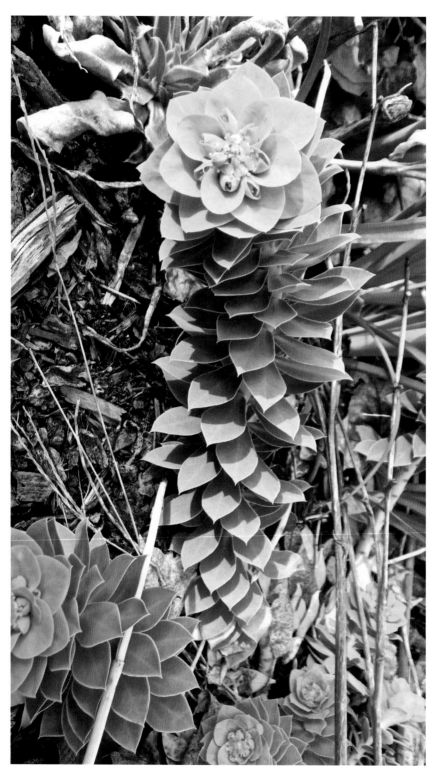

Rhodiola rosea

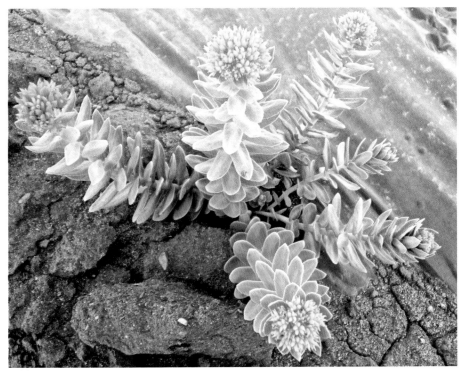

Alberta grown Rhodiola rosea.

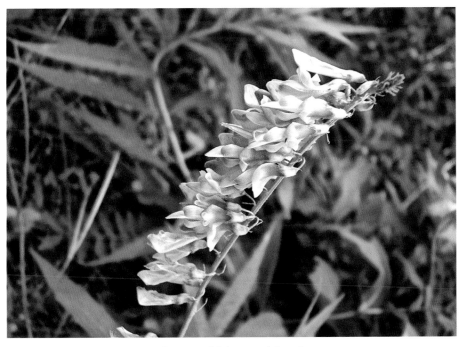

Bear root (Hedysarum alpinum)

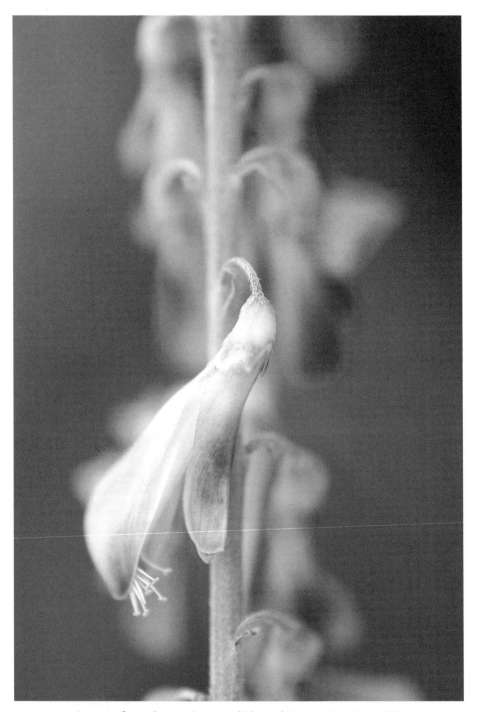

Bear root flower close up. Courtesy of Glen and Maureen Lee, Regina SK.

8

Molting Moon Herbal Allies

Ghost Pipe

Ghost Pipe ✦ Indian Pipe ✦ Ghost of Summer's Woods ✦ Fairy Smoke ✦ Corpse Plant—*Monotropa uniflora* L.

Pinesap ✦ Fringed Pinesap ✦ Yellow Bird's Nest ✦ Dutchman's Pipe—*Monotropa hypopitys* L. ✦ *Hypopitys monotropa* Crantz

Pine Drops ✦ Giant Bird's Nest ✦ Dragon's Claw—*Pterospora andromedea* Nuttall

> *It is the weirdest flower that grows, so palpably ghastly that we feel almost a cheerful satisfaction in the perfection of its performance and our own responsive thrill, just as we do in a good ghost story.*
>
> —Alice M. Earle

> *No wonder this degenerate hangs its head, no wonder it grows black with shame on being picked, as if its wickedness were only just then discovered.… To one who can read the faces of flowers, as it were, it stands a branded sinner.*
>
> —Neltje Blanchan

> *[It] must have been imbued by some evil genius with the idea that the world owed it a living … forthwith it began its search for a way to get its living through the work of others.*
>
> —Arthur C. Quick

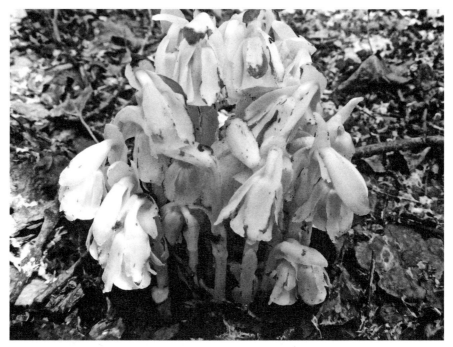

Ghost pipe

The first time I met this herbal ally, I will admit I looked it up in a book. I use the word *plant* consciously because ghost pipe contain no chlorophyll and thus cannot photosynthesis sugars. It appears in a ravine near my home every second year at least, more recently on a regular annual basis. Sometimes I smell them before I see them, exuding a faint urea or ammonia scent. I will often bike down to the area, and as soon as I see the white heads popping out of the soil, I wait about five days and then go harvest them. I cannot help but hum the tune of "A Whiter Shade of Pale" by Procol Harum as I pick the juicy, white stems. I immediately race home and immerse the stems in 70% alcohol at about a 1 to 3 ratio. When tinctured, it initially turns a light turquoise and then deep purple, with a faint chocolate-coffee smell. After two weeks it is ready to press and strain.

Monotropa is derived from *mono*, meaning "one," and *tropo*, "turn," referring to the facing of the flower. *Uniflora* means "one-flowered." The name Indian pipe is from the pipe-bowl shape of the flowers. *Hypopitys* means "under" or "beneath" a pine tree. Linnaeus originally misspelled it as *hypopithys*, and many taxonomists continue to recognize the mistake. *Pterospora* means "winged seed"; *Andromedea* alludes to its resemblance to flowers of the *Andromeda* genus from the Ericaceae family. I don't see it. Andromeda is the Greek goddess of dreams.

After pollination, the flowers rotate upward to form a seedpod. Pine drops may derive from the unopened flowers, resembling resin droplets, or from the sticky surface of the stems. Early students of the plant considered it to be a parasite. Later, Ghost pipe was thought to be a saprophyte, which feeds on dead organic matter containing carbohydrates. The root is a round mass encased in a layer of fungus that easily crumbles into sand. It was thought the fungal mycelium helped in the absorption of carbohydrates.

Erik Björkman (1960), from Stockholm, pointed out mushrooms cannot break down cellulose but rely on dissolved glucose already in the soil. "How can a plant possessing no nutritional store of its own, and no possibility of producing one, grow so rapidly during late summer that it reaches its full development in a week or so?" He noted the fungus on ghost pipe roots was similar to a fungus on the tree root and asked if the plant may well be dependent on the trees. He injected the pines and spruces with radioactive glucose and found that four or five days later, the *Monotropa* showed similar signs of contamination. His work proving the parasitic nature of ghost pipe was published over half a century ago, but many wildflower books still call it a saprophyte. *Sapro* is from the Greek, meaning "putrid," and *phyte* means "plant."

All is not clear, however, as a true parasite is a one-way relationship. Radioactive phosphorus injected in ghost pipe winds up in the neighboring trees. It also produces chemicals that have a powerful stimulating effect on the growth of fungi. I have noted *Russula* species of mushrooms are found in the same proximity. A number of botanists now use the term *epiparasite*, or *mycoheterotroph*, to describe the tripartite relationship between ghost pipe, mycorrhizal fungi, and host trees. Work by Bidartondo and Bruns (2001) has helped clarify

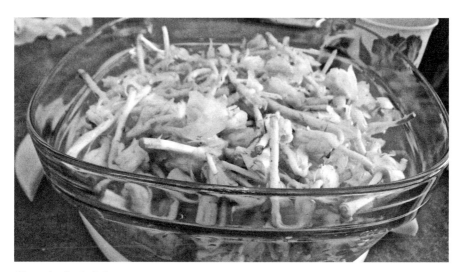

Ghost pipe in alcohol

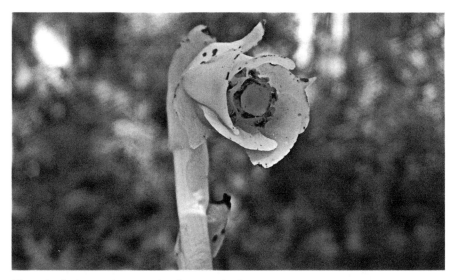

Ghost pipe begins turning upward to form a seedpod

all of this a bit. The roots of *Monotropa* species have a fungal mantle outside and a Hartig-type net of fungal hyphae inside. It appears the plant is taking food from the *Russula* fungi, but how and why? The trees, usually conifers, make sugars and pass them to *Russula*, which translocates them through mycelium in the soil and for some unknown reason hands over part of their food to *Monotropa*.

Ryan Drum shared the work of a team of researchers who watched regeneration of New England land cleared in 1700s and farmed, mowed, and grazed for two hundred years. They found ghost pipe grew in new forest within the first decade, before mushrooms had even appeared. Parasites are supposed to be opportunistic, but here it was growing back before the host community had developed. I attended a talk he gave at the Montana Herb Gathering and wrote this down: "I suspect that *Monotropa* may be far more than just a botanical curiosity, and actually a critical factor or component in long-term forest health." He once ate one ounce of the raw tops and felt nauseous. It is said to taste a bit like asparagus when cooked, but I have never had the desire to try it. It has a waxy, blue-white coloration that appears eerily out of place in the plant kingdom.

Traditional Uses

The Cree call it *mipitahmaskihkih*, meaning "teeth medicine." They chewed the flowers for toothache. It was considered sacred by many tribes and used for various inflammatory afflictions. The clear juice was mixed with water to soothe sore eyes and rubbed into persistent wounds that would not heal. The Cherokee call it *unesdala* and traditionally used the pulverized root as an aid for convulsion and epilepsy in children. The Nlaka'pamux (Thompson) name is "wolf urine" or "wolf's pipe" in the belief that the plant grew wherever wolves relieved themselves. They considered it very valuable for sores that would not heal. I believe the name derives from the ammonia-like smell of the herb. This tribe and other First Nations people believed Ghost Pipe was an indicator of many wood mushrooms in the coming season.

It was used for fevers, insomnia and other nervous irritation; and combines well with willow bark for this purpose. It was placed in the *Canada Pharmacopoeia* in 1868, one year after the birth of the country. The plant shows insecticidal activity. It produces a multitude of seeds with no stored food. When the seeds hit the ground, mushroom hyphae enter them and are then coerced into providing the seeds the nutrients needed to grow.

Pinesap looks similar but is multiflowered and a tawny yellow color. The Thompson tribe called it hummingbird's sucking substance, a term also given to harebell, Indian paintbrush, honeysuckle, and beard's tongue. It yields, upon distillation, a volatile oil containing methyl salicylate. Gerard (1633) wrote that pinesap

> *hath many tangling roots platted or crossed one over another very intricately, which resembleth a Crowes nest made of sticks; from which riseth up a thicke soft grosse stalk of a browne colour, set with short leaves of the colour of a dry Oken leafe that hath lien under the tree all the winter. On the top of the stalke groweth a spikie eare or tuft of floures.*

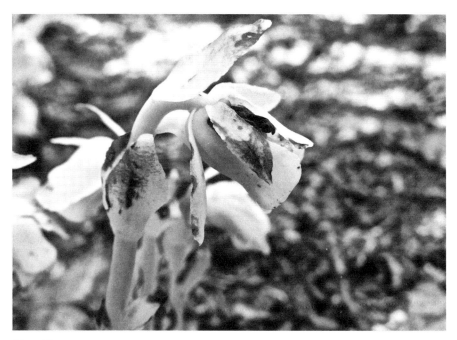

Ghost Pipe

Pinesap shares a complex fungi, tree, and saprophytic system. Some studies suggest substances from these plants help trees fight disease. In the summer of 2002, Laurie and I

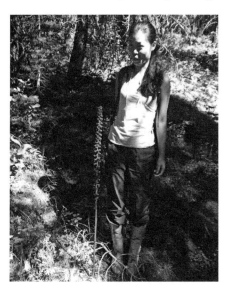

made a family reunion trip to Nova Scotia. One night while mushroom picking with my cousin Gary, I saw the largest ring of pinesap in my life. There were at least forty individual heads in a twenty-five foot diameter circle under a two-hundred-year-old pine tree.

They tend to correspond with *Tricholoma* genus fungi, rather than *Russula*, associated with ghost pipe.

Pinedrops are known as giant bird's nest and called nosebleed medicine by the Tsitsistas (Cheyenne). The flowers resemble drops of resin, hence the name. Or perhaps it comes from the sticky surface of the stems. They are considered mycohetero-trophic and live in association with *Rhizo-pogon* fungi. Pinedrops are rare in eastern North America and should be protected.

Pinedrops

On the west side of the continent, they are abundant. A large plant can hold up to 128 capsules, each containing up to four thousand seeds. Tsitsistas used cold infusions of the powdered stems and berries for bleeding lungs as well as nosebleeds, due to its astringent nature. The Nlaka'pamux of British Columbia used root infusions for gonorrhea. Grinnel (1905) wrote that pinedrops were

> used to prevent nose-bleeding and bleeding from the lungs. Grind the fresh stem and berries together, make an infusion in boiling water, and let it cool. When cold, snuff some of the infusion up the nose and put some of it on the head for nosebleed and drink it for bleeding at the lungs.

The dry powder was used at one time as a snuff for nosebleeds. The Salish (Flathead) of Montana boiled pinedrops with clematis vine (*Clematis columbiana*) as a hair shampoo.

Medicinal Uses

Constituents: *M. uniflora*: various glycosides, gaultherin, andromedotoxin, and salicylic acid.

M. hypopitys: gaultherin, precursor to methyl salicylate.

William Cook, in *The Physio-Medical Dispensatory* (1869), wrote of ghost pipe:

This root is a pleasant-tasting and nearly pure relaxant, with only a modicum of stimulating action, and a little demulcent property. Very diffusive in action, and perhaps unsurpassed for the promptness with which it secures a profuse perspiration. As a diaphoretic, it is of the first value in all febrile cases—relieving arterial excitement and abating nervous irritability. It is of equal service in erysipelas, measles, pneumonia, pleurisy, phrenitis, and other acute inflammations; soothing the patient and restoring the capillary circulation without depressing the system. The uterine organs feel its action promptly; and it promotes the catamenia and lochia, relieves painful menstruation, acts to fine effect in acute ovarian and uterine inflammation, and is of value in after-pains and puerperal fever. Dose, ten to twenty grains every two hours or oftener; usually given in warm water, but not often made in infusion because of the great loss of strength occasioned by heat.

Ghost pipe is a sedative, cooling, and drying tonic with antispasmodic properties. The tincture is valuable for nervous irritability, restlessness, epilepsy, and other neuromuscular disorders. I have used it in combination for issues such as painful dysmenorrhea or fibromyalgia. A douche can relieve vaginal infection and irritation. It can be added in small amounts, the equivalent of four to six drops per dose. The fresh juice can be used to treat blepharitis or conjunctivitis. Gently rub the base of the eyelid with juice to liquefy the oil glands.

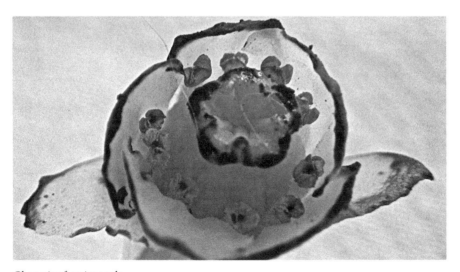

Ghost pipe forming seeds

Its action is similar, according to herbal colleague David Winston, to the effect of nitrous oxide at the dentist: "You are conscious and aware of the pain, but distant from it." It therefore raises pain tolerance and is used with anodyne and anti-inflammatory herbs in combination. He suggests combining it with *Dicentra canadensis* for the chronic pain of cancer. Traditional herbalist and friend Sean Donahue believes:

> Ghost pipe is not disorienting or intoxicating in the ways that nitrous oxide is. Indeed, so far, when I've given Indian pipe for physical pain, I've seen the person become more lucid, present, and grounded. It's a horizontal shift, a refocusing of attention away from the pain.
>
> Ghost pipe helps to manage the flow of sensory information, easing panic. In all but two cases I have seen one or two 30-drop doses of ghost pipe tincture allow a person have a "bad trip" to calm down within a few minutes, and then go to sleep within fifteen to thirty minutes, waking up completely lucid several hours later.
>
> Ghost pipe seems to work by helping a person better manage the onslaught of sensation in an intense situation—be it physical pain or emotional trauma—just as the plant maintains the integrity of the chemical and electromagnetic signals sent within its own body that are necessary to its functioning even while remaining tapped into the torrents of information moving across the networks of roots and mycelia beneath the forest floor.
>
> The second is that ghost pipe is probably not operating on a purely physiological level. Our language is inadequate to describe exactly what is happening, but, at the risk of anthropomorphizing the process, I would say that at some level the plant communicates a way of relating to the flow of information that another organism can integrate and make its own.
>
> Ghost Pipe shows us ways to maintain our sense of self while connecting with all that is within and around us, reconnecting with the world beneath the surface of our consciousness—making it safe for what has slept below to emerge into the world again.

Ryan Drum suggests its use as a psychiatric nervine. He cautions that 15 ml or more at a time induces a deep sleep and ultravivid dreams that are frequently erotic. The fresh or preserved juice is specific for all acute and chronic ophthalmic disorders. It may be combined with and preserved by the addition of rose water. Ulcers and inflammations of the bladder are treated with the juice internally.

The dried root, combined with fennel seed, can be used as a decoction for easing vaginal irritation and infection. The root may be dried and powdered. It is used for restlessness, muscle pain, intermittent fever, and nervous disorders. Dr. Stewart considered the dried herb an excellent opium substitute for "easing pain, comforting the stomach, and causing sleep" (Millspaugh 1887, 412).

Ghost pipe and pinesap contain gaultherin, a natural salicylate derivative found in wintergreen (*Gaultheria*) and birch species. It is analgesic and anti-inflammatory and does not cause the stomach bleeds associated with aspirin. Gautherin releases salicylate slowly, but not in the stomach, and leaves COX-1 unaffected. Williamson (2011) writes, "Indian pipe may be employed instead of quinine in treating conditions such as malaria and West Nile virus. Administer a dose of 1 dram the powdered root in warm yarrow tea … 2 or 3 times a day." Of course, this does not account for its total effect, and some unknown compound or compounds, as yet unidentified, may play a role. I do not harvest the root, preferring to harvest the aerial parts on a regular basis, and not destroy the plant.

Recent studies indicate significant antibiotic activity from the aerial parts of Indian pipe against MRSA. Water, acetone, ether, and alcohol extracts of the fresh stem all show activity against gram-positive bacteria. Yellow Bird's Nest tincture was recommended for whooping cough and spasmodic coughing without expectoration (Steinmetz 1954).

In Europe, pinedrops are used as a sedative and induce perspiration as a diaphoretic.

No record exists of homeopathic provings, but due to the relative rarity of this beautiful plant, it would be worthy of trial.

Flower Essence

In 1992 I made an essence of ghost pipe. Here is a summary of my travels with the plant. It is a research essence of Prairie Deva Flower Essences.

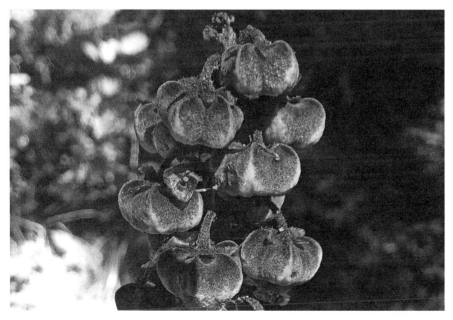

Pinedrops

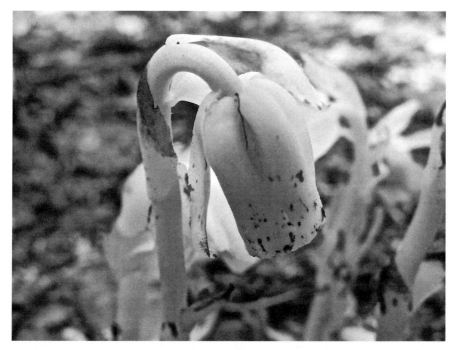

Ghost pipe

Indian pipe flower essence is for those who suffer love sickness. The breaking up of an intimate relationship is similar to the grieving process from the death of a loved one. Indian pipe helps one move through the stages necessary to begin loving oneself again. It brings light to darkness, particularly in those with one foot on the earth and the other underground.

Personality Traits

The plant reveals its personality to a number of studied authors. Neltje Blanchan (1917) contributed these observations:

> *Among plants as among souls, there are all degrees of backsliders. The foxglove, which is guilty of only sly, petty larceny, wears not the equivalent of the striped suit and the shaved head; nor does the mistletoe, which steals crude food from the tree, but still digests it itself, and is therefore only a dingy yellowish green. Such plants, however, as the broom-rape, pinesap, beech-drops, the Indian pipe, and the dodder—which marks the lowest stage of degradation of them all—appear among their race branded with the*

mark of crime as surely as was Cain. No wonder this degenerate hangs its head; no wonder it grows black with shame on being picked, as if its wickedness were only just then discovered! To think that a plant related on one side to many of the loveliest flowers in Nature's garden—the azaleas, laurels, rhododendrons, and the bonny heather—and on the other side to the modest but no less charming wintergreen tribe, should have fallen from grace to such a depth! Its scientific name, meaning "a flower once turned," describes it during only a part of its career. When the minute, innumerable seeds begin to form, it proudly raises its head erect, as if conscious that it had performed the one righteous act of its life.

A previously unpublished collection of Emily Carr (2006) was published as *Wild Flowers*. I was fortunate to find this at the Royal BC Museum on one of my visits to teach about medicinal mushrooms in Victoria.

The necks look like corpulent maggots whose heads and tails are still below ground. When Ghost has hooked herself about an inch above the soil she straightens one end of the hook. There is a nobble on the top, and this she pokes into the air, and it swells and swells, then it unfolds into a flower something like the old-fashioned columbine before they glorified her spurs and petals. The ghost flower is fleshy in texture and dead white, stalk, leaf, and flower. Her leaves climb the stalk clinging like scales. She stands rigid like gobs of milk that have frozen on the purplish floor of the forest.... There is within her the quality of illumined tranquility which you see in the afterglow that sometimes lights the face of a corpse.

Henry David Thoreau wrote:

August 10, 1858. I see many tobacco-pipes, now perhaps in their prime, if not a little late, and hear of pinesap. The Indian pipe, though coming with the fungi and suggesting, no doubt, a close relation to them—a sort of connecting link between flowers and fungi—is a very interesting flower, and will bear close inspection when fresh. The whole plant has a sweetish, earthy odor.... I see them now on the leafy floor of this oak wood, in families of twelve to thirty sisters of various heights—from two to eight inches—as close together as they can stand, the youngest standing close up to the others, all with faces yet modestly turned downwards under their long hoods.... Springing up in the shade with so little color, they look like the more fragile and delicate. They have very delicate pinkish half-naked stems with a few semitransparent crystalline-white scales for leaves, and from the sinuses at the base of the petals without (when their heads are drooping) more or less dark purple is reflected, like the purple of the arteries seen on a nude body. (Searls 2009)

Myths and Legends

One of my favorite legends is from a book by Hamel and Chiltoskey (1975):

> *Before selfishness came into the world, the Cherokee people were happy sharing their hunting and fishing places with their neighbors.… All this changed when Selfishness came into the world.… Finally the chiefs of several tribes met in council to try and settle the dispute. They smoked the pipe and continued to quarrel for seven days and seven nights. This displeased the Great Spirit …[who] decided to do something to remind people to smoke the pipe only at the time they make peace. The Great Spirit turned the old men into grayish flowers we now call Indian pipes and he made them grow where friends and relatives have quarreled. He made the smoke hang over these mountains until all the people all over the world learn to live together in peace.*

RECIPES

Infusion: Ghost pipe does not dry well, turning completely black. Fresh infusions can be made, or use the dried, blackened aerial parts to make into a tea. This is not recommended due to inefficiency.

Dose: 1 teaspoon to 1 pint of water. Drink 1–2 ounces as needed.

Tincture: The fresh plant tincture is a brilliant dark-purple color from the flowering tops. It has a smell reminiscent of Tia Maria liqueur. Make at 1:3 ratio of 70% alcohol. There is no need to harvest the roots.

Dose: 1–20 drops up to 3 times daily. It is a most unusual sedative and relaxant. More than 15 ml per day can result in disturbing dreams. Note the huge variation in dosage. Many people, including herbalists, find low doses of 1–4 drops work well in many cases. My observation from working with this herb is that people have a wide range of pain thresholds, as well as the manner in which they hold pain in their body or are able to release it. It is totally subjective and wonderfully so.

Fresh juice: Mix with equal amounts of water or rose water. A small amount of vegetable glycerin will help preserve. Use external applications for eye inflammation. Internally, use for the bladder. You can also freeze in ice cubes.

Scullcap

Marsh Scullcap—*Scutellaria galericulata* L.

Blue Scullcap—*Scutellaria lateriflora* L.

Marsh scullcap is one of my favorite herbal allies. My nervous system is sensitive, and no other herb works so well for me, helping restore a calm nature. It also helps extinguish the fire of my choleric constitution that is far too reactive when under stress and deadlines. Like editing a book.

Marsh scullcap is common in wet places, shorelines, and streambeds throughout the prairies. It often appears in the same areas as wild mint and bugleweed, which likewise prefer wet feet. However, it has no scent, narrower leaves, and blue flowers at the leaf axils. Bugleweed has white flowers at the axil. It is properly spelled *scullcap*, not *skullcap*.

Another scullcap, naturalized farther east on the prairies, is blue scullcap (*S. lateriflora*). In the summer of 2007, while on a mushroom foray near Lac La Biche, Alberta, I came upon a mature blue scullcap that looked like a three-foot-tall by five-foot-in-diameter bush,

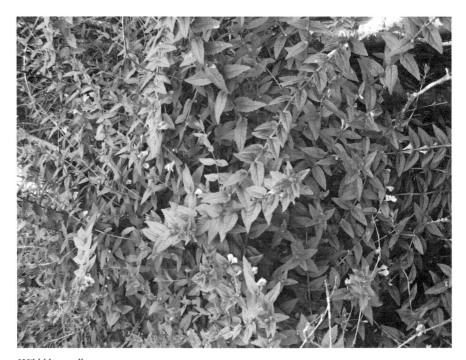

Wild blue scullcap

239

composed of over seventy stalks. I gave thanks and immediately harvested and tinctured it fresh, of course. But why the emphasis on fresh? Because dried aerial parts of scullcap are practically devoid of benefit in comparison to the freshly prepared tincture. Traditionally, herbs were dried for preservation and transport. The term *drug* is derived from *droge*, meaning "to dry." It was the only widespread approach to preserving and transporting herbs in the past.

James Duke (1985) writes that "in commenting on its toxicity, the FDA said, 'As destitute of medicinal properties as a plant may be.'" Today, the FDA suggests large doses can cause dizziness, erratic pulse, mental confusion, twitching of the limbs, and other symptoms indicative of epilepsy. The U.S. *Dispensatory* from 1926 to 1944 said the same thing, noting it "not even being aromatic." It should simply be noted the fresh plant extracts have significantly greater therapeutic value.

Both species are similar in action and were traditionally associated with Saturn, water, and feminine energy. *Scutellaria* is from the Latin *scutella*, meaning "little dish," "tray," or "saucer" and referring to the bell-shaped, lipped calyx or scute at the base of the flower. *Galericulata* means "helmet-shaped," another reference to the flower's appearance. Scullcap is named for the flower's resemblance to a head or skull with a hood; think of a helmet with a raised visor. After going to seed, the inverted calyx closes over it, and hence a cap fitting the skull. This became the plant's doctrine of signatures, suggesting its use for ailments of the skull.

Traditional Uses

Ancient pagan customs used potions of scullcap to be exchanged between those wishing to reconnect in the afterlife. The Cree and other Boreal native healers used the marsh scullcap leaves and flowers as a tea for healing ulcers and fevers. An unusual name for this species by the Cree of southern Saskatchewan is beaver sweetgrass, *amisk(i)-wistak*. The Cherokee used aerial parts of blue scullcap as infusion to suppress menstruation and relieve diarrhea. Decoctions of the root and stem were used to treat breast pain, nerves, and as a postpartum sedative. It is called *gŭ'nïgwalïskï*, meaning "it becomes discolored when bruised." The roots were combined with bear grease to treat skin sores and inflammation.

Tela Star Hawk Lake (1988, 201), a female shaman, notes scullcap is known to treat infertility and "helps regulate sexual desires that may occur in some women whose hormones and sensitivity might increase during menses, and who according to the natural law, custom, beliefs, and practices should abstain from sex during this time." Many other tribes used the plant for diarrhea and various nerve problems. The Ojibwe used scullcap as a heart medicine and poultice for breast pain.

Marsh scullcap (*S. galericulata*) was traditionally used in Europe for intermittent fevers that skip days and cause restless sleep. The number of days between intermittent fevers is an important indicator, helping herbalists pinpoint what organ systems are at play. Scullcap was used in spells of relaxation and peace. Traditionally, a woman would wear a scullcap to protect her husband against the charms of other women.

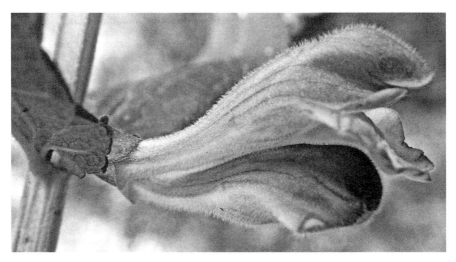

Marsh scullcap flower close-up

Medicinal Uses

Constituents: *S. galericulata*: diterpenes such as jodrellin A and B, 14,15-dihydrojodrellin T, catapol, scutellaine, iridoids, galericulin, scutellarein, two baicaleins (baicalein-7-O-glucuronide and 5,6,7-trihydroxyflavone), baicalein 7-O-beta-L-rhamnofuranoside (galeroside), dihydrobaicalein, 7-O-glucuronide, wogonin, dihydro-norwogonin, scutellarin (scutellarein 7-O-glucuronide), scutellarein (5,6,7,4f-tetrahydroxy-flavone), apigenin 7-O-glucuronide, cosmosiin (apigenin 7-O-glucoside), various waxes (C31, C33, and C35 hydrocarbons), galerosides (baicalein-beta-L-rhamnofuranoside), chrysin (2.7%) and luteolin and their 7-O-glucuronides, oroxyloside (oroxylin A 7-O-glucuronide), oroxylin A, 6-hydroxyluteolin and its 7-O-glucuronide, dihydro-norwogonin-7-O-glucoronide, calcium, potassium, and magnesium phosphate and various flavonoid glycosides, eriodictyol and luteolin glycosides, various neo-clerodane diterpenoids, scutegalerins A, B, C, and D, scutecolumin C, neoajugapyrin A, and tannins 3.5%.

S. lateriflora: catalpol; various flavonoid glycosides, including baicalin, dihydrobaicalin, lateriflorin, ikonnikoside I, scutellarin, and oroxylin A-7-O-glucuronide; the aglycones baicalein, oroxylin A, wogonin, apigenin, hispidulin, luteolin, scutellarein, scutellaric acid, caffeic acid, pomolic acid, ursolic acid, palmitic acid, scutellaterins A–C, acteoside (verbascoside), ajugapitin, scutecypyrol A, 2-methyl alkanes, 3,9-diemthyl alkanes, 3-methyl alkanes, scuteflorins A and B, decursin, chrysin, dihydrochrysin, dihydrooroxylin A, lupenol, volatile oils, lignins, beta-sitosterol, daucosterol, resins, and tannins. Plant is 86% water. As well as baicalein and baicalin, associated with the nervine and sedative effects of Baikal scullcap (*S. baicalensis*) root, the aerial parts contain GABA and glutamine as well as smaller amounts of

241

tryptophan, proline, melatonin, and phenylalanine. 10.9% protein, 102.5 mg vitamin C, and a variety of minerals per 100 grams: aluminum 25.8 mg, calcium 455 mg, chromium 0.7 mg, cobalt 1.1 mg, iron 25 mg, magnesium 113 mg, manganese 4.7 mg, potassium 2,180 mg, selenium 8.3 mg, silicon 4.8 mg, tin 1.2 mg, and zinc 102.5 mg.

Scullcap is foremost a nervine and antispasmodic. In cases of nervous overexcitement, or whenever restlessness accompanies acute or chronic illness, scullcap excels. In children it soothes the nervous system and reduces teething pain. Marsh scullcap is more bitter than its cousin, but both are astringent, cool, dry, relaxing, and restorative. Consider scullcap as a modulator of life energy and flow, useful when emotions and body feel stuck. It combines well with California poppy, wild peony root, or black cohosh for muscle tension. But while relaxing the nervous tension, it revives and fortifies the central nervous system. It is a specific for seizures and epilepsy, and combines well with cow's parsnip for sciatica, trigeminal neuralgia, and fascial pains.

Zhang et al. (2009) identified ten flavonoids and two phenylethanoid glycosides that show anticonvulsant and acute seizure amelioration in a rodent model. Scullcap plays an important role in regulating the balance of adrenaline and noradrenalin, a hormonal function that appears as a nervous disorder. This may explain in part its usefulness in reducing PMS symptoms. It encourages the brain to produce endorphins, which not only promote sleep but ease worry and anxiety. It may be useful when experiencing anxiety and agitation while taking entheogens such as marijuana, psilocybin, and other psychoactive substances. Older studies in Russia have confirmed the plant's usefulness as a sedative and stabilizer of stress-related cardiovascular problems.

Usow (1958) found the herb lowers blood pressure and blood cholesterol levels. It has a cardiotonic action that clinically reduces heart rate and both systolic and diastolic blood pressure. Scullcap helps reduce chest pain and heart palpitations, combining well with motherwort, and it reduces irritability and nervous stress due to nervous tension and unrest. Sean Donahue combines the herb with passionflower "when circular thinking or spiraling thoughts are part of the picture." I have not tried smoking the dried herb, but Sean believes it works more quickly this way.

Noted herbalist 7Song thinks along the same lines, using the herb for those who think too much or overthink and have trouble initially getting to sleep. They tend to go over the past day and how they might have done things differently. This reminds me a lot of White Chestnut, the flower remedy developed by Edward Bach for helping quiet a racing mind at bedtime. As a brain tonic, it calms the mind and reduces hot emotions like anger, jealousy, and hatred, thereby promoting clarity, detachment, and calm awareness. I have studied and practiced iridology for over forty years. I would suggest scullcap is well suited to the neurogenic genotype, with its attendant hypersensitivity to allergies and the environment in general.

By calming the fetus, it may prevent miscarriage or premature birthing. Matthew Wood (2009, 325) suggests it may be useful in gestational diabetes with an agitated fetus and when the mother's skin is somewhat irritated. It combines well with other herbs for oversensitivity of peripheral nerves and relieves sciatic, neuralgic, and shingle pain. It calms incessant hiccups and coughing related to sensory overload and irritability. One of my herbal students asked me about her husband's prolonged eighteen-day hiccup issue and found that scullcap resolved the issue permanently within twenty-four hours.

Scullcap is useful in the motor symptoms associated with Sydenham's chorea (formerly Saint Vitus' dance) and the nerve pain associated with early stages of MS. It may have application with other herbs in anorexia nervosa, mild cases of Tourette's syndrome, and pain associated with fibromyalgia. Dr. Christopher, an early teacher, combined equal parts of scullcap, feverfew, and lady's slipper for chorea, taken as a cold infusion. For insomnia and nervous sleepers, he suggested equal parts of scullcap, lady's slipper, skunk cabbage, and pleurisy root as fluid extract or tincture. Lady's slipper is rare and endangered in my part of the world, so I substitute small amounts of corydalis (*C. aureum*), which is plentiful. California poppy would be another suitable companion herbal ally.

For treating delirium tremens of alcoholism, combine 2 parts of herb with 1 part American ginseng root. The fresh plant tincture of scullcap is preferred, but in the case of alcohol addiction, the freeze-dried aerial parts would be a good solution. A fresh glycerite may also be appropriate. Warm infusions keep the skin moist via diaphoretic action, while cool infusions are more toning.

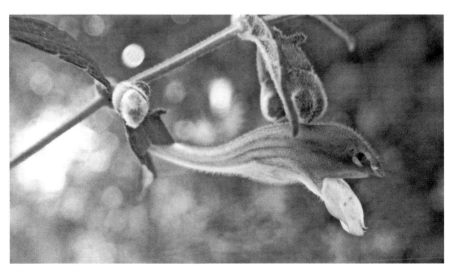

Blue scullcap flowers

Many of the compounds found in aerial parts of marsh and blue scullcap are found in the root of *S. baicalensis*, widely used in TCM. Trembling limbs, spinal meningitis, epilepsy, convulsions, tetanus, and various localized paralytic conditions, including pain associated with MS, respond well to scullcap. Shingle pain may be relieved by internal use of the fresh tincture. Its bitter properties may be helpful in irregular heartbeat associated with alcohol, cigarettes, and hypertension. Heart and kidney yin-deficient symptoms may include afternoon flushes or heat, night sweats, ringing in the ears, and general irritability.

In vitro studies have found scullcap possesses antibacterial and antihistamine activity. Clinical studies by Stefan et al. (1995) indicate that flavonoid glycosides of *S. galericulata* possess antihistaminic activity. Barberan (1986) found flavonoids such as baicalin present in *S. galericulata*. This may explain in part the anti-inflammatory, diuretic, and antiallergic properties of the herb. Baicalin-7-rhamnoside inhibits glyoxylase I and platelet lipoxygenase, while baicalein, in high levels, prolongs the clotting time of fibrinogen by thrombin. It is also an antipromoter in carcinogenesis.

Chrysin, present in poplar buds and bee propolis, is found in its 7-glucuronidein form in marsh scullcap. This compound is anti-inflammatory and antibiotic, reduces lens aldose reductase, induces estrogen synthetase and hemoglobin, and inhibits iodothyrine deiodinase. Chrysin taken daily for six weeks reduced elevated blood pressure and cardiac hypertrophy due to antioxidant activity (Villar et al. 2002). Chrysin also appears to activate GABA(A) receptors (Zanoli et al. 2000). The *Physician's Desk Reference (PDR) for Herbal Medicines* suggests blue scullcap (*S. lateriflora*) shows lipid peroxide inhibitor effects, suggestive of antioxidant activity.

Stefan Gafner et al. (2003), at the University of Ottawa, discovered blue scullcap contains the flavones baicalein and baicalin, long associated with the nervine and sedative properties of more famous Baikal scullcap of China. This study found a 70% ethanol extract contained various compounds, one of which, ikonnikoside I, showed the highest inhibition of [³H]-LSD binding as well as activity on 5-HT receptors. Until recently, almost all research on scullcap focused on the Chinese herb, probably the main reason much more is known of that species. See Awad et al. (2003) for more constituents of *S. lateriflora*.

Another paper by Makino et al. (2008) found baicalin and other flavonoids in the leaf similar to the constituents found in root of *S. baicalensis*. The authors suggest the classification of aerial parts of *S. lateriflora* as nonactive needs reconsideration. Really? Do you think? The reality is scutellarein wogonin, baicalein, and baicalin all contain phenylbenzopyrone nuclei and bind to the benzodiazepine site of the GABA receptor (Hui et al. 2000). Baicalein is a potent inhibitor of GABA transaminase, and scutellarein inhibits succinic semialdehyde dehydrogenase, both of which increase GABA levels in the brain (Tao et al. 2008). That is, scutellarein can assist the brain to produce more endorphins and thereby enhance awareness and calmness. This suggests use in panic attacks, stress-induced headaches, and emotional trauma.

Scutellarin possesses both estrogenic and neuroprotective properties. This may have benefit in postmenopausal symptoms as well as Alzheimer's disease due to in vitro inhibition of beta-amyloid and prevention of neuron cell death (Zhu et al. 2009). It also enhances uptake of niacin. Scutellarin may be helpful in MS by protecting neural stem cells (Wang et al. 2016). Blue scullcap and its flavonoids baicalein and baicalin were found in vitro and in vivo to inhibit accumulation of encoded prions associated with spongiform encephalopathy. The tea prolonged incubation time of scrapie-infected mice upon oral treatment (Eiden et al. 2012). The best-known prion disease is Creutzfeldt-Jakob disease, but new variants are emerging. Bovine spongiform encephalopathy (BSE) or mad cow disease may be a far greater and more widespread issue than revealed to the general public.

Blue scullcap exhibits significant antioxidant activity and has great therapeutic potential against stress associated with mental disorders. Scutellarin inhibits cancer cell metastasis and attenuates development of fibrosarcoma in vivo (Shi et al. 2015). Baicalin is an effective antianxiety flavonoid that works synergistically with other herbs and drugs. Scullcap is quite useful in those individuals suffering nervous tension from withdrawal of tobacco or opium-derived drugs, combining well with hops, lady's slipper, black cohosh, and catnip as both a nerve tonic and sleep aid. Green flowering oats may be a useful addition for opiate withdrawal.

It is worth noting that scullcap is a cooling herb and works best for those individuals with a hot or warm constitution. Valerian root, on the other hand, is a warming herb, and more useful to those with cool or cold constitution. This is a vast generalization and not a hard and fast rule. Dosage is equally important, especially with valerian root. Scullcap combines well with vervain for insomnia in some individuals.

A double-blind placebo-controlled crossover study of 19 healthy volunteers involved subjective rating of energy, cognition, and anxiety associated with three different doses of freeze-dried scullcap or placebo. The effect on anxiety was most pronounced in all three preparations, with 200 mg dosage having the greatest benefit (Wolfson and Hoffmann 2003). A recent randomized double-blind placebo-controlled crossover study with *S. lateriflora* in 43 healthy volunteers found no significant difference for the mildly anxious (81%) group. However, there was a highly significant difference in anxiety levels from pretest scores with the herb but not placebo. The authors suggest that because scullcap enhanced global mood without a reduction in energy or cognition, a future study should look at notably anxious subjects with comorbid depression. The aerial parts were freeze-dried, and the placebo was freeze-dried nettles (Brock et al. 2014). Maybe nettles was not the best placebo, for several reasons.

Baicalin is active against *Chlamydia trachomatis* via protease-like activity and may be worth trialing in chlamydia infections (Hao et al. 2009). Qian Wang et al. (2004) found coupling baicalin with zinc is a far more effective inhibitor of recombinant reverse transcriptase and HIV-1 entry into host cells, reducing the EC_{50} by threefold. A combination of baicalin and catechin derived from two plant sources has been found to demonstrate significant COX-1 and COX-2 inhibition. An in vitro study on human cells found it was more effective than ibuprofen in acting as a LOX pathway inhibitor and suppressed the gene expression of key pro-inflammatory cytokines. The antioxidant activity is nearly four times more powerful than vitamin C.

Baicalin modulates Th1-Th2 balance of the immune system by increasing IL-10 production and may be of use in treating asthma (Huang et al. 2009). Th-1 cells protect against bacterial and viral diseases. A Th-2–stimulated immune system protects from parasites and worms and helps produce antibodies against pathogens. The dark side is that Th-2 dominance creates a predisposition to allergies and asthma. Most people are Th-1 dominant, and these cytokines protect us against viruses, cancer, and certain mycoplasma bacteria that get into cells. The bad side of this dominance is that it can launch an attack against your own cells and create autoimmune response, organ transplant rejection, and even fetal rejection. In fact, women switch from Th-1 dominance to Th-2 dominance during pregnancy. This is why sashimi is not recommended for pregnant women.

In countries with good hygiene, vaccination, and antibiotics, a low level of Th-1 stimulation results in an increase in Th-2. This triggers exaggerated mucus production and contraction of muscles in the airways that can cause allergies and asthma. In the reverse scenario, where pathogens are abundant and vaccination and antibiotic use is low, Th2 responses are activated, leading to repeated cycles of infection and inflammation, the latter countered with natural antiallergic reactions. It is as if Th-2 has learned to recognize an innocuous but foreign substance and respond, but does not produce a panic response with swollen tissue and dripping glands. Zinc supplementation supports Th-1 but diminishes protection against worms and parasites. Insufficient zinc and poor nutrition means that worm defense flourishes and defense against pathogens like viruses grows weaker. Vitamin A has the opposite effect, boosting protection against parasites and decreasing cell-entry defense. Baicalin stops hormonal reactions that constrict the bronchial tubes, causing asthma, and prevents DNA damage caused by dexamethasone, a drug used to treat asthma.

Baicalin has been found to potentiate the effectiveness of beta-lactam antibiotics against MRSA and other resistant strains (Liu et al. 2000). Baicalin has been found in laboratory studies to be effective against human T cell leukemia virus and Epstein-Barr virus and protects liver tissue from free-radical damage associated with iron excess. It may be worthy of a trial in preventing organ damage in patients with hemachromatosis. Baicalin induced apoptosis of several prostate cancer cell lines, suggesting adjuvant therapy in prostate cancer or chemoprevention (Chan et al. 2000). Scullcap and fireweed may be a useful combination for this issue. Baicalin, in low concentrations, has been found to increase the uptake of nimodipine across the blood-brain barrier. Berberine, found in Oregon grape root and goldenseal, does the same thing. Baicalin shows anti-fibrotic activity on liver cells. Baicalin and baicalein show potent inhibitory effect on amyloid-beta

246

protein induced neurotoxicity, suggesting possible use in chemoprevention of Alzheimer's disease (Heo et al. 2004).

Baicalin is transformed to baicalein by intestinal bacteria, absorbed in the intestine, and conjugated back to baicalin in the blood plasma (Akao et al. 2000). Baicalin is a strong glycation inhibitor, suggesting benefit in type 2 diabetic conditions (Grzegorczyk-Karolak et al. 2016). Baicalein appears to protect against and possibly treat Parkinson's disease (Mu et al. 2009). It inhibits prolyl-oligopeptidase associated with bipolar, schizophrenia, and other related neurodisorders (Tarragó et al. 2008). It appears to protect SH-SY5Y cells and be a potent inhibitor of alpha-synuclein and amyloid beta-peptide–induced toxicity in PC12 cells, suggesting benefit in Alzheimer's and Parkinson's diseases. It blocks activation of the aryl hydrocarbon receptor, suggestive of protection from environmental pollutants. Baicalein is highly active in neutralizing, for example, the harmful effects of cigarette smoke. This flavone blocks the action of phospholipase. It seems that baicalein lessens the influx of calcium through the cell membrane and inhibits the release of calcium from the sarcoplasmic reticulum inside the cell. This decreases activation of phospholipase and inflammatory response.

Baicalein prolongs clotting time of fibrinogen by thrombin, acting on thrombin protease activated receptors. Baicalein inhibits osteoclast and bone resorption, suggesting possible use in the prevention or treatment of osteoporosis (Kim et al. 2008). Research has shown baicalein-induced apoptosis or cellular suicide of four pancreatic cancer cell types. It down-regulates antiapoptoic Mcl-1 protein associated with pancreatic cancer cell lines. Baicalein inhibits cancer cell multiplication and induces cancer cell death in vitro. Scullcap appears to be synergistic with cyclophosphamide and 5-fluorouracil (5FU) by decreasing tumor-cell viability and improving tolerance to cytostatic agents (Razina et al. 1987). Baicalein nearly doubles the bioavailability of doxorubicin, suggesting dosage changes and effectiveness (Shin et al. 2009).

Baicalein reduces the gastrointestinal distress associated with ritonavir, a protease inhibitor taken by some AIDS patients. Baicalin and baicalein are antiviral, antioxidant, antitumor, and anti-inflammatory, and reduce blood pressure and relax arterial smooth-muscle cells. Both compounds have been found by Huang et al. (2004) to inhibit endothelial aortic relaxation via inhibition of cyclic GMP accumulation in vascular smooth-muscle cells. This suggests its benefit in acute edema and inhibition of lipoxygenase, involved in inflammation. Baicalein and baicalin inhibit alpha-glucosidase, suggesting use in blood sugar issues (Kuroda et al. 2012). Baicalin inhibits sucrase activity in the small intestine and may play a role in antidiabetic activity.

Chrysin is found in decent amounts in marsh scullcap. More information on this compound can be found in the section on poplar in Chapter 5. Chrysin, baicalin, baicalein, and wogonin all show activity against the H1N1 virus, and all are more potent than the drug oseltamivir phosphate (Ji et al. 2015).

Scutellarein was tested in a clinical trial of 634 patients with cerebral embolism, cerebral thrombosis, or stroke-induced paralysis. The compound improved blood flow in more than 88% of patients, either ingested or injected (Xiao and Chen 1987). Scutellarein inhibits proliferation of cells associated with diabetic retinopathy and inhibits hypoxia (Rong Gao et al. 2008). The compound inhibits new DNA synthesis catalyzed by Rous-associated virus-2 reverse transcriptase, an additive benefit to baicalin activity. Scutellarin increases cerebral blood flow and inhibits ADP-induced platelet aggregation (Xiao and Chen 1987). Scutellarin may be helpful in postmenopausal symptoms and Alzheimer's disease (Zhu et al. 2009). Scutellarin, according to Williamson (2011), helps stimulate the brain to produce more endorphins and enhance awareness and calmness.

Wogonin is present in blue and marsh scullcap. Baicalin and wogonin inhibit basal mucin release and increase ATP-induced release, suggesting a mucoregulation that may be useful in various respiratory conditions, including chronic and genetic defect diseases (Heo et al. 2007). Active metabolites of baicalin and wogonin glucuronide (baicalein and wogonin, respectively), as well as isoscutellarein-8-O-glucuronide, are potent inhibitors of the enzyme sialidase (Nagai et al. 1989). Sialic acids are present in mucous secretions and cell membranes and are thought to be the sites at which viruses attach to cell walls.

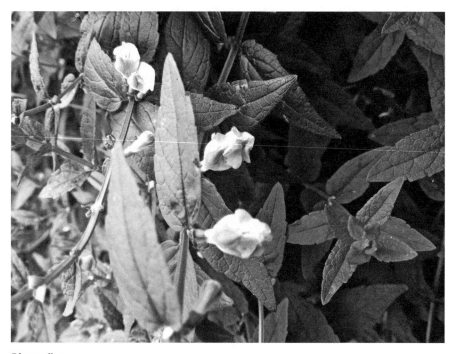

Blue scullcap

Serum sialic acid increases in certain cancers, infections, inflammations, and rheumatic disease. Inhibition of sialidase may have therapeutic use in these conditions. Wogonin, baicalin, baicalein, and oroxylin A affect different brain receptors in vitro. It exerts an antianxiety effect in mice without sedative or muscle relaxant activity. Wogonin inhibits the growth of *Vibrio cholerae*, the gram-negative bacillus responsible for cholera. It also inhibits collagen and arachidonic acid–induced blood platelet aggregation and triglyceride deposition. Wogonin inhibits tumors associated with estrogen-positive and negative breast cancer cell lines, especially the more aggressive latter (Chung et al. 2008).

Scutellaria species appear to be tumor-specific to malignant glioma as well as breast and prostate cancers. Parajuli et al. (2009). Interesting work by Huang et al. (2009) found scutellarin and wogonin significantly inhibited MCF breast cancer cells in vitro, but scutellarin and baicalin increased cancer growth. Somehow this became translated, by pharmaceutical reductionists, that scullcap without baicalin may be better for treating human breast cancer.

Wogonin acts on androgen receptors and lowers PSA levels, suggesting benefit as well in prostate inflammation and cancers (S. Chen et al. 2008). Wogonin can suppress HBV surface antigen production without any evidence of cytotoxicity. A more recent study on the hepatitis B virus confirmed potent activity of wogonin, at least in vitro. Wogonin inhibits COX-2 and inducible nitric oxide synthase and inhibits IL-6–induced angiogenesis by down-regulating VEGF and VEGFR-1. Wogonin inhibits COX-2 by inhibiting c-Jun expression and AP-1 activation in A549 cells. Wogonin inhibits osteoclast formation induced by lipopolysaccharide. It helps prevent glucocorticoid-induced thymocyte apoptosis without diminishing anti-inflammatory efficacy. Wogonin inhibits migration of gallbladder GBC-SD cancer cells by inducing expression of maspin (Dong et al. 2011). Work by Lee et al. (2009) found wogonin potentiates action on cancer cells but not normal cells. Wogonin reduces the damage of etoposide in normal cells and potentiated activity against tumor cells (Enomoto et al. 2011).

Catapol is found in scullcap species and mullein. It possesses an antidepressant-like effect mediated through the serotonin pathways (Wang et al. 2014). Cosmosiin may be helpful in diabetic complications through enhanced adiponectin secretion, tyrosine phosphorylation of insulin receptor-beta, and GLUT4 translocation (Rao et al. 2011).

Scullcap is somewhat interchangeable with hops in cases of panic attacks, night sweats, insomnia, and more kidney yin deficiency conditions. But that is where the comparisons end. For skin itching associated with menopausal hot flashes, or that crawling skin irritation associated with insomnia, combined with lady's mantle and/or St. John's wort. Scullcap tincture helps depress uterine activity, and can be used in cases of threatened miscarriage. For muscle cramping, combine equal parts of crampbark, skunk cabbage root, and blue scullcap as a hot infusion. For nerve pain, consider combining with corydalis or California poppy. Taken at first symptoms, the fresh tincture can relieve shingle pain (herpes zoster).

Take 20 to 40 drops 3 to 4 times daily at onset. Noted herbalist Daniel Gagnon recommends blue scullcap for phantom limb pain, quickly relieving shingle, and other herpes-related pain, when the patient "wants to crawl out of their skin."

Research by Peredery and Persinger (2004) found no seizure after inducement following administration of blue scullcap. It is worth a trial when Dilantin has been given for cases of idiopathic epilepsy with no brain lesions, and based on a single childhood episode. I used it with good success in several cases of misdiagnosed epilepsy, sometimes combining the herb with passionflower leaf when the pattern fit. Take 40 drops of fresh tincture at the aura phase of epilepsy, and it will often prevent developing into seizure. The same dose in water before bedtime may prevent petit mal while sleeping in affected individuals.

Scullcap flavonoids help strengthen collagen and protein in fibroblasts, suggesting use in periodontal disease. Gargle, swish, and swallow the tea or diluted tincture. Interesting work by Cole et al. (2008) found melatonin, serotonin, baicalin, baicalein, scutellarin, and wogonin in clonal plants. Serotonin levels were fivefold higher in *S. lateriflora* than *S. baicalensis*. Baicalin content was similar but baicalein content was higher than two other species tested.

Jiayu Gao et al. (2008) analyzed a number of blue scullcap commercial preparations. They found a wide range of active ingredients, including a number with 0% of the three most studied constituents. Ranges included 0–12.6 mg/mL for baicalin, 0–0.63 for baicalein, and 0–0.16 for wogonin. This may reflect the difference between various harvesting, drying, or preparation techniques, or it may reflect on poor manufacturing and

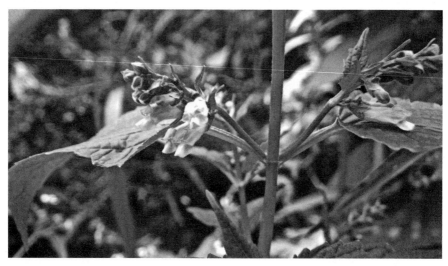

Blue scullcap

adulteration. I like to prepare my scullcap as fresh as possible. Michael Moore (2003) wrote, "Some peculiar observations I have had about our scullcaps: *S. galericulata* is the strongest, most anti-inflammatory, and least complicated." Insist upon fresh plant tinctures, or prepare them yourself.

Scullcap prevents a rise in serum cholesterol in animals on high-cholesterol diets. This might be helpful in miniature schnauzers and beagles prone to cholesterol problems. Scullcap works well in veterinary applications for panic, meningitis, nervous spasms, lack of appetite, and gastroenteritis. This includes dogs and cats as well as farm animals. The herb may benefit animals suffering epilepsy or seizure activity. Ask your holistic veterinarian for advice in such matters.

Homeopathy

Homeopathic scullcap is a nerve sedative that relieves cardiac irritability as well as nervous muscle twitching. There is often a mental expectation of calamity, with restless sleep and frightful dreams. Males may be prone to seminal emissions or impotency, with fear of it never improving. There may be migraine or dull frontal headaches over the right eye. All symptoms are exaggerated with noise, odors, and light but see improvement from rest and are better in the evening. Hiccups, fear of snakes, and constant dry cough may be present, with symptoms worse from lying down at night.

I have noted improvement in cystic fibrosis muscle and nerve irritability from use of homeopathic scullcap. Nickel allergy may be present, a craving for vinegar, or a sensation of a lump in the throat so one cannot swallow. Recurrent tonsillitis responds well, and the thyroid gland may be swollen or enlarged.

Dose: 5 drops of the mother tincture to lower potencies. The mother tincture is made from *S. lateriflora* aboveground plant in its prime. Provings originated with self-experimentation by Gordon with tincture in 1865 and Royal with nine provers at 3X and 30X in 1897. Hale, Boericke, and Mangialavori have added additional clinical observations.

Essential Oils

Although a member of the mint family, the plant has no perceptible scent. However, upon steam distillation, a low yield of interesting essential oils occurs. The hydrosol may be of interest. Note the significant difference of oil constituents between the two species.

Scullcap (*S. galericulata*) yields an essential oil upon distillation composed of caryophyllene (30%), beta-farnescene (17%), menthone (10.4%), 1-octen-3-ol (8%), and other monoterpenes, including limonene, germacrene D, gamma-humulene, and beta-cubebene.

S. lateriflora has a different essential oil composition: mainly sesquiterpenes (78%), including delta-cadinene (27%), calamenene (15.2%), beta-elemene (9.2%), cubebene, and humulene (8.4%). At least 73 compounds have been identified in the oil.

Leaf Oil

Scullcap leaf oil can help relieve uterine cramping as well as vaginal burning and itching associated with viral infection. Prepare at 1:5 ratio weight to volume with freshly wilted herb and good quality carrier oil. Sun infusions work in warmer climates, but it is better to use a crock pot in cooler settings.

Flower Essence

Many years ago I prepared marsh scullcap flower essence. It is a research essence in the Prairie Deva line. The essence is related to acceptance toward the nature of the bureaucratic world. By allowing release of anger, frustration, and bitterness associated with passive-aggressive positions, a deeper level of understanding will come. On a physical level, gall bladder irritation is relieved and mental patterns of blame are released.

Emotionally, the essence brings a heightened sense of calm and detachment from tilting at windmills. On a spiritual level, a sense of nurturance and renewal of soul purpose is brought to manifestation.

Spiritual Properties

Laura Aversano (2002), in her wonderful book *The Divine Nature of Plants*, relates her experience with scullcap.

> *In calling the spirit of the plant, a male spirit appears to me. He completed life on earth many years ago, and before his passing, he left many things incomplete. From the moment he crossed over into the spirit world, he made a vow to assist others to uncover the truth in their lives and to bring light and completion to their experiences…. He will only help when he is called upon, acknowledging each person's free will to live their lives as they choose. Call on the spirit of the plant to help open the throat chakra. It gives one the courage to speak. It helps to heal the energetic trauma around deafness [and] cerebral palsy.*

Personality Traits

Dorothy Hall (1998) wrote a great personality profile on Scullcap.

> *Classical scullcaps are tall and intellectually brilliant. At school, they are the daydreamers, or written off by teachers as too smart for their own good. Their quick minds can easily become agitated, irritable, and self-pitying. They constantly need new input and new ideas generated. They often seem bone-tired and at times have shaking hands. The most extreme types will have an upper eyelid that droops sharply over the outside corner.*

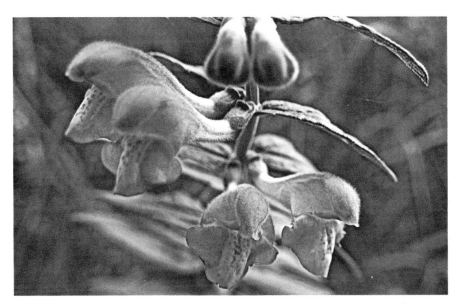

Marsh scullcap

They tend to burn the candle at both ends, as a negative trait. They are walking nervous breakdowns waiting to happen. The adrenal glands pump adrenaline to fight real or imagined challenges. In the process, the muscles harden and the blood is sent to the heart and head, ignoring the digestive system. When they become exhausted, individuals will rely on cigarettes, coffee, alcohol, and stimulants. They suffer insomnia tension and migraine headaches.

The positive scullcap regulates the flow of adrenaline with practical action and real performance. Scullcap tea helps level ups and downs. Ideas are put into practical form. At times shock, anxiety, and stress make urgent demand on the adrenal system; and this is the time for a nervine like scullcap. It is not a tranquilizer that blunts our sensitivity, or reduces stress reaction, but balances the adrenal hormones.

Vermeulen and Johnston (2011) record notes from Neil Tessler on three cases of *Scutellaria* in 1994.

I noticed that all three of my cases were individuals with difficult backgrounds. In all three cases there was estrangement from their parents at a young age.... The nervous tension these children suffer binds their energy inwardly, a contraction onto their own inner resources. They develop something of a survival mentality.... The nervous system is weakened by the sustained tension of grief, fear, uncertainty.

Botanica Poetica

SCULLCAP

If you were bit by rabid dog
And were not feeling great
This bitter tasting herb
You'd absolutely take
Or if perhaps of alcohol
You needed to be through
And you felt rather shaky
Scullcap would be for you
Here's the classic nervine
(That means it acts on people's nerves)
Brings on a calm and makes serene
Your restlessness to curb
For neuralgia and sciatica
But do not overuse
Scutellaria lateriflora
Can make you giddy and confused
But if you cannot sleep
Overwrought with stimulation
Its tinctures and its tea
Will bring you relaxation.

—Sylvia Chatroux (2004)

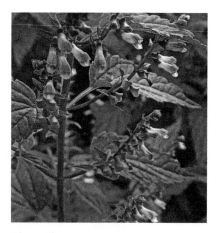

Cultivation

For commercial purposes, blue scullcap (*S. lateriflora*) continues to have the better market. It prefers moist, fertile soil with sufficient water being key. Harvest is best at the beginning of flower. In the first year, only one crop is possible, but in subsequent years you can cut twice a summer. Pruning shears work well. Yields of two tons per acre of fresh plant material can be realized. Seeds are plentiful and have been used as bird feed in the past.

Blue scullcap

RECIPES

Infusions are next to useless, except for fresh plant or well-dried plant material used within six months. Drink 3 ounces cool, as a nervine and relaxant up to 3 times daily. Freshly juiced herb, frozen in ice cubes, is a good alternative method of storage.

Tincture: 10–40 drops at time of fresh plant 1:3 tincture at 60–70% alcohol. For childhood epilepsy without lesions, particularly when there has been a single childhood seizure event, try 5–10 drops. For teething pain, try 10–20 drops three times daily. For control of tremors associated with Parkinson's disease, try 60–120 drops four times daily, as suggested by professional herbalist David Winston. For insomnia, use up to 180 drops before bedtime, according to Mitchell. Some herbalists believe a fresh plant tincture will enter your bloodstream quicker if you put it in several ounces of hot water. This may be true. It is also advisable for treating young children or alcoholics to place drops of tincture in recently boiled water to evaporate off any alcohol.

Powdered capsules: 2–3 after heavy or fatty meals, up to 4 capsules 2 times daily for arthritis.

Fluid extract: 5 drops at a time.

Periodontal disease: Combine equal parts of scullcap, Oregon grape root, self-heal, and American ginseng tinctures. Add 100 drops to water 2 times daily before meals. Gargle and swallow.

Caution: Long-term use of the herb has been shown to diminish sexual desire, at least in males. This may be due to scutellarin and its mild phytoestrogenic effect. Maybe. Aerial parts are safe to use during pregnancy. Do not take repeatedly in high doses as dizziness or irregular pulse may occur, as well as numbness of the fingers, toes, and lips. It should not be combined with blood thinners or sedative pharmaceuticals. Baicalin reduces hepatotoxicity of acetaminophen, at least in mice. Adulteration with various germander species (*Teucrium canadense, T. chamaedrys*) in the early 1990s gave a bad reputation to scullcap; hepatotoxicity and deaths occurred from adulteration with the "pink scullcap." I also recall one Canadian herb company receiving aerial parts of Baikal scullcap and marketing the product before becoming aware of the error. Oops! Curcumin, from turmeric root, inhibits absorption of baicalein (Fong et al. 2012).

Cow Parsnip

Cow Parsnip ✦ Indian Celery ✦ Beaver Root—*Heracleum sphondylium* ssp. *montanum* (Schleich. ex Gaudin) Briq. ✦ *H. lanatum* Michx. ✦ *H. maximum* Bartr. ✦ *H. sphondylium* var. *lanatum* (Michx.) Dorn

Siberian Cow Parsnip ✦ European Cow Parsnip ✦ Hogweed—*Heracleum sphondylium* L. ✦ *H. sphondylium* ssp. *montanum* (Schleich. ex Gaudin) Briq. ✦ *H. sphondylium* ssp. *sibiricum* (L.) Simonkai

Giant Hogweed—*Heracleum mantegazzianum* Sommier & Levier

Whoever eats hogweed, moistens his living.

—Marcin of Urzędów, 1595

Mighty hogweed is avenged
Human bodies soon will know our anger.
Kill them with your hogweed hairs.

—Genesis, "The Return of the Giant Hogweed"

Most of these umbellifers are biennial, and they express the dynamic force of Mars. Thus the shoots of the second year grow especially high, as in the cow parsnip...

—Ernst Michael Kranich

Cow parsnip has been an herbal ally of mine for several decades. It is little discussed in most medicinal herbal books. The cow parsnip genus refers to Hercules, an obvious comment on the plants size. *Lanatum* is derived from the Greek, meaning "woolly." Hairy may be more accurate. *Maximum* is obvious, as is *sibiricum*. *Sphondylium* means "vertebrate," in reference to the shape of the segmented stem.

Recent taxonomic work classifies common cow parsnip, Siberian cow parsnip, and European cow parsnip under the same binomial. *Heracleum sphondylium* ssp. *montanum* (Schleich. ex Gaudin) Briq. is presently accepted as the proper name for all. This is hard to understand, as the Siberian version seed head looks distinctly different. I have left above the nonaccepted synonyms for herbalists wishing to do your own research.

This bamboo of the north is familiar in meadows and roadsides, growing up to ten feet tall in a summer. Parsnip River, in northern British Columbia, is so-named for the profusion of plants along the bank of the river. In the area around Lesser Slave Lake it is one of the most dominant plants in summer.

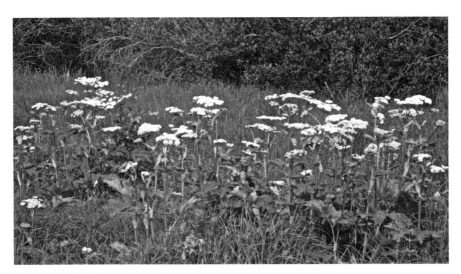

Cow parsnip field

The stems, when cooked and limp, taste like celery with a rhubarb texture. They are over 18% protein and full of nourishment. The stems contain furanocoumarins that cause photosensitivity in some individuals. Use gloves to gather. The stems are best before flowering, later becoming more bitter. The stem is split open and then bent back upon itself to separate the stringy outer peel from the edible and fleshy inner portion. Peeling the stems helps prevent this sensitivity. Some native people believe the plants growing in shade are edible, while those in full sun should be avoided, probably due to this phototoxicity. If you look closely at the stems in the shade, the irritating hairs are largely absent, compared to plants in full sunlight. Kuhnlein and Turner (1987) found peeled stalks contain only half the furanocoumarin content.

The leaves are slightly aromatic, a little sweet and slimy, but after a while become hot and bitter in the mouth. I have not steamed nor eaten the leaves so cannot comment on their suitability as an edible. Mors Kochanski, noted survivalist and good friend, told me about a case of photosensitivity observed during one of his famous nine day summer training course. One of the participants got into the habit of nibbling on the unripe flower buds during the day.

These are my favorite part of the plant, steamed in tinfoil over a bed of coals with a little salt. Delicious. But in this case, the buds were being eaten raw. About day five, he was walking the trail with bare arms, and he brushed against the plant. Soon after, his skin began to itch, and by nightfall he had a severe rash on his right arm. By morning it was a wet, oozing, eczema-like, very painful skin condition that later required cortisone cream to bring it under control.

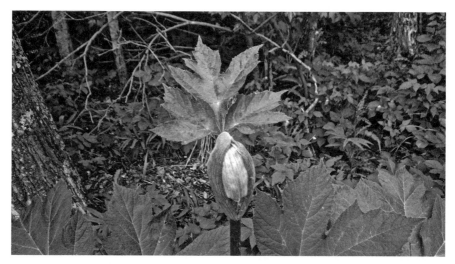

Cow parsnip flower bud

The roots are mashed when fresh or roasted over hot coals and taste somewhat like turnip or sweet potato. I have found the first-year roots most tasty and the least trouble to prepare. Mors compares the small roots to ginseng in flavor. The side roots so resemble ginseng that native peoples in the East would use them to adulterate the ginseng roots sold to European or Chinese buyers.

Traditional Uses

Cow parsnip was widely utilized by the Cree for food. They call it *pukwan-ahtik*, meaning "tent-like leaf wood" or "tent wood." I have also heard *piygwanatik* or *pagwanatik*, meaning "hollow inside." Another Cree name is *manitoskatask*. The Cree applied mashed roots to boils or glandular swellings. The Blackfoot call it *po-kint-somo* and roasted the stem over coals. Decoctions of the root were drunk for intestinal pain or cramps, or applied externally as a fomentation for arthritic and rheumatic pain. Young stems, when fresh, were boiled as a tea for treating diarrhea, or to remove warts.

The Kainai (Blood) call it "wild rhubarb," which it resembles as young growth. They distinguished between male and female plants. The male *napim* (uncovered umbel) was peeled before roasting, while the female *skim* was split open, cut into small lengths, and dipped in animal blood for winter use. The larger diameter stems are segmented, like bamboo. Fresh stems were filled with animal blood and sealed for later use. In winter, a few dried blood and vegetable stems were added, along with hot rocks, to a birch bark vessel filled with water.

I find the large stems useful in wilderness hiking. Insects, bees, earthworms, and other creatures can be tossed into a temporarily sealed segment in case they are needed as fish

258

bait. You never know. The dried plant was taken, with water, in the treatment of a broken leg. This is probably as much based on the doctrine of signatures as anything else. The juice of a fresh plant can be applied to warts. The Cree of Saskatchewan call it *askiwiskatask* or "earth carrot." The root was combined with calamus and water lily roots for external relief from painful limbs and severe headaches. The raw root may be pounded as a poultice and applied to swollen glands, or combine the raw root with water as a gargle for sore throats. A small piece of raw root was placed in tooth cavities, but the saliva was spit out. It stings a bit and is not as powerful as yarrow root, but it does the job.

The Dene (Chipewyan) crushed the root and mixed it into bait for trapping bears. Some tribes call it beaver root, although I'm not sure why. Assigning animal totems to various plants is common in First Nations medicine. The qualities of the plant speak to the healing power of the plant, or the manner in which the condition manifests or is cured. The Dene Tha (Slavey) call it either *etsoh*, "Indian rhubarb," or *deko naydi*, "cough medicine." Indigenous residents of Haida Gwaii know the plant as *hik'iid*. The Dena'ina people of Alaska call it *ggis*, meaning "stem," or *buchgi*, a word derived from Russian. The root is used for colds, sore throats, mouth sores, and tuberculosis in the form of tea. For a stronger medicine, it is cooked with aged beaver castor. Cetyl myristoleate is a fatty acid found in the musk gland of beavers. Research has shown it effective in relieving the pain of chronic fatigue syndrome, fibromyalgia, and osteo- and rheumatoid arthritis. It also helps improve efficacy of the immune system. The Met'suwet'en name is the very similar *ggus*. They used root decoctions for cough medicine. The Carrier name is *goos*. The root was heated wrapped and placed around the throat for swollen glands and tonsillitis. The Gitksan name is *hamook*. The root is one ingredient in a combination of herbs for soul retrieval in individuals affected by dark or evil sorcerers. The mixture is burned as a smudge to turn the evil back on its initiator.

The root is decocted and the water used as a wash for swellings, aches, and sores, or mashed as a poultice applied to affected areas. A piece of heated root is jammed into

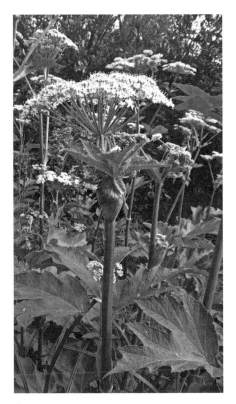

Cow parsnip stems

259

tooth cavities to kill the nerve pain. A small piece of dried root is smudged on top of wood-stoves to keep sickness out of home. Small pieces of root are added as worm medicine to meat fed for sled dogs. The Omaha and Ponca call it beaver medicine, or *zhaba-makan*. The Omaha people boiled the root for intestinal pain. The dried, pounded roots were mixed with beaver dung and placed in the hole dug for ceremonial poles.

In Alberta, the raising of the central pole for the Sun Dance is preceded by staking a single stalk of cow parsnip, with an eagle feather attached to the top, toward the west. These are considered symbols of lightness and are believed to ensure a safe raising of the center pole. The Huron of Eastern Canada used hot infusions of the plant during the influenza epidemic of 1918 with good success. Farther west, *Lomatium* was the herb of choice for this devastating event. The neighboring Chippewa, or Ojibwe, used *bi'bigwe'wunuck*, "flute reed," for indigestion, sore throats and boils. The Mesquaki used the root tea internally and externally to treat erysipelas, a painful staphylococcus infection of the skin.

Natives of Alaska chew the raw root or drink decocted root tea for colds and sore throats, while the heated leaves are applied to sore muscles. The Kwakiutl dried and pounded the root, combining it with fish oil. This was rubbed on the scalp as hair ointment, or ceremonially rubbed on the face and waist of girls at puberty. The northern Dene decocted the fresh or dried root and drank up to two ounces at a time for coughs.

Kids made the hollow, bamboo-like stems into peashooters, using chokecherry pits as the projectile. They also make very good flutes and whistles. The hollow tube is also a handy wilderness storage vessel for horseflies and other insects used as live fishing lures. They are simply placed in the tube and the other end is sealed with mud or leaves until needed. The tubes are also useful for storing earthworms, which favor living around the roots of this particular plant. Natives of British Columbia used the hollow stalks as breathing snorkels for underwater swimming. The Menomini used the plant as part of protection ceremony. Huron Smith (1923) wrote:

> *This plant [cow parsnip] and the leaves of Cynthia are burned in the smudge to take out the charm by which the hunter was enabled to kill the deer. This smudge is also to drive away the evil spirit called* sokenau, *whose special mission is to steal one's hunting luck. On a deer hunt, as soon as the camp is established and the fire built, some of this cow parsnip is thrown on the fire, and the odor and smoke permeate the air for great distances, making it impossible for the* sokenau *to approach too closely under ordinary circumstances. But if the* sokenau *is desperate and determined to steal one's hunting luck, he may come right into camp, but the smoke of pikiwunus (cow parsnip) will cause him to go blind. In case a person is afflicted with bad hunting luck, a medicine made of pikiwunus seeds ... is used.*

260

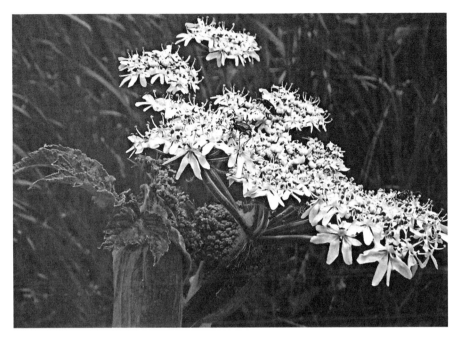

Cow parsnip flower head

In parts of Lithuania and Russia, the stems are distilled or mixed with bilberry to make a popular alcoholic beverage. One species found in Yukon and other northwest sites, *H. sibiricum*, has been used in the past as perennial animal fodder, particularly for ewes. Another species, *H. sosnowskyi*, produced one hundred tons per acre of fresh fodder in the first year, and more than two hundred in the second and third years. No word on photosensitivity in animals is found.

In Mexico, the root powder is used for sore throats and to tighten loose teeth. The root powder is combined with lard and rubbed over the entire body for reducing fever, rheumatic pains, or heart tremors. The seeds are used to relieve toothache pain or gum abscess. The plant is known in the U.S. Southwest as *yerba del oso*, herb of the bear. The root was dried and smudged as part of hunting rituals. The root was ground into small pieces and then sprayed into the throat of those suffering from diphtheria. Another method is to prepare a gargle of ½ teaspoon powdered root into 1 cup of hot water.

Young flower heads may be added to your wilderness salad or rubbed on the body as a mosquito or insect repellant. Keep in mind the photosensitivity factor. The dried, green seeds are abundant and add zest when used to spice soups and stews. They have a substantiated aphrodisiac activity, according to some books. I have not noticed, or I did not eat enough of them. The taste is somewhat like a cross between cumin and coriander, with touch of fennel. The stems have a high sugar content. If opened and set in the sun to dry, little honey-like droplets will form that are very sweet.

Gerard (1633), the English herbalist, called it "cow persnep" or "madnep":

> *If a phrenticke or melancholicke mans head bee anointed with oile wherein the leaves and roots have been sodden, it helpeth him very much, and such as be troubled with the head-ache and the lethargie, or sicknesse called the forgetfull evill."*

In Europe, a traditional name was "poor man's beer." The stems were boiled in water and steeped a few days. Yeast was added and allowed to ferment. The Eastern Europeans called this *parst*. Maybe. If anything, a native yeast would have been introduced from the plants. In Eastern Europe the leaves, stems, and fruit were covered with water in a large barrel, and after a few weeks of lactic-acid fermentation, were cooked and eaten as soup. This was known as *bartsch* or *bortch* (Polish *barszcz*). This sound a lot like the beet soup borscht, a personal favorite of mine. This was eaten every Wednesday during Lent, and also to treat fever and alleviate thirst. The plant can be preserved as food for several months throughout the winter in this way.

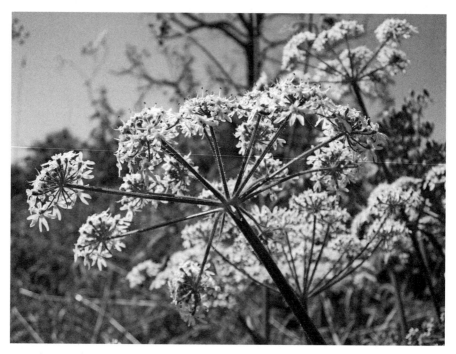

Giant hogweed

The Kamtschadalis of eastern Russia combined the sweet stem with fireweed pith infusions for a fermented liquid, later distilled. See "Fireweed" in Chapter 7 for a beer recipe that includes *Amanita muscaria* and unripe bog blueberries. The stems and leaves make excellent and inexpensive rabbit food where found. Dry them in full sun or mold will take hold. I have done this. The leaves, like those of *Petasites*, can be squeezed into round balls and allowed to dry. These are later burned to produce a white ash with a high content of potassium chloride. Siberian cow parsnip has been found in Yukon and throughout parts of North America. It has distinct clustered flower head.

The parsnip webworm feeds on the seeds and sequesters lutein that protects it from the linear furanocoumarins. This allows them to ingest the food without accumulating phototoxins. It is a major spring food for bears, accounting for up to 12 percent of their caloric intake in some areas.

Giant hogweed (*H. mantegazzianum*) has been introduced to North America. It causes serious inflammation of the skin when juice is applied and then exposed to sun. This species is to be avoided, as touching the juice to the eye can cause blindness. It should be carefully removed where found.

Medicinal Uses

Constituents: *H. lanatum* aerial: apterin, vaginidiol, isobergapten, xanthotoxin (8-methoxypsoralen), scopoletin, umbelliferone, lanatin, pimpinellin, isopimpinellin, coumaric and ferulic acids, bergapten, sphondin, xanthotoxol, psoralen, heraclenin, amino acids glutamine and arginine, essential oils, and resins.

Root: coumarins, apterin, bergapten, ferulic acid, angelicin, isobergapten, iso-pimpinellin, para-coumaric acid, scopoletin, sphondin, (3R, 8S)-falcarindiol, 6-isopentenyloxyisobergapten, 7-isopentenyloxycoumarin, umbelliferone, and vaginidol.

Stems: 40 grams contains 11 g calcium, 0.1 mg iron, and 1 mg vitamin C.

H. sibiricum: roots: furanocoumarins, including bergapten, isobergapten, umbelliferone, angelicin, isopimpinellin, pimpinellin sphondin.

Fruit: bergapten, phellopterin, xanthtoxin, isopimpinellin, heraclenin, byakangelicol, imperatorin, byakangelicin.

H. sphondylium: aerial parts: xanthotoxin, bergapten, imperatorin.

Root: oroselol.

H. mantegazzianum: angelicin, bergapten, isobergapten, isopimpinellin, methoxalen, osthole, pimpinellin, sphondin, umbellliferone, imperatorin, psoralen.

Fruit: bergapten, xanthotoxin, isopimpinellin, imperatorin, pimpinellin, limettin (5,7-dimethoxycoumarin).

The dried roots are decocted and tea consumed for persistent nausea, heartburn, and indigestion. It is a very useful remedy for elderly women suffering from hiatus hernia and other digestive disorders. The fresh seed tincture works just as well. Stronger decoctions are used in bathwater of the recently paralyzed. Topical application of the tea is very valuable for trigeminal neuralgia, Bell's palsy, or any temporary viral or mechanical paralysis of the face, mouth, tongue, neck, or limbs. I have found it particularly useful in treating pain associated with TMJ disorders. I would also refer these clients to a holistic dentist for a fitted mouth guard.

Internal use will help as well, keeping in mind the photosensitizing aspect of outdoor exposure. I used the fresh green seed tincture with good success in my eighteen years of clinical practice for all the conditions above. The roots and seeds contain antispasmodic properties that quiet cramps of the ileum and large intestine. Cramping of the uterus and bronchial tubes, or any other smooth muscle, is also relieved. The seed tincture in water may help relieve symptoms of hiatus hernia. The powdered root or ground seeds are used as a poultice on sore muscles and joints, with mild rubefacient effect. Both seed and root are warm and drying. Maria Treben (1982) recommended leaf poultices for nerve pain associated with MS.

The leaf is used in combinations to reduce hypertension. The root stimulates the spinal cord and medulla centers—vascular, respiratory, and vagus—in small doses, however causes an elevation of blood pressure. Dr. Vassar wrote of this plant, and the information was passed on by Ellingwood (1915):

> [Heracleum] *acts upon the nervous system as an antispasmodic. It produces, when taken in the mouth, a sensation of tingling, prickling, a benumbing sensation upon the throat, fauces, and tongue, similar to that of echinacea, aconite, and xanthoxylum.… It stimulates the pulse, and strengthens the capillary circulation. With the tingling and numbness of the throat, is difficult deglutition.… It exercises an influence upon the capillary circulation of the spinal cord and upon the capillary circulation in general.*

Eclectic physicians looked for symptoms to its use, including a heavily coated tongue with halitosis, a pulse that is full and sluggish, or a feverish state, when the pulse is quite slow. For gum conditions like gingivitis, gargle with water and fresh-seed tincture drops. For loose tooth and attendant pain, apply freshly pressed seed to the affected area. A piece of fresh root can be placed in tooth cavities in emergency situations. It is nearly as effective as yarrow root for immediate pain relief.

Early Eclectic physicians, including Felter and King, believed the root of *H. lanatum* to possess stimulating, antispasmodic, and carminative properties. They suggested decoctions for flatulence and dyspepsia, and 2–3 drams of the dried and powdered root taken daily for epilepsy. They combined this with a strong infusion of the leaves in the evening. The tinctured root was recommended in asthma, colic, amenorrhea, dysmenorrhea, palsy, apoplexy, and intermittent fever in doses of 5–60 minims. The root was officially in the U.S. *Pharmacopoeia* from 1820 to 1863.

In India, the roots of cow parsnip are used for leukoderma and psoriasis, and the flowers and leaves are made into a paste applied to the forehead for headaches. The root contains a polyacetylene compound and a number of furanocoumarins. These compounds exhibit strong inhibition of *Mycobacterium tuberculosis* (O'Neill et al. 2013; Webster et al. 2010). The authors suggest this knowledge supports the traditional use of herb by First Nations and Native American communities to treat infectious disease, including tuberculosis.

Sphondin isolated from the root suppresses COX-2 expression, rather than inhibiting COX-2 enzyme activity. This suggests an anti-inflammatory nature that may help respiratory inflammation, as suggested by early Eclectic physicians (Yang et al. 2002). Sphondin is a potent inhibitor of nitric oxide production that plays a role in reducing inflammation (Wang et al. 2000). Sphondin, bergapten, isobergapten, and xanthotoxin show antitumor activity against melanoma cell lines (Sumiyoshi et al. 2014). Bergapten is found in a large number of fruits and vegetables. Bergapten exhibits antispasmodic activity and inhibits production of pro-inflammatory cytokines, mainly TNF-alpha and interleukin 6.

Matthew Wood (2009) noted one of his early teachers, William LeSassier, used the herb for its neurological applications. He passed on to Matt that the seeds have a "revelatory aspect." Chewing a few seeds "opens the third eye," heightens sensitivity to nature, and confers psychic benefits. I do enjoy chewing on the fresh green seeds partly for this effect but also to discern the right time to pick them to make a tincture. The seed should squirt when you bite into it, releasing a most unusual flavor. Some compare it to cumin, or carrot seed, or parsley, but it is unique unto itself and makes a great culinary herb for soups and stews. Only a few are needed to spice up a dull-tasting dish.

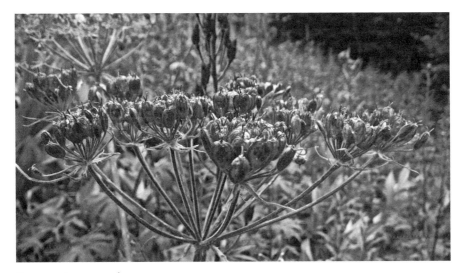

Cow parsnip green seeds

The seeds contain byakangelicol, a compound shown to significantly inhibit beta-secretase (BACE1) associated with the onset of dementia (Marumoto and Miyazawa 2010). They also contain (+/)byakangelicin, an agent showing protection against sepsis, albeit in vivo in mice (Song et al. 2005). Byakangelicin is considered an inhibitor of aldose reductase, a marker suggesting prevention or treatment of diabetic cataracts and neuropathy (Shin et al. 1998). It helped reduce histamine response in one mouse study.

The root, used in TCM, is known as *duhuo* or *niu fang feng*. It relieves headaches, itchy skin, swellings, and helps remove corns from the feet. Various laboratory studies in China confirm its analgesic, sedative, and anti-inflammatory effects. It is sometimes substituted for *Ledebouriella* species and other members of Umbelliferae family. *Fang feng* means "wind-protecting," referring to rheumatic pain and wind associated with the onset of influenza. The roots, like the rest of the plant, are photosensitizing. One clinical study found xanthotoxin increased plasma copper levels in patients suffering vitiligo. Matsuda et al. (2005) found ethanol extracts possess potent stimulation on melanin production with significant enhancement of cell proliferation. The furanocoumarin methoxsalen is used in the treatment of psoriasis. Caution is advised as UV radiation, in combination with cow parsnip, can cause burning instead of tanning. Root tinctures increase delayed menstrual flow when scanty or painful and help relax uterine cramps. It combines well with crampbark tincture for the latter, 1 tablespoon every 15 minutes.

One compound, 7-isopentenyloxycoumarin, inhibits phospholipid metabolism and Epstein-Barr virus activation and may have application in the treatment of skin tumors (Baba et al. 2002). It shows selective toxic effects on bladder cancer cell lines, inducing apoptosis and cell cycle arrest (Haghighi et al. 2014). The root may work well in combination with roseroot (*Rhodiola rosea*), which also helps prevent bladder cancer recurrence (Yang et al. 2007). This compound suppressed seizures in mice, but the relevance to humans is presently unknown. The compound is found in other members of the Umbelliferae and Rutaceae (citrus) family.

Angelicin, from cow parsnip root, shows antiviral activity against gammaherpes viruses, including Epstein-Barr, and Kaposi's sarcoma–associated herpes virus (Cho et al. 2013). It is an effective apoptosis-inducing compound of human SH-SY5Y neuroblastoma cells, suggesting possible use in human cancers (Rahman et al. 2012). Various angelicin derivatives have been studied for anti-influenza drug development. Various furanocoumarins reduce gastric ulcers, particularly bergapten and pimpinellin. Pimpinellin and isopimpinellin show strong activity against tuberculosis mycobacterium. Xanthotoxol, from the root of cow parsnip and edible garden parsnip, inhibits HeLa (cervical) cancer cell proliferation. Imperatorin, found in Siberian cow parsnip root, exhibits anticancer activity against human colon cancer cell lines (Zheng et al. 2016). Umbelliferone is anti-inflammatory and induces self-programmed death (apoptosis) in colorectal cancer cell lines (Muthu et al. 2015). The seeds of Siberian cow parsnip show apoptosis against human leukemia cell line C8166 (91%) and six other human leukemia cell lines.

Umbelliferone is both antifungal and antibacterial. Ramesh and Pugalendi (2006) found this compound to possess antihyperglycemic effects comparable to glibenclamide at 30 mg/kg in diabetic rats. Umbelliferone is found in many members of the family, including wild carrot, parsnip, dill, caraway, and cumin. Umbelliferone ameliorated insulin resistance in chronic mildly stress-induced rats (Su et al. 2016). Xanthotoxin, bergapten and umbelliferone all inhibit CYP2A6, a liver enzyme involved in 70–80% of the initial metabolism of nicotine. By slowing down the breakdown, they may prolong the antidepressive and procognitive effects of nicotine (Budzynska et al. 2016). Maybe.

Psoralen inhibits lung cancer and osteo-sarcoma in vitro. Apterin, a glucoside of vaginol, is found in the root of angelica, gout weed, lovage, and meadow parsnip (*Zizia aptera*). It helps dilate coronary arteries and block calcium channels, like other members of the family. It is little realized that common celery has six different compounds that block calcium channels and reduce hypertension. Aerial parts were found to exhibit antihypertensive activity through in inhibition of Ca^{2+} mobilization and changes in Kv channel conduction (Senejoux et al. 2013).

Tincture of the seed is so powerful that a few drops on the tongue will settle the most unruly stomach. It is a valuable analgesic gargle for sore teeth, cavities, and gum problems. Angelicin has a muscle relaxant effect on smooth muscle (not heart or skeletal) and is as potent as papaverine, derived from the opium poppy. McCutcheon et al. (1994) confirmed the antifungal activity of cow's parsnip root. All nine species tested showed inhibition. An endophyte found in *H. maximum* showed significant activity against *Mycobacterium tuberculosis* H37Ra (Clark et al. 2015). Some researchers believe the medicinal aspects of most herbs are due, in part, to their endophytic compounds. They may be right. Work by McCutcheon et al. (1992) found methanol extracts of the aerial parts active against *Mycobacterium phlei, Pseudomonas aeruginosa*, MRSA, and *Salmonella* species. The root showed weak activity against *Bacillus subtilis* and *Staphylococcus* strains, but stronger activity against *E. coli* and *Salmonella*. The seed heads and stems are slightly stronger than leaves, but all parts possess activity against *Staphylococcus aureus*.

The root may well possess antiviral activity, as it stimulates IL-6 production (Webster et al. 2006). Work by Tkachenko (2006), in fact, found the root essential oil more antiviral than the fruits. See "Essential Oils" below. Cow parsnip (*H. sphondylium*) contains hormone-like substances analogous to testosterone. Root extracts containing heraclenin show activity against various nematodes, suggesting water decoction soaks may be useful against garden pests. This compound is a mild anticoagulant. Furanocoumarins from the related *H. crenatifolium*, show anti-acetylcholinesterase and anti-butyrylcholinesterase activity, suggestive of benefit in Alzheimer's disease and related neuronal health conditions (Orhan et al. 2008).

To recap, *H. lanatum* is antispasmodic, carminative, and stimulant; *H. sphondylium* is stimulant, digestive, and hypotensive. And, to confuse us all further, some taxonomists believe they are subspecies of the same plant.

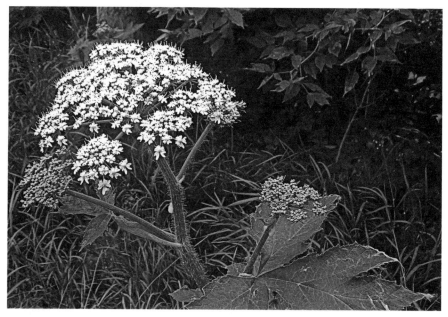

Cow parsnip flowers

Homeopathy

Heracleum has been studied for homeopathic use. Heracleum (*H. sphondylium*) is a valuable spinal stimulant and may be used in epilepsy. It is equally valuable for abdominal and spleen pains, gouty arthritis, and such. The person that benefits will have fatty perspiration on the head, accompanied perhaps by violent itching of the skin. The head is drowsy and aches, and this is relieved by wrapping it in a cloth. Excessive oily scalp with itching is a specific. Unhealthy skin, seborrhea, and acne on the face, back, and chest are other indications.

Tscherteu, in his proving, found sadness with the desire to weep, and inexplicable anxiety and lack of confidence in a crowd, as if being amidst strangers. Tendency to bulimia is noted in evening, especially toward bread and cheese. Desire for sweets and aversion to smoking are noted. Symptoms become worse from coffee. There is a sensation of an empty stomach. Exhaustion, indolence, and weakness are worse in the morning or after dinner, but better from lying down, after sleep and some motion. Vertigo may occur while reading and sitting. Limbs are heavy and feel full of lead. Eyes become worse from reading. Symptoms are worse from cold damp weather and cold wind, with offensive perspiration, especially at night.

Dose: 3rd potency. The mother tincture is prepared from the fresh seeds. The original proving was by Rosenberg and three others, using the tincture around 1838. A more recent proving in 1987 by Tscherteu in Austria involved 14 provers. Caution is advised if you choose to make your own mother tincture.

Essential Oils

Constituents: *H. sphondylium*: seed: ethyl butyrates, caproic esters, bergaterpene, octyl acetate (55–60%) and butyrate (10–13%), (furano-coumarin), pimpinellin, *n*-octyl acetate, iso-pimpinellin, and sprondrin. Steam and hydro-distillation give different essential oil composition. In the former, the oil is 42.9% octyl butyrate, 30.9% octyl acetate, and 9% octanol. With hydro-distillation, the results are 39% octanol, 10% octyl acetate, and 27% octyl butyrate, suggesting hydrolysis of octyl esters, and steam-distillation is the milder, preferred method. A clear oil is distilled from the seeds and yields from 0.5–3%. The specific gravity is 0.865 and it has an optical rotation of 0–+2 degrees.

H. lanatum: flowering aerial parts: beta-phellandrene (14.1%), lavandulyl acetate (8.87%), bicyclogermacrene (7.94%), germacrene D (6.75%), sabinene (6.75%), (E)-beta-ocimene (6.45%) and gamma-eudesmol were among the 65 compounds identified.

H. mantegazzianum: seed: isobutyl isobutyrate, isoamyl butyrate, hexyl hexanoate, 1-hexadecanol.

Essential oils from various *Heracleum* species show antimicrobial and antifungal activity against *Staphylococcus aureus* and *Candida albicans*. Essential oils from roots have been extensively studied in Europe, Russia, and India. One study by Tkachenko (2006) looked at the essential oil from the seeds of 18 different Heracleum species and their antiviral and antibacterial properties. Essential oils derived from roots are more antiviral than those distilled from fruit (Tkachenko 2009). Essential oil from seeds of *H. sphondylium* possess activity against A375 human malignant melanoma and HCT116 human colon carcinoma cells lines. Octyl acetate is the compound believed responsible (Maggi et al. 2014).

The essential oil from aerial parts of *H. sibiricum* consists of octyl butanoate (36.82%), hexyl butanoate (16.08%), 1-octanol (13.6%), and octyl hexanoate (8.1%). The oil shows activity against gram-positive bacteria (Miladinovic et al. 2013). A volatile oil from *H. lanatum* was used in 112 cases of soft-tissue damage with a marked effective rate of 76.52%. Pain was reduced, swelling subsided, and functions recovered.

In a study by Kharkwal et al. (2014), the essential oil of the flowering aerial parts showed significant inhibition of *Klebsiella pneumoniae* as well as *Staphylococcus aureus, E. coli, Salmonella enterica, Pseudomonas aeruginosa*, and *Proteus vulgaris*. Octyl butyrate is a wasp attractant, and may be useful in leading them to death traps.

Hydrosol

Cow parsnip hydrosol (1 dropper to 1 pint) is used for nausea and morning sickness, according to Darcy Williamson (2011), a noted herbalist from Idaho.

Seed Oil

Take one part of freshly crushed green seeds to five parts of a good-quality monosaturated oil and simmer at 115°F for four hours. Press and strain well. This oil is excellent for nerve pain, including neuralgia and sciatica, as well as numbness of the legs associated with MS and paralysis of affected limbs. It is better when slightly warmed and combines well with Saint John's wort carrier oil for nerve-related conditions.

Spiritual Properties

Grohmann (1989) follows the original concepts of Goethe and looks at plants from a cosmic and anthroposophic perspective.

> In the Umbelliferae, the cosmic-astral principle is inhibited and restricted in a certain way, and just as the flower are only poorly developed, so likewise is there no proper connection with the earthly element.... The cosmic-astral forces work in the middle region of the plant. Our human feelings are less involved with the Umbelliferae than with other flowering plants. There is nothing poetic about them.

Flower Essence

Darcy Williamson (2011) uses cow parsnip flower essence for those "feeling cut off from one's roots; unsure of one's inner direction; difficulty connecting with or adapting to new surroundings after a move."

Myths and Legends

The following legend is from the Menomini people.

> An evil medicine used by the sorcerers, this herb is always found in the hunting bundle. It is a very personal sort of deer charm as only the owner of the bundle can handle it. If others touch it, they will turn black and die. After the deer is killed, then it must be hung up and smudged for four days, after certain parts are removed. This plant and the leaves of Cynthia are burned in the smudge to take out the charm, by which the hunter was enabled to kill the deer.
>
> This smudge is also to drive away the evil spirit called sokenau, whose special mission is to steal one's hunting luck.
>
> On a deer hunt, as soon as the camp is established and the fire built, some of this cow parsnip is thrown on the fire, and the odor and smoke permeate the air for great distances, making it impossible for the sokenau to approach too closely under ordinary circumstances.

But if the sokenau is desperate and determined to steal one's hunting luck, he may come right into camp, but the smoke of pikiwunus (cow parsnip) will cause him to go blind. In case a person is afflicted with bad hunting luck, a medicine made of pikiwunus seeds is used. The whole hunting paraphernalia is smoked and smudged to drive away bad luck. The hunter must not eat any of the meat during this four day's smudging process. If he did, the Menomini believe that he would turn black and die. Wild ginger root is boiled with deer meat to remove the hunting charm. (Smith 1923)

In Tlingit mythology, cow parsnip was formerly a person who offended Raven by speaking angrily and was transformed into food (Swanton 1905).

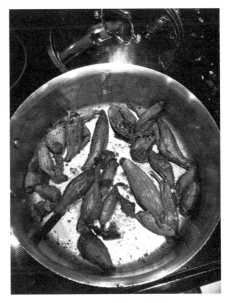

Cow parsnip unripened flower bud sautée

RECIPES

Decoction: 1 teaspoon of dried root to 1 pint of water. Simmer for 20 minutes. Drink 2 ounces cold up to 4 times daily. For external use 1 tablespoon. Never use fresh root.

Tincture: The tincture is made by immersing 4 ounces of fresh crushed green seed and/or dry root slices in 8 ounces of 60% alcohol. Shake daily for 2 weeks and strain. Take ½ teaspoon internally when needed or apply externally. Take up to 30 drops in lots of water as a prophylactic against threatened epilepsy or convulsions.

Insect repellant: Soak flowers in oil for 7–10 days. Strain and use as needed.

Salve: Place 2 parts dried root and 1 part seeds in a crock pot. Cover with 5 times by volume of canola or olive oil and gently simmer for 4 hours. Strain and add beeswax to desired thickness. This is a great salve for rheumatic pain.

Caution: Cow parsnip contains a number of photosensitizing compounds. Care must be exercised when ingesting tea or tinctures for any period of time, especially with exposure to the sun. Pale skin and red-haired individuals may be more at risk of sunburn and exposed skin pigmentation. Do not use in early pregnancy (speculative) due to its empirical emmenagogue effect (Brinker 2010).

9

Flying Moon Herbal Allies

Buffalo Berry

Thorny Buffalo Berry ♦ Silver Buffalo Berry ♦ Bull-Berry ♦ Rabbit Lip Tree—*Shepherdia argentea* (Pursh) Nutt.

Canadian Buffalo Berry ♦ Soapberry ♦ Russet Buffalo Berry ♦ Rabbit Berry ♦ Mouse's Hand ♦ Snake Willow—*Shepherdia canadensis* (L.) Nutt.

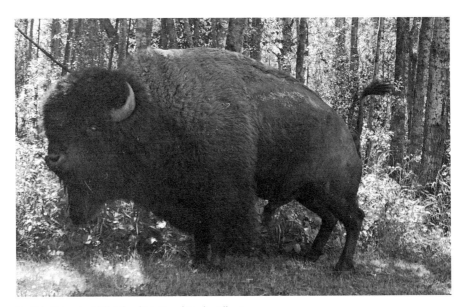

Buffalo (bison) at Elk Island National Park, Alberta

A clump of bull-berry bushes in bloom along the moist edge of a brown pool of freshly melted snow, looks for all the world like a ruffle of time-yellowed lace from grandmother's attic.

—Annora Brown

Buffalo berry is an amazing plant. It is one of only two plants that I am aware of recorded on videotape actually growing at −22°F. It is one of the first plants in the boreal forest to produce small greenish-yellow flowers, sometimes in the frigid cold of late March or earlier.

Shepherdia is named after John Shepherd, an English botanist and horticulturalist of the late-eighteenth and early-nineteenth centuries. He was curator of the Liverpool Botanical Garden and the first horticulturist to raise ferns from spores. *Argentea* means silver, referring to the silvery star-shaped exudations on the under leaf. *Canadensis* means "from Canada." Buffalo berry was misnamed, due to its use as condiment jelly or sauce served with native bison meat. In 2016 the United States declared the bison its national mammal. Great choice! Some individuals believe the small brown dots on the underside of the leaf represent herds of bison (buffalo). Quite imaginative!

Soapberry (*S. canadensis*) is common to subalpine forests and clearings where you would also find fireweed and other earth regenerators. The undersides of the leaves have tiny conspicuous brown scales, or a polka-dot appearance. The youngest leaves, at twig tip, look like hands folded in prayer. I often see it flowering while snow is still on the ground. The flowers are inconspicuous, yellow-green, appear in early spring, and are followed by yellow (rare) to red berries. In most areas it is a shrub, but in some places it can grow up to eight feet tall.

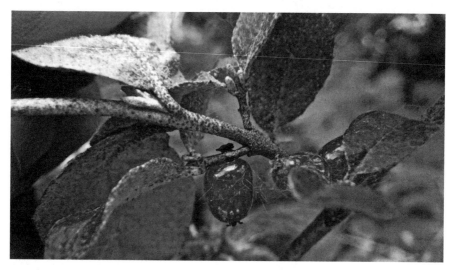

Canadian buffalo berry

S. argentea is much more tree-like, up to 15 feet tall. It bears spines and prefers moister terrain near rivers and coulees. The berries contain up to 0.74% saponins. Soapberry has brownish flowers and orange-red berries.

Traditional Uses

Various indigenous peoples collected the berries by beating the branches over a hide with a stick. They were either eaten raw or dried for future use. This is a good way to collect them, as hand-picking is tedious, juicy, and ineffective. Preserving was accomplished by placing the ripe berries in a basket, heating them with hot rocks, and then spreading out the juice on mats of timber grass to dry. This part of the process was performed in the open when windy or near a campfire to speed up the drying. Sometimes the juice from boiled berries was poured over the drying cakes a little at a time. If the berries were dried on grass, they would store them that way. Later, when they whipped them into Indian ice cream, the grass would assist in raising the foam, and the grass could be scooped off the top.

They contain a bitter saponin that will cause severe blood problems if injected directly into the blood stream, so don't do that. Upon eating, the saponins are converting into steroids and other substances by our digestive juices. This saponin makes the berries quite soapy and foamy when whipped, hence the common name soapberry. The Chinookan name *soopolallie* derives from "soap" and "berry." Thorny buffalo berries will also froth but contains less saponins. Traditionally, the berries were whipped into a dessert called Indian ice cream. When honey or sugar became more readily available, it was the addition of choice.

The Gitxsan of northern British Columbia call the treat *yal is*. It can be made instantly with ripe berries, the seeds being squeezed out and the juice and a little water whipped by hand into a thick creamy mixture. Green berries were cooked before whipping, giving a chartreuse-colored foam, while the ripe berries make a delicate pink fluff. Special spoons carved from caribou ribs were reserved and used for this ceremonial dessert. Recipes varied throughout our western region, but generally they were boiled overnight in some wooden container with hot rocks, mashed up, and spread out to dry on thimbleberry leaves.

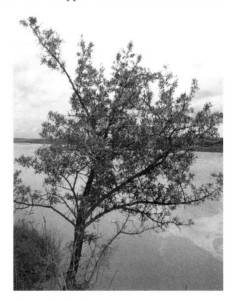

Thorny buffalo berry

275

The dry cakes were about ¼ inch thick, 1 foot wide, and up to 9 feet long. They used infusions of the dried leaves, picked after the berries were ripe, as a diuretic for bladder and uterine infections. The berries are said to increase labor contractions by stimulating the uterus. Other reports by Leslie Johnson (1997), in her doctoral thesis, mention using the whole plant, including roots, as a decoction for chronic coughs, and the root only, combined with spruce twigs and needles, for rheumatism.

The Dena'ina of Alaska call it *dlin'a lu,* meaning "mouse's hand," referring to the hands-together appearance of the winter buds. They use the stems and branches for tuberculosis, cuts, and swellings. Dena'ina means "the people." Buffalo berries are added to stews or made into jellies, jams, fermented drinks, and syrups. The Dene Tha (True People) mixed the berries with cooked moose liver or animal tallow. The term *Slavey,* applied to this indigenous group by ethnobotanists, is derived from a Cree word meaning "servile one." It is considered derogatory.

The fruit of *S. argentea* is sour but good raw, while those derived from *S. canadensis* are insipid and quite bitter. Both improve in flavor with the first frost. The berries are rich in iron and vitamin C, but in excess will cause diarrhea, vomiting, and cramping of the intestines. The berry froth can be used as a soap substitute, especially for shampoos, and

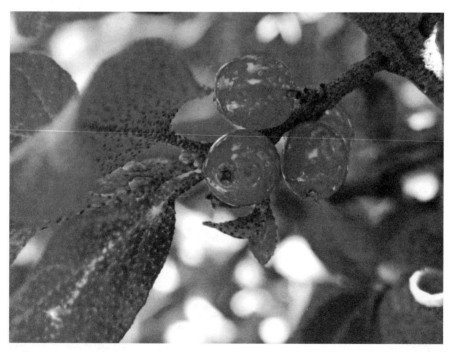

Soapberries

combines well with horsetail for washing pots and pans during camping trips. The saponins of berries combine with the silica coarseness of horsetail for a thorough, ecological, nonpolluting cleaning job. The berry juice was a natural type of perm for hair used by pioneer women. The branches can be decocted for dark brown water that dyes the hair and gives it more body.

The Woods Cree of Saskatchewan know soapberry as *kinipikominanahtik*, meaning "snake berry tree." It is also called *kinipikomina*, "snake berry plant." The Cree healer Russell Willier calls it snake willow, or *kinipiknipsi*. He suggests its use for skin problems, such as psoriasis, probably due to the saponin content of berries. The snake symbolizes healing and rebirth to native people. The Cree used plant decoctions externally for aching limbs and arthritis. The stem was considered important in the treatment of venereal disease, while the inner bark was infused as a reliable laxative. The most recent twigs were used in decoction to prevent miscarriage.

A decoction of the fresh split-peeled roots and split twigs reduced fevers in babies. This was also used as a rub or rinse for the sore mouth and teething. The Tanana Athabaskans boiled soapberry root, or *hooshum*, for stomach and gallbladder complaints. Adults used a wash for cuts, swellings, and skin sores like impetigo. The root has been added to heart medicines in an unspecified manner. The roots are strongly laxative and were used traditionally for chronic coughs and tuberculosis.

The neighboring Gwich'in on the Mackenzie Delta call it "mooseberry," *dinjik jàk*. They ate the raw berries for colds or sore throats, and decocted the stems and roots for stomach aches and diarrhea. The roots were sometimes combined with juniper berries and decocted as a laxative, one cup taken before each meal. The boiled berries were said to increase appetite. Sophie Thomas, a native elder and healer from Stoney Creek, British Columbia, knew the bush as *nuwuschun*. The berries helped kill parasites in the gastrointestinal tract, and the stems were decocted and taken internally for cancers. The branches were decocted as a wash for sore legs or to soothe mosquito bites and subsequent infections that resulted from scratching. For fevers, especially in children, the roots and lower stems were decocted for up to two hours, until the water was red. Two to four ounces were taken at a time.

It would be wise, however, to avoid burning the wood in fires, as some tribes called it "stinkwood," *miss-is-a-misoi*. Like its close relative, wolf willow, the green wood gives off an odor similar to human feces when burned. One of my favorite campfire tricks is to sneak a stem into the nighttime gathering and watch everyone turning their heads and sniffing the air.

The Athabaskan peoples used soapberry decoctions for tuberculosis and as a wash for cuts and swelling. Be careful with open wounds, as the saponins can be very reactive with blood. The Wet'suwet'en use *niwis* berries for stomach ulcers, while a decoction of the inner bark of branches was used as a laxative or for sore stomach. The Nlaka'pamux (Thompson) used the stem and leaf decoctions in sweats to help purify them for hunts or before raiding parties. A leaf and fruit tea is good for ulcers and is a sedative. The branches and leaves were decocted to treat cancer of the stomach and high blood pressure. The neighboring Dakelh (Carrier) used the branches in a similar manner. They know the plant as *nuwus chun*.

Decocted soapberry, willow, balsam poplar, or cherry bark were used as a poultice wrap for broken bones that hardened solid. Hawthorn bark was considered the best but was not always available. The Secwepemc (Shuswap) boiled the twigs and sticks as a laxative tea. The Dine'e (Navajo) ate buffalo berries to help bring down fevers, whereas the Dakota (the allies) used the fruit in ceremonial feasts during female puberty rites. This is possibly related to the red color of berries and blood. The Arapaho name is *auch ha hay be na*, the Paiute call it *wea pu wi*, the Shoshone *weyumb*, and the Siksika (Blackfoot) of Montana know it as *me e nixen*. The Tsitsistas (Cheyenne) call it *mat'si ta si'mins*, or red-hearted, and collected the berries after the first frost.

The Anishinaabe and other eastern peoples used the bark as a medicinal tea. They also used the bark, softened in hot water, along with pin cherry bark as a type of plaster cast for broken limbs. When dried, the bark strips would shrink and stiffen, helping hold fractures together. Hawthorn bark, when available, makes the best wilderness cast for fractures. The Siksika (Blackfoot) name for thorny buffalo berry is *miksin-itsim*, or "bull berry." The Lakota know it as *mas'tinca-pute'can*, or "rabbit lip tree." The Plains Cree name, *mihkominsa*,

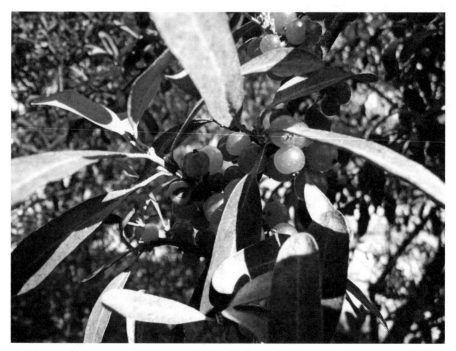

Thorny buffalo berry

278

is very similar to the Blackfoot name and means "blood berry" or "red berry." Early voyageurs called it *graisse de boeuf*, or beef fat, a welcome accompaniment to a monotonous diet of bison tongues and steaks.

The trees have large thorns on the branches, making berry collection difficult by hand. A large hide was placed under the tree after the first frost, and the tree was shaken and beaten with wooden poles to release the berries. The Blackfoot would sometimes mash them in a buffalo horn with a stick and drink the juice for stomach problems, or as a mild laxative. Various British Columbia tribes, including the Nlaka'pamux, Stl'atl'imx, and Secwepemc, made a type of lemonade from soapberry juice. This was a refreshing tonic but also used for acne, boils, and digestive problems, including gallstone pain.

The saponins were used as poison on the arrows and spears of hunters. If the wild game was not initially killed, they would track it, and it would slowly die from blood hemorrhage. John Richardson, best known for his search for the Franklin expedition, wrote a book, published in 1851, in which he noted buffalo berries make a quick and excellent beer that ferments in twenty-four hours into a beverage "most agreeable in hot weather."

Mors Kochanski, a personal friend and world-renowned survival expert, considers the winter tips of buffalo berry an endorphin inducer, used by indigenous people to fend off hunger pains and other discomforts of winter living. Harmine alkaloids may be responsible, in part, due to monoamine oxidase (MAO) inhibition. A whole class of older antidepressant prescription medications was based on the inhibition of MOA. They are rarely used today, with SSRIs and other antidepressants filling the void. The drugs rarely address the underlying issues for many patients.

In early fall, the bears begin to fatten up for winter. They have a couple of goals in mind to help them through the rough times of hibernation with no food and loss of weight. One of their great concerns is their load of intestinal parasites. Both grizzly and black bears cannot afford to lose nutrition to these freeloaders, so a mechanism of action is required. Bearberry (*Arctostaphylos uva-ursi*) is a well-named plant. The berries, which are somewhat dry and mealy, are eaten in massive amounts by the magnificent mammals. This is not just for food but mainly for the intestinal paralyzing seeds in the fruit. Their whole digestive tract becomes stagnant and constipated. The bears then go down to the swamp and seek out various *Carex* species. These three-sided grasses are sharp, like a razor or barbed wire. In fact, razor grass is the common name for one particular sedge

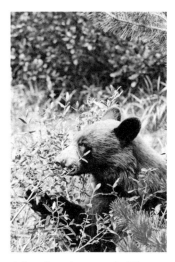

A bear fattening up on buffalo berries

species. As we say in botany, "sedges have edges." The bears eat and eat. And then they wait. The large evacuation of stool that follows is accompanied by a plethora of parasites, impaled upon the sharp grasses that penetrated their armor. And now, the bears are ready to fatten up. A favored food is buffalo berry. These orange-red berries are rich in protein, fats, and saponins. Saponins are soap-like molecules that have an influence on hormones but also act as building blocks for the production of fat. In a few weeks of nonstop feeding, a large grizzly may gain up to four hundred pounds additional weight on their already sizeable frame.

The mention of saponins reminds me of a funny incident that happened some 30 years ago at the University of Alberta. Ironically, I am now an assistant clinical professor in family medicine at my alma mater. I was invited to present a ninety-minute lecture on herbal medicine to a group of third- and fourth-year medical students. I was moving through the different constituents in plants and how they impact the human body. As I was getting close to the end of my presentation, I noted that the professor, sitting nearby, was becoming more and more agitated and looking somewhat irritated and hostile. I asked at my conclusion if there were any questions, and he immediately jumped up.

"Mister Rogers," he said. For those of you not familiar with the ways of academia, the term Mister is meant to be derogatory. As in, you do not have a doctorate, so your credibility is diminished, and anything you say cannot be accepted at face value or lacks credibility.

"Mister Rogers. Are you aware that if you take saponins and put them into a hypodermic syringe, and inject them into the bloodstream, they will destroy red blood cells?"

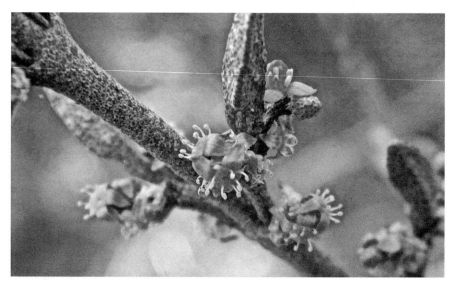

Buffalo berry flowers

I was well aware of this, but waited for a good ten seconds to respond.

"Well," I replied. "What idiot would do that?"

At which time, all the students in the room burst out in loud laughter. It was pretty funny.

Medicinal Uses

Constituents: *S. argentea* leaves: caffeic, chlorogenic, coumaric, ferulic, sinapic, gallic, syringic, and ellagic acids; isoquercitrin, catechol, tetra-hydroharmol, shephagenins A and B; N,O-diacetyl-tetrahydroharmol, various kaempferol and quercetin rhamnosides.

Berries: 12–21% sugars; up to 250 mg ascorbic acid, beta-carotene, lycopene (0.27 g/kg fresh), methyl apo-6f-lycopenoate (0.32 g/kg fresh) leucoanthocyanins, catechols, flavonols.

S. canadensis: root bark: serotonin, shepherdine, tetrahydroharmol.

Berries: 1% carotenoid, of which 42% is lycopene and 45% methyl lycopenate.

Twigs and leaves: harmine, harmaline, harmane, harmol.

The root bark of both contains shepherdine, tetrahydroharmol, and N,O-diacetyltetrahydro-harmol. Both *Shepherdia* plants have been studied for medicinal benefit. One study by Ritch-Krc et al. (1996) looked at the medicinal effects of soapberry (*S. canadensis*). They reported anticancer activity against mouse mastocytoma cells in a methanol extract derived from the stems. The IC_{50} value was 76 mcg/ml and indicates a need for further research. Shepherdin inhibits human tumor growth via apoptotic and nonapoptotic mechanisms (Plescia et al. 2005).

Canadian buffalo berry, the shrub, is being promoted more actively by Extropian Agroforestry Ventures of Lake Alma, Saskatchewan. Over the past ten years they have planted one hundred thousand shrubs on their plantation. Research indicates the leaves, branches, and bark contain compounds able to neutralize 93% of free radicals. According to Morris Johnson, Extropian's research director, the plant exhibits anticancer, cardioprotective, antiviral, and phase 2 enzyme oxidative stress-reducing factors. The berries contain components shown to work in conjunction with colostrum in maintaining intestinal health.

Saponins froth in water like soap due to half of the molecule being water insoluble. Saponins don't enter our body's cells but attach themselves to the outside. Saponins help improve our digestive function, control appetite, and regulate what nutrients are absorbed, including glucose. Patients suffering hypoglycemia may benefit, as saponins help prevent our pancreas from producing too much insulin. They inhibit the growth of viruses and aid in regulation of abnormal cell growth, including apoptosis, or self-programmed death, of cancer cells. Saponins stimulate the immune system by hooking onto receptor sites of immune cells, turbocharging the immune cell's response. They help stimulate lymphocyte production and regulate production of bile. Too little is associated with constipation and inability to metabolize cholesterol, and too much is associated with development of colon cancer.

On average, the Japanese eat three times the amount of saponin-rich food as North Americans. Strong root infusions were traditionally used to aid childbirth and treat tuberculosis, while the berry tincture was recommended by midwives to induce parturition. Give up to 1 tablespoon per hour. Stem decoction may be used as a stomach tonic, taken in small doses. Berry tinctures benefit the heart, particularly for hypertension, combining well with hawthorn berry. The berries contain lycopene, associated with supporting prostate health and anti–platelet aggregation (Sawardekar et al. 2016).

Thorny buffalo berry (*S. argentea*) has been studied for medicinal value by a team of Japanese researchers led by Yoshida et al. (1996). The leaf tannins show remarkable inhibitory activity against HIV-reverse transcriptase and deserve additional study. Burns Kraft et al. (2008) found the berries inhibit aldose reductase, improve glycogen accumulation, and reduce expression of both IL-1-beta and COX-2, suggesting protection from diabetic microvascular complications, countering metabolic syndrome, and reducing inflammation. Harmine and harmol alkaloids decrease cardiac heart rate and myocardial contractile force and show vasopressin-like effect. Harmaline and related alkaloids induce smooth-muscle relaxation and have therapeutic activity in treating amoebic dysentery, acting as an anthelmintic.

Harmine increases insulin sensitivity and blocks a pathway that normally encourages fat-cell production. Pancreatic beta cell deficiency is linked to type 2 diabetes. Work by

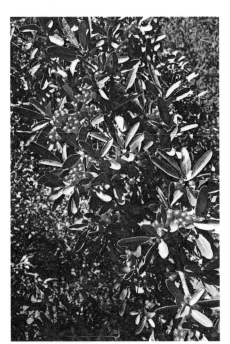

Peng Wang et al. (2015) found analogues of harmine induce regeneration and expansion of adult human beta cells in the pancreas. This is very exciting news. James Shapiro at the University of Alberta has been working on islet transplant for some twenty years. He led the Edmonton Protocol team in 2000. His research team has found a way to harvest beta cells and place them in a plastic insert that prevents transplant rejection, hoping in time the body comes to accept and utilize the cells to produce insulin in type 1 diabetics. It is very exciting work. Using a harmine analogue to increase beta cell replication would be a great step forward.

Harmine and paclitaxel, found in hazelnut twigs, leaves, and husks, when combined, appear to inhibit the migration and invasion of gastric cancer cells via downregulation of COX-2 expression (Sun et al.

Thorny buffalo berry

2015). Buffalo berry and hazelnut are common and easily accessible shrubs in the boreal forest. Pacific yew was the original source of paclitaxel, but the needles of this tree are considerably more toxic due to other constituents. Harmine and harmol are moderately potent haspin kinase inhibitors, a potential anticancer pathway (Cuny et al. 2012). Laboratory studies show rats influenced by harmaline display greater speed in achieving erections and increased frequency of copulation. Human application is unknown.

Harmine is a reversible MAO inhibitor and is the very same psychoactive compound, banisterine, found in a South American rainforest vine, used in the preparation of ayahuasca. Banisterine was one of the first alkaloids investigated for the possible treatment of Parkinson's disease. Harmine targets DYRK1A, which may reduce cardiac toxicity associated with the cancer drug doxorubicin (Atteya et al. 2016). Harmine appears to help treat Parkinson's disease, but the dimethylated harmine is a potential causative agent of the condition. Harmine and berberine show potential therapeutic use in myotonic dystrophy (Herrendorff et al. 2016). It may protect and regulation metabolism of osteoblasts, osteoclasts, and chondrocytes associated with osteoporosis, osteoarthritis, and bone fractures (Hu and Xie 2016).

Harmine was previously named telepathine, and was used by the Germans in World War II as a truth serum. Harmala alkaloids vary in potency. The equivalent of 100 mg harmine is 50 mg harmaline, 35 mg tetrahydryaharman, 25 mg harmalol or harmol, and 4 mg methoxyharmalan. Overdoses can cause progressive CNS paralysis. Not only does harmine act as a MAO inhibitor, but it was used in herbal smoking combinations by northern Cree to extend the activity of other herbal smoking mixtures. It would be combined with red osier dogwood bark for analgesic and anti-inflammatory activity, and with other herb combinations where there was a need to extend the "half-life" for healing purposes.

I spent a good part of 1982 to 1984 in Peru and had the opportunity to participate in ayahuasca ceremonies. I also spent time with Eduardo Calderón, near Trujillo, where he conducted healing ceremonies utilizing mescaline-rich San Pedro cacti. Upon my return to northern Alberta, I asked several Cree elders if they used combinations of plants as entheogens. The answer was typically no. With one native healer that I met on an annual basis, I asked the same question each time we met, and he always replied in the negative. About twelve years later, I asked the same question, bringing up the use of buffalo berry. He sat me down and revealed that they used the root of reed canary grass in combination for those individuals that

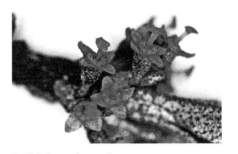

Buffalo berry flower close-up

felt stuck in a depressing mindset or were not comfortable in their own body. That interested me, and sure enough, when I looked at the chemistry of reed canary grass rhizome, it contains di-methyl tryptamine (DMT). Combining the two botanicals would be the equivalent of an ayahuasca analogue, but what are the dosage and ratio of each? This has yet to be fully determined. The ratio of 4 parts harmine to 1 part DMT is a good place to start. This is not a recommendation.

It is worth noting that harmol and other beta-carboline derivatives are present in the bark of Russian olive, wolf willow, sea buckthorn, and other members of the Elaeagnaceae family.

Flower Essence

Darcy Williamson (2011) suggests the flower essence "relieves the fear of the power of nature, fear of one's own power, using one's power in irresponsible, inappropriate, or unbalanced ways."

Myths and Legends

Annora Brown (1970) recorded the following legend.

> [There is] a Blackfoot legend of Old Man, in the days when he had ceased to be a god and had become a poor, foolish, irrational trickster. Old Man wandered through the woods one day feeling very hungry. He came to a deep, still pool, and stooping for a drink, he beheld, lying at the bottom of the pool, a cluster of bright red berries. These were just what he wanted, so he tried to reach them by diving after them.
>
> Again and again he dived into the clear water, but could not reach the bottom. Each time he stood on the bank he saw them there in the transparent depths. At last he conceived a plan that could not fail. Tearing strips of bark from trees along the bank, he bound heavy stones about his wrists and neck and waist. Then he dived again.
>
> This time, he reached the bottom—but there were not berries there. When he decided to return to the surface, however, the stones still held him to the bottom, head down, feet floating far above. He had a desperate struggle to unloose the strings of bark, but at last he threw himself half-drowned on the soft bank of the pond. As he lay there, gasping and choking for air, he looked up into the tangled branches above and there, scarcely higher than his own head, was the cluster of berries he had been diving after. Furious at being so deceived, he seized a stick and beat the bushes until the branches were broken and the berries dropped to the ground. "Your branches will always look broken and people will always gather your berries by beating you," he told the tree. And people always have.
>
> This story recalls another use for the shrub. The strips of bark which Old Man used to tie the stones about his wrist and waist were from the bush for whose berries he was diving. The Indians used it as a substitute, if raw hide were not available.

Having given its bark for strings and its berries for food, this strange tree turned perverse and refused its wood for firewood. Miss-is-a-misoi, or stink wood, the Indians called it, and you have only to try burning it on your camp fire to understand the reason.

Early work by Thomas McIlwraith (1948) recorded much of the way of life of the Bella Coola of British Columbia. This story tells of how buffalo berry was introduced to the west coast.

Long, long ago, Slexlekwailx, a mountain in the Carrier country above Burnt Ridge, was a chief, possessing human characteristics. Buffalo berries [soapberries] flourished on his slopes and he wanted to keep these for food for his guests. On one occasion he invited all the animals and birds, including Raven, to a feast and dance. His house was the interior of the mountain, and when all had assembled, he carefully closed every opening so that none of the berries could escape. Raven determined to obtain some of this food for the Bella Coola, and accordingly, used his power to force one of the guests to go outside. As soon as a door was opened to let him out, Raven seized some of the whip and flew away, scattering drops of it in his flight. Berries grew wherever the drops fell, and since that time, everybody has been able to make this luxury. Slexlekwailx was very angry but could do nothing.

RECIPES

Indian ice cream: Add ¼ cup water to each quart of fresh berries, or 2 tablespoons of dried powdered berries. Beat the mixture into light foam, until the consistency of egg whites. You can add some sugar as the foam is forming if you like (3–4 tablespoons per cup of berries). Traditionally, saskatoons and other berries were added as sweeteners. Green soapberries make white foam, the ripe berries a pink or salmon color. Do not allow any grease or oil to contact the berries or they won't whip up.

Dandruff shampoo and conditioner: Combine equal parts of dried buffalo berries and dogwood berries in water and decoct for 10 minutes. Allow to stand until cool, strain, and use immediately or store in the fridge.

Infusion: 1 tablespoon of dried leaf to 1 pint of boiled water. Steep for 10 minutes. Drink ½ cup several times daily.

Decoction: 1 tablespoon of dried, cut, and sifted root or bark to 1 pint of water. Simmer for 15 minutes, cool, and drink. ½ cup twice daily is a good place to start.

Tincture: Prepare the fresh leaves, picked before berries appear, at 1:5 in a 40% alcohol tincture. Take 10–20 drops up to 4 times daily as required. Dried bark or root tincture is prepared at 1:5 and 40% alcohol.

Crampbark

Crampbark ♦ High Bush Cranberry ♦ Pembina ♦ Kalyna ♦ White Dogwood—*Viburnum trilobum* Marsh ♦ *V. opulus* ssp. *trilobum* (Marsh.) R. T. Clausen ♦ *V. opulus* var. *americanum* Ait.

Low Bush Cranberry ♦ Squashberry ♦ Mooseberry—*Viburnum edule* (Michx.) Raf.

My love for you is filled to the brim with the bitterness of the kalyna.

—Liubov Zabashta

The kalyna's *blood, as a singular song, burns in my heart with bitter stars.*

—Ivan Drach

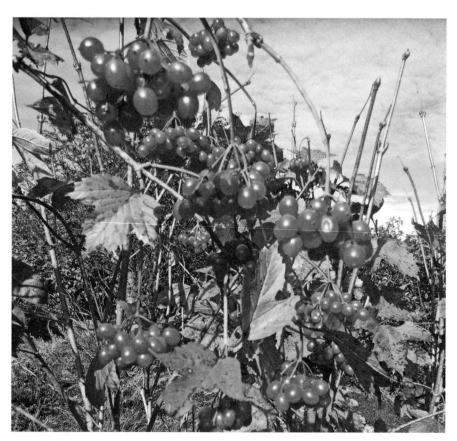

Crampbark shrub

Viburnum may derive from the Latin *vieo*, "to tie," referring to the use of flexible stems for tying bundles. Cranberry was originally "craneberry" in reference to the bird connection. *Opulus* may derive from the same root as *opulent*, meaning "generous," "extravagant," or "showy." *Edule* means "edible." Both low and high bush cranberry are similar in appearance and properties. In autumn the leaves turn a brilliant red, and the first frost brings out the distinct smell of the berries that defines an Alberta fall for me. High bush cranberry symbolizes growing old and a birth date of July 9.

The berries (drupes) are rich in vitamins C and K and are used for coughs, colds, or a daily cordial that helps keep hypertension in check. The berries are tart but delicious and can be preserved as a jam or ketchup for wild game. Both Siberians and Scandinavians prepare a liqueur, a wine with a honey paste, from the fruit. The collection of the berries and preparation into ketchup is one of my favorite activities in fall. I love the smell that emanates from the first touch of frost, a mild pungent valerianic scent that is somewhat pleasing. In some years the branches are hanging low with the weight of the fruit, making for easy picking. I have constructed a large basket that is supported by my back and shoulders so I can accomplish two-fisted harvests.

In Russia the berries are used as part of a brandy preparation called *nastoika*, used for treating peptic ulcers. Early Slavic settlers in Alberta called the plant *kalyna*. The term is the ethnic and national symbol of Ukraine, the color of the nation's soul. Just northeast of Edmonton is found the Kalyna Country Ecomuseum, an area of interesting natural and historic sites traveled by early explorers such as Anthony Henday, Peter Pond, and David Thompson.

The berries turn black when dried and make a fabric dye, and were once used to make ink. The Cree call High bush cranberry *nipin minan*, meaning "summer berry," while *mongsoa-meena* or *mosomina*, meaning "mooseberry," is reserved for the low-bush variety. Russell Willier, noted herbalist and friend, calls this plant *nêpiminana*. He uses it in combinations to remove a curse. This name was believed corrupted by traders and voyageurs in Pembina, hence the name of the plant and river. In some books you will read that Pembina or Pimbina is derived from the Cree *nipiminan*, for "berry growing by the water." An 1853 journal from the Red River suggests the name comes from *anepeminan*, with *nepen* meaning "summer" and *minan* "berry." I believe the latter is correct (Young et al. 2015).

In some parts of the prairies, the low-bush form is referred to as mooseberry. In Yukon, the lower form is known as high bush cranberry to distinguish it from lingonberry and bog cranberry. Confused yet? High bush cranberries are easier to pick, hanging like clusters of grapes, whereas low bush berries are more spotty and tedious to gather. The local river valley, on most years, produces an abundance of fruit.

Bark tea was prepared by Cree healers as a diuretic and taken to prevent postpartum infections in new mothers after birth. That is, the bark decoction will help expel any retain afterbirth and placenta, ensuring sepsis does not occur. The bark tea was traditionally used for insomnia. This may be due in part to the content of valerianic and baldrianic acids. The Chippewa (Ojibwe) call the plant *nipinminan,* nearly the same as the Cree name. They traditionally used the root tea for prolapsed uterus. The Innu (Montagnais) used the bark tea for swollen glands and mumps. *Montagnais* is French for "mountain people." *Innu* means "the people." The term *Naskapi,* a band name, is sometimes used and means "bad dressers" in the Innu language.

Ukrainian settlers used bark infusions to stop hemorrhages after birth and to slow heavy menstruation as well as bleeding hemorrhoids. It was used to stop spontaneous abortions and used in the form of a sitz bath for vaginal problems. A decoction of twigs was used to treat uterine infections and sepsis related to the incomplete removal of afterbirth.

The flowers were dried and used for coughs, colds, asthma, sclerosis, tuberculosis, and stomach problems. It was used as a throat gargle and wash for wounds. The berry was eaten for anxiety, arteriosclerosis, and blood vessel spasms. They were cooked with honey for cough, laryngitis, asthma, liver complaints, and diarrhea. The berry juice with honey was specific for breast cancer and as a prophylactic for stomach cancer in patients with hyperacidity and gastritis. A berry infusion was used as a diaphoretic when taken hot, and as a relaxing agent when drunk cool for eczema, carbuncles, acne, and blackheads.

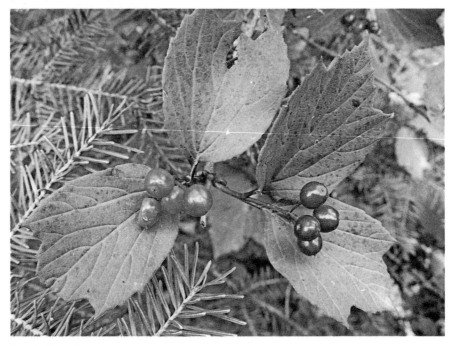

Low bush cranberry

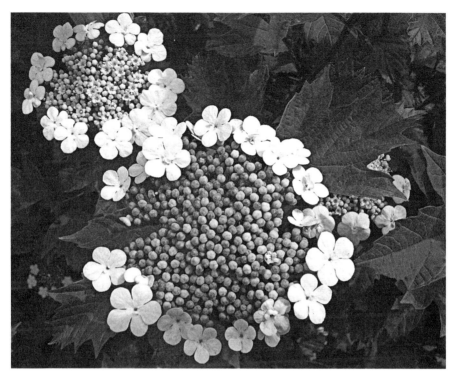

Crampbark flowers

Low Bush berries were used as fish bait while the inner bark was scraped out, dried, and included in smoking mixtures with bearberry (*A. uva-ursi*) leaves and dogwood inner bark. The unopened flower buds were chewed and plastered on lip sores. For sore throats, they chewed the twigs and swallowed the juice. The roots were boiled to treat teething problems. Cree women boiled the fresh or dried bark to relieve menstrual cramping. Other northern tribes drank the hot leaf tea for sore backs, cold in the kidneys, or sore-throat gargles. The Dene (Chipewyan) of Northern Alberta called the edible berries *denijie*, or mooseberry. A few tribes, including the Carrier of British Columbia, smoked the inner bark to relieve muscle spasms. The Gitksan made dry cakes for winter, like many other indigenous peoples, combining the fruit, called *ts'idipxst*, with blueberries or rosehips. The leaf and twigs were decocted with devil's club bark for those patients unable to urinate, or to treat hernias. The low bush cranberry is called *'mii oot*.

The twigs are strong enough to tie logs for rafts together if first twisted and the fiber broken. It is easy to do; simply take your twig and while holding it down with your foot, and start twisting, first in one direction and then the other. They make superior arrows as the material is stiff and resists the archer's paradox for a more efficient and quiet release from the bow. It is not often thought of, but an arrow flexes upon release, and not just any stick will do.

The Dena'ina boil the stems for stomach problems, or to make a gargle for colds, sore throats, and laryngitis. The Haida believe the fruit is the food of supernatural beings, the plant being the most frequently mentioned in their "myths." In several of them, the heroes are given a small piece of salmon and a single cranberry by a supernatural helper. No matter how much they eat, they can never finish either. It is a legend somewhat reminiscent of a story in the Bible, where Jesus, the fishes, and the loaves fed everyone.

The Shishalh (Sechelt) used the plant as a diuretic and blood purifier. The Nlaka'pamux (Thompson) call the plant *q'ep'/q'epkwle*, an onomatopoetic term which refers to the click-click sound produced from the chewed seeds. Indigenous people of New Brunswick used infusions of the fruit to reduce swollen mumps. A poultice of the berries has an astringent effect on skin problems.

Medicinal Uses

Constituents: *V. opulus* bark: amentoflavone, alpha- and beta-amyrin, arbutin, hydroquinines, chlorogenic acids, caffeic acid, p-coumaric acid, ferulic acid, gallic acid, syringic acid, protocatechuic acid, 3,4,5-trimethoxybenzoic acid, chlorogenic acid, ellagic acid, arbutin, scopoletin, scopoline; capric, baldrianic, valerianic, oleanolic, and ursolic acids; 3,4-dihydroxyphenylacetic acid, homogentisic acid, vibutin, viburnin, valeric acid, catechins, viopudial, opulus iridoids, esculetin, and calcium oxalate. Bark is 8.6% protein and contains 115 ppm cobalt. Specific anthocyans are cyanidine-3-arabinosylglucoside and cyanidine-3-glucoside, with minor amounts of malvidine-3-glucoside. Both the berries and leaves contain 7 monosaccharides, and 5 neutral sugars. The berries are also rich in vitamins C and K, viburnin, anthocyanins and leucoanthocyanins (up to 2.3% of fresh fruit), pectin 5%, paeoniside, cinnamic acid, ursolic acid. Also contain phenolic acids (up to 1,400 mg/100 g), including caffeic, chlorogenic, and hydroxybenzoic acid. Anthocyanins include cyanidin 3,5-diglucoside, cyanidin 3-glucoside, and petunidin 3-glucoside/galactoside. Also contain lycopene and beta-carotene.

flowers: astragalin (kaempferol-3-O-glucoside).

V. edule: fresh fruit: flavonoids (4.89 g/kg), vitamin C (1.64 g/kg), polyphenolics, including gallic acid (8.29g/kg).

William Cook (1869), one of the great physio-medicalists, praised the low bush cranberry, or mooseberry, as it is known. He recommended an infusion of the branches and twigs for bronchial irritation and coughs due to nervine and antispasmodic properties. Also for various form of indigestion, irritable stomach, and "in cases of uterine sensitiveness, with leucorrhea and nervous irritability, I am confident it will be found of significant benefit."

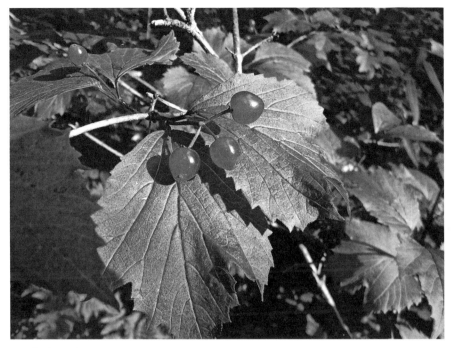

Low bush cranberry

Crampbark combines well with mullein and a small amount of lobelia for asthma, either in a tincture combination or a smoking mixture. The inner bark of crampbark contains the properties leading to its name. Collected in May or June, the vibrant green inner bark possesses antispasmodic and nervine properties useful smooth and striated muscles. Why early in spring? The sap is rising, and the inner bark peels most easily at that time. A little tip that I pass on to my herbal students is to peel one side of a stem and lay the bark side down on a flat surface, and then wait. It may take a beer or even two, but within a few hours, depending on the heat and sun of the day, the outer and inner layers will begin to separate at the ends. You can then just peel the inner part off and save a lot of scraping.

Crampbark helps relax the uterus, relieving period pains and combining well with valerian root when pain is more severe. Crampbark combines sour, bitter, and acrid properties that help reduce both heat and tension. The bark is somewhat astringent, slightly sweet and cool, and dry as well. Relief of tension in the body is helped by this herb, including digestive, respiratory, and urogenital tissue. Although primarily considered in cases of uterine issues, it also works well in asthma and irritable bowel syndrome.

When teaching herbal students about herbs, I will often ask them to first experience a plant tincture without attaching a name. Just three to five drops are ingested, and then students are given time to experience its action. Terms such as *cooling, relaxing, softening,* and *healing* consistently come up.

These qualities of moving, relaxing, and cooling tissue make it most useful in menstrual pain and excessive menstrual bleeding. The bitterness and acrid nature moves blood and the slight sweet nourishes the blood and muscles. It relieves pain of ovaritis, endometriosis, and orchitis. Threatened miscarriage in the third trimester with rhythmic cramping and little or no spotting may be abated. A combination of partridge berry, false unicorn, and possibly ginger may be useful for acute threatened miscarriage. Contact your midwife, herbalist, or other health practitioner immediately.

In habitual miscarriage, the herb tincture can be taken, 1 to 2 teaspoons daily, well into the second trimester if needed. Crampbark, partridge berry, false unicorn and red raspberry leaf in equal parts by weight may be useful. I have found chasteberry very reliable for preventing first trimester miscarriage, as it helps promote the mild progesterone influence necessary to retain uterine lining.

In threatened miscarriage, 1 teaspoon every hour is taken until the crises has passed. Later, the herb is given prior to labor, preparing the uterus for the vigorous activity to come. Ellingwood (1915) suggests crampbark is inferior to black haw for this purpose, but I found it worked well in my clinical cases. I would say crampbark is relaxant to both smooth and striated muscle, but not greatly restorative, via phytoprogesterone pathways, to uterine tissue. It combines well with partridge berry *(Mitchella repens)* to strengthen uterine tissue during pregnancy. And finally, it is given to reduce the severity of after-pains and uterine spasms and help prevent painful involution. Consider a dose of crampbark before gynecological procedures such as Pap smears, to help relax the muscles. Middle-age males scheduled for their annual prostate exam may also find a relaxing benefit. I have noticed that in patients helped by crampbark, the herb works more quickly in subsequent doses, as if the body anticipates the relief to come.

It can be used to treat excessive blood loss and muscle pain that sometimes accompany menopause. Combine the herb with black cohosh for muscle spasms, with motherwort for painful cramping and PMS, and with goldenseal for postnatal pain and bleeding. The cramping relief extends to all manner of spasm, be it convulsions, restless leg syndrome, epileptic seizures, and even lockjaw. Combine with cow parsnip root or green seed tincture for these affections. It is useful in chronic lower back pain, associated with weak kidneys and an inability to remove waste efficiently. Combine with birch leaves. For muscle cramping and cold extremities, combine with prickly ash bark.

Sharp bladder pain or dysuria may be relieved, combining well with mullein root where the picture fits, especially in cases of spasmodic bladder. Spasms of all smooth and striated muscles such as the bladder and lungs, as in whooping cough, are helped by crampbark. Scopoletin and esculetin have shown antispasmodic action one-eighth to one-tenth the strength of papaverine. Godfrey and Saunders (2010, 336), in their somewhat spotty botanical book, suggest empirical evidence of its efficacy as an adjuvant for opiate addiction. Consider combining it with scullcap and green flowering oats for soothing withdrawal anguish. Scopoletin is involved in the secretion of serotonin, helping to reduce anxiety and depression. The herb nourishes the heart, quiets the spirit, and clears heat from the heart, making it a useful addition with scullcap for insomnia, anxiety, and depression.

I make a flower tincture in season. It combines well with hawthorn flower for addressing cardiovascular issues. Astragalin, a major component of the flowers, has been found cardioprotective, via antioxidant, antiapoptotic, and anti-inflammatory activities (Qu et al. 2016). This compound is also found in astragalus root. Astragalin relieves allergic inflammation in mouse models of allergic asthma. Again, the flower and bark tinctures combine well for respiratory conditions (Liu et al. 2015).

For migraines associated with stress, combine crampbark with hawthorn, linden, marsh hedge nettle, or scullcap, depending upon the picture pattern. Crampbark is useful for treating seizures during pregnancy or in young children, combined with marsh or blue scullcap.

Crampbark was an official drug in the U.S. *Pharmacopoeia* from 1882 to 1916 and the *National Formulary* from 1916 to 1960. Ellingwood (1915), the great Eclectic physician, wrote over a century ago that "the specific influence of the agent is exercised in relieving irregular spasmodic pains of the womb and ovaries. It is antispasmodic in its action upon the entire pelvic viscera, influencing spasmodic contractions of … the bladder."

Decoctions of the inner bark can be applied to streptococcus infections of the skin. Likewise, warm douches for vaginitis, enemas for diarrhea, and gargles for gingi-

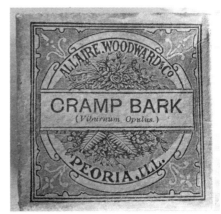

Crampbark packaged on June 30, 1906

vitis and loose teeth produce the desired result. It combines well with mullein root and St. John's wort in some cases of bed-wetting in children. Medical research has validated viopudial as an antispasmodic useful for hypotension and bradycardia. It seems to possess activity on cholinesterase, influencing myocardial contractions (Nicholson et al. 1972). The bark also possesses anti-inflammatory properties.

Scopoletin has been identified as one of the main antispasmodic components (Jarboe et al. 1967). Crampbark is primarily a B_2 agonist, with action primarily on the uterus but on all muscular vascular tissue to a lesser degree. It varies from black haw, which is more of a restorative, phytoprogesteronic, and autonomic nervous relaxant that helps reduce smooth muscle spasms. Crampbark is a better neuromuscular relaxant that inhibits both smooth and striated muscle spasms. Think of this herb for cases of arthritis with painful joints that have caused the muscles to contract and become painful due to their constant contraction. A lotion can be made from the inner bark for application to the joints, helping restore normal blood flow and relax the muscles. Combine the external application with internal use. Historically, black haw (*V. prunifolium*) root bark was used more during pregnancy and crampbark during menstruation. In the northern part of the continent we only have crampbark, and if I had to choose between these two great herbs, I would prefer the one we have in the north.

Paul Bergner, noted herbalist, conducted a double-blind challenge with his students who had training in pulse diagnosis. Nine students took ten drops of crampbark tincture and eight took same amount of black haw. After ten minutes, eight of the nine stated that crampbark created a reduction of tension in pulse or a slight sinking effect. In the other group, all eight found tension in the pulse increased or became more elevated. The fact that black haw bark does not contain viopudial and contains less potassium chloride may account in part for the difference.

Water extracts of the bark, leaves, fruit, and flower—the bark being most active—of *V. opulus* have shown digitalis-type cardiotonic action in work conducted by Vlad et al. (1977). The glycoside concentrates of the bark have cardiotonic action up to a dilution of 1 part in 250,000. Amentoflavone, a bioflavonoid, inhibits human platelet cAMP phosphodiesterase. Amentoflavone, in the presence of prostaglandin E1, induces a 3.7-fold increase in total platelet cAMP (Beretz et al. 1986). Amentoflavone, also found in the medicinal

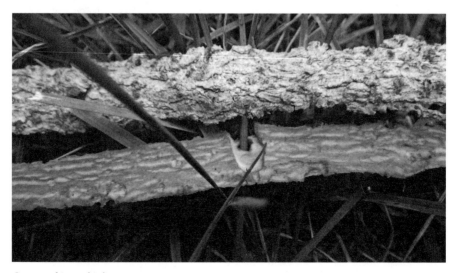

Outer and inner bark

herb St. John's wort, is a negative modulator of GABA at GABA(A) receptors, suggesting a benefit in mood enhancement (Hanrahan et al. 2003; Baureithel et al. 1997). Amentoflavone is a potent caffeine-like Ca^{2+} releaser in skeletal muscle, but twenty times more potent than any coffee derivative (Suzuki et al. 1999). Amentoflavone suppresses NF-kappa-B–mediated inflammation and induces apoptosis in keratinocytes, suggesting its use in psoriasis (An et al. 2016). The same mechanism may induce antiangiogenic and antimetastatic effects in MCF-7 breast cancer cells (J. H. Chen et al. 2015). Amentoflavone shows activity against influenza A and B viruses, and moderate activity against herpes viruses HSV-1 and HSV-2 (Lin et al. 1999).

The bark was used traditionally for its uterotonic, sedative, and diuretic properties, and modern science appears to validate these uses. One compound in the bark has a most unusual effect. Homogentisic acid accumulates in the body of those individuals suffering the rare metabolic condition alkaptonuria. In this condition, ochronotic pigment is deposited in cartilage and attacked by homogentisic acid. This in turn causes the cartilage matrix to stiffen, causing osteoarthritis and joint destruction. This compound is also implicated in kidney and prostate stone formation in those suffering the enzyme defect. On the other hand, a study by Szwajgier (2015) found homogentisic acid the most active phenolic acid tested for anti-acetylcholinesterase activity. This suggests benefit in the amelioration or treatment of Alzheimer's disease.

Both fruit and leaves contain enough polysaccharides to be considered in the class of pectin substances. Work by Ovodova et al. (2000) found the water-soluble polysaccharides from fresh berries possess immune-stimulating activity. They enhance phagocytosis and in particular the phagocytic index and the secretion of lysosomal enzymes with peritoneal macrophages. Calcium ions have been found necessary for the appearance of this stimulating effect.

Pound the berries to pulp them and spread on a cloth for application to malignant ulcers, erysipelas, or to treat the increasingly rare scarlet fever. The berries can be used fresh or dried for hypertension and minor heart problems. Tuglu et al. (2014) suggested the berry juice, being high in citrate and potassium and low in calcium and sodium, could be used by people suffering mild to moderate hypocitraturic stones.

High bush cranberry fruit inhibits aldose reductase, improves glucose uptake, reduces inflammation, and modulates energy expenditure. This suggests a role for the berries in preventing diabetic microvascular complications such as retinopathy and may have a role to play in insulin resistance and metabolic syndrome (Burns Kraft et al. 2008). Recent work by Zaklos-Szyda et al. (2015) concludes crampbark may be a promising source of compounds with anti-diabetic properties. The fruit juice, in a mouse study, was found to significantly prevent colon cancer (Ulger et al. 2013). Human implications are unknown. Work by Saltan et al. (2016) found *V. opulus* fruit extracts may be useful to treat endometriosis, albeit in a rat study.

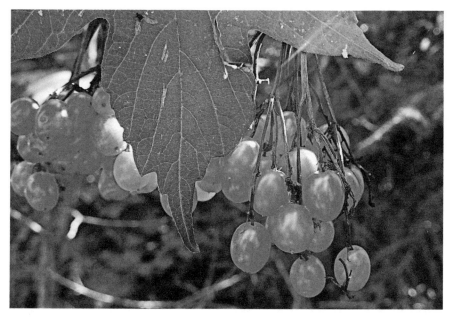

High bush cranberries

Homeopathy

The fresh bark was made into a mother tincture and proved for homeopathic usage in late 1800s. *Viburnum opulus* is considered mainly a female remedy, useful in cases of false labor pain or threatened miscarriage. The head may be irritable, or there may be persistent dizziness with a tendency for the patient to fall forward. The patient is very nervous and excessively irritable. There is awakening with a start from sleep, or a sensation as if falling.

Menstruation may be delayed, but when menses finally come, they may be scanty and only last a few hours. However, the ovarian region feels heavy and congested with frequent urging of pale urine. The bladder will not hold water when coughing or even walking. The lower limbs may feel weak and heavy. Vertigo may be present in the afternoon upon closing the eyes, but is made worse descending stairs or walking in a dimly lighted room. One may be disoriented and can't tell where he or she is. There may be crampy, colicky pain in the ovaries, extending down the thighs.

The mother tincture and lower potencies are used. The mother tincture is prepared from the fresh bark. First proving was conducted by Allen with 12 provers with tincture, 1X, and 30X in 1879 and 1881. Hawkes used seven provers with tincture in 1880. Fenton used six female provers with tincture (potencies produced no symptoms) in 1895.

Note: This is prepared from the related European *V. opulus*, which has naturalized in parts of the northeastern United States. The fruit is very acidic but can be prepared by cooking. The bark can be used for the medicinal purposes above. If you look carefully at the petiolar glands, you will note the European shrub has flat or slightly indented buds, while the American buds are convex or club-shaped.

Sun-Infused Oil

The flowers from the high bush cranberry have a peculiar scent, somewhat like the dirty sock aroma of valerian. The scent is very noticeable in early fall after the first frost.

Sun-infused oil can be made from the fresh blossoms; shaking the jar daily and straining after 10 days. Use a 1:5 ratio of blossoms by weight to carrier oil by volume. In a colder climate like northern Alberta, I find a low-temperature crockpot a quick and handy method. You may find your cat attracted to the oil, first being stimulated and then relaxed, similar to the effect of honeysuckle wood or catnip herb. An oil may be prepared from the dried inner bark as well and applied externally for joint and muscle pain. Use the same 1:5 ratio.

Flower Essence

I prepared a high bush cranberry flower essence in the 1980s and found it is associated with flexibility on the spiritual plane. Rigid, religious attitudes tend to have us put blinders on with regard to our own spiritual connections on earth. This flower essence helps us to examine and be self-critical with regard to seemingly contradictory messages we may receive in the dream state. It is considered a research essence in the Prairie Deva Essence line developed by Laurie Szott-Rogers and me.

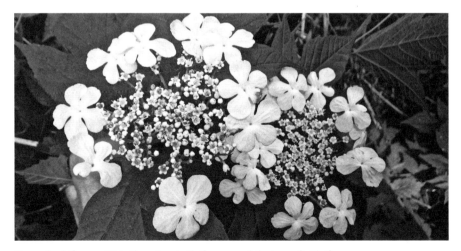

Crampbark flowers. Note the outer sterile flowers and the inner fertile flowers.

Bits and Pieces

Orysiz Tracz (2001) is a noted scholar and author. She wrote about the high bush cran-berry in The Ukrainian Weekly:

> Kalyna, *the high bush cranberry, is not merely a plant. It has become a symbol, a legend, so deeply has it been intertwined into Ukrainian culture and into folklore.... To every Ukrainian, it symbolizes beauty, love, purity, and Ukraine itself. The kalyna's bitterness is cited in both folksongs and poetry. In his book* Chervona Kalyna: an Ethnobotanical Study, *Hordiienko theorizes that in ancient times, the habitat of kalyna was the gathering place of people worshipping pre-Christian god and spirits. During the feast of Kupalo (summer solstice), young people spent the night pairing up and merrymaking. The young women wore wreaths of fresh flowers, including the kalyna, which blooms at that time. Eventually, Hordiienko thinks, the flower came to symbolize a maiden's beauty as well as her innocence. And it is the leaves, rather than the blossoms, that are the important symbol in Ukrainian culture.*
>
> *First love, lovemaking, and losing one's virginity are part of many folksong lyrics, but they are couched in such beautiful symbolism that most Ukrainians today do not realize how explicit the songs really are. Kalyna is another word for the hymen, so to lose one's wreath, or to break the kalyna, means to lose one's virginity. The kalyna was mentioned in almost every wedding song, especially after the couple's first night, when proof of the bride's virginity on her nightshirt was paraded around to show the guests. This red stain on the shirt looked very much like a crushed kalyna berry and was called "kalyna."*
>
> *The mythical kalynovyi mist (bridge made of kalyna branches), mentioned in song and poetry, is a symbolic Rubicon between single and married life. Therefore, it also symbolizes all that will never return. Many songs are about the kalyna growing on a grave. The anthem of Ukrainian soldiers of World War I, "Oy, u luzi chervona kalyna," clearly shows the connection.*

The Russian composer Ivan Larionov released the musical piece Kalinka in 1860. It is a very popular and frequently performed song.

Myths and Legends

There are many interesting myths and legends surrounding *Viburnum* species. Here is one preserved by Guillet (1962):

> *In the beginning, the Great Father gave the snake woman all the seeds. She sorted them and gave many to her two sons to distribute. "Plant the Arrow wood seeds everywhere," she told them. Every day her sons came back with empty sacks and she gave them more seeds. But after a time they grew tired of planting and she made a new plan: "Go everywhere and give six seeds of each plant to a person. Tell the person to plant them and water them and*

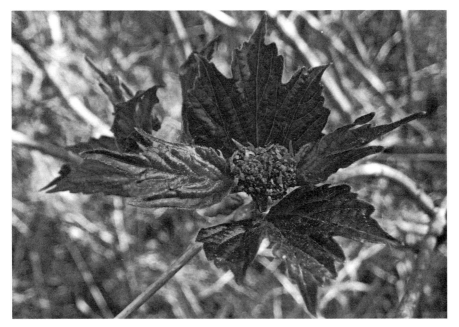

New leaves and unopened flower bud

give them loving care." Then she commanded the people, "Tell your little children that they must not touch the seeds or even point at them. And if any one gathers the seeds before they are ripe, a poisonous snake will come out and bite him."

So, to this day, Indian women tell their children: "Don't go near the growing plants. If you touch them the snake will bite you." The Snake Woman's sons are still traveling all over the world, giving seeds of new plants to the people. Those who plant them and water them and care for them have the approval of the Great Father, and they are given more seeds to plant.

An old Montagnais tale was recorded by Norman (1990):

The High and Low Bush Cranberries were hunting companions and neighbors. They could look out and see Moose swimming across the lake. They were best of friends, and were known far and wide as the cranberry partners. All through winter, spring, and summer it was impossible to embarrass them, but now it was fall and both were ripe. They were fat and full of juice.

One day they heard the sound of a moose passing by. Both jumped up and grabbed their bow and arrow. They ran to the door, but being so fat they all got jammed in the doorways so that none of them could get out. They couldn't get to the moose in time. Because of this, the cranberries were embarrassed.

299

Swanton (1905) preserved this story about Raven and high bush cranberry:

Raven was visiting the Beaver People. Two days in a row he was served salmon, high bush cranberries, and the inside parts of the mountain goat. On the second morning, Raven was taken behind a screen where there was a fish trap in a creek filled with salmon and several points on a lake which were red with cranberries. After the beavers had gone for the day, Raven ate the usual meal. Then he stole the salmon-filled lake and the house, rolling it up and hiding it under his arm, and climbed a tree with it. When the beavers returned, they tried to catch him by chewing down the tree, but Raven simply flew to another. Finally they gave up, and Raven flew inland and unrolled the lake there and kept the fish trap and house to teach the people of Haida Gwaii and the mainland how to live. Since then, there have been many high bush cranberries in Haida Gwaii.

The Cree of northern Canada also share a legend preserved for us by Tamra Andrews (2000):

According to Cree legend, a man perceived to be a magician cursed the berries and made them sour. This hungry man was sitting on a riverbank one day when suddenly he saw bunches of ripe, red cranberries floating in the water. He jumped into the water and tried to reach them, but they vanished just as quickly as they had appeared. The magician dove deep into the water, over and over again, but never found the cranberries. Then he realized that it was only the reflection of the cranberries he saw in the water; the real fruit hung from a tree overhead. The cranberry bush, which had a mind of its own, decided to trick the foolish magician by moving up higher and higher and staying just out of his reach. This so frustrated the man that he cursed the cranberries. From then on, this high bush cranberry produced only berries that were bitter to the taste.

Here is another, about moose. A Cree legend tells of the trials of Wesakechak, son of the west wind. After he had finished creating all the animals, he had some spare parts left over. He found a large coat with long dark hair, two floppy ears, long legs, and flat antlers. He wasn't sure, but after putting them together, he had created a moose. Moose was teased by the other animals, and so he went to live in a dark, swampy place all by himself.

RECIPES

Decoction: 2 ounces of dried inner bark to 1 quart of hot water. Simmer down to 1 pint and drink cool, 1 ounce 3–4 times daily. Collect the bark in spring before the leaves have budded. If you let the bark sit in a warm setting for 4–6 hours, the inner bark will peel away nicely from the outer bark that is composted.

Tincture: 1 teaspoon 3–4 times daily. The tincture is made from the fresh inner bark at 1:4 at 40% alcohol, or dried inner bark at 1:5 and 30%. Standardized extracts are measured using viopudiol content. You can also make a flower tincture. Collect the fertile and sterile flower heads and prepare fresh at 1:4 and 40% alcohol. For threatened miscarriage take 1 teaspoon of bark tincture every hour. To prevent seizures during third trimester, take 1–2 teaspoons daily. Women and children, including teenagers who are allergic to aspirin (Reye's syndrome), should avoid *Viburnum* species. In some individuals it may aggravate tinnitus, or ringing in the ears. It may lower blood pressure, so be cautious. Avoid use with blood thinners.

Cranberry ketchup: Place 4 cups of ripe berries in 1 cup of water and ½ cup of good-quality apple cider vinegar. Bring this to boil and then lower heat to simmer until soft. Process with a food mill or blender to remove the seeds.

To this puree add 1 cup of honey and assorted spices like nutmeg, cinnamon, wild ginger, allspice, or calamus root. Cook slowly until thick. Remove and preserve. Serve with wild game or roasted potatoes.

Note: Cranberry is rich in pectin. The cooking berries smell like dirty socks, but the final product does not.

Mullein

Mullein ✦ Hare's Beard—*Verbascum thapsus* L.

Where mullein grows in abundance, the maidens are poor.

—Polish folk song

I have been a practicing herbalist for over forty-three years and have used various parts of mullein with good success during my eighteen years of clinical practice. On a plant video trip to the interior of British Columbia, I noted the massive amount of naturalized mullein on the dry hillside around Kamloops and the vicinity. But I never saw it around Edmonton, Alberta, my home for the past thirty-some years. One hot August day I was driving north from the international airport on a busy divided highway parallel to railroad tracks. I looked over and saw a large stand of what looked like mullein, with its large seed heads. Risking a traffic snafu, I pulled onto the shoulder and scrambled over to the rails. Sure enough, mullein was growing happily beside the tracks, probably the result of some seeds hitchhiking across the mountains and falling off as the trains slowed down at their final destination. Feeling pretty lucky, I quickly harvested a dozen fully mature seed heads and headed home.

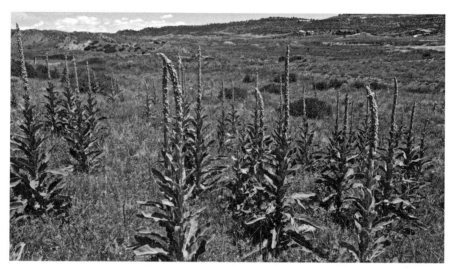

Mullein field in northern Colorado

My beautiful wife Laurie wanted to know what I was planning to do with this large bag of black seeds. I replied that I was not sure, but later took a handful of seeds and spread them over half the lawn on our corner lot in suburbia. It had become a household joke that I would only mow half the lawn at a time. It was true the south facing part was always dry and parched, and I was not about to get into watering grass.

The next summer a number of the seeds sprouted, and by mid-summer I had a great supply of large furry leaves that I promptly tinctured. And then I mowed the lawn for the first time that summer. Mullein is a robust biennial and started to shoot skyward the next summer. I was really enjoying them and decided to see how things developed. As the mullein reached five and six feet tall, it began to produce beautiful yellow flowers with bright orange stamens. I picked new flowers daily and added them to my jar of olive oil, sitting in the sun. This is a great medicine, as I will explain later. For the next three weeks, once or twice daily, neighbors would walk by and comment how beautiful they were, what is it called, and where can they get them. I asked if they would like seeds, and many replied in the affirmative. Within a few years, mullein (rated in Alberta a prohibited noxious weed) was happily growing throughout the whole neighborhood. Since each plant may produce up to one hundred and eighty thousand seeds, there was plenty for all.

Verbascum is derived from the Latin *barbascum*, meaning "bearded," in obvious reference to the hairy orange stamens, three of which have small hairs that exude a sweet sap. Kahlee Keane (2012), known as Root Woman, wrote, "to me, mullein's Latin name, *Verbascum*, spoken slowly and deeply, holds just the right resonance: this might well be this plant's Soul Song." *Ver-bas-cum. Thapsus* is from the Greek island Thapsos or

Tunisian island Thapsus, now Magnise, where, in ancient times, mullein was gathered in abundance. It may derive from the Greek *thapsinos*, meaning "yellow," referring to the yellow flowers or to dyeing one's hair yellow using mullein flowers steeped in lye. Mullein is believed to be the *phlemos* described by Hippocrates. Note the resemblance to phlegm.

An ancient Greek myth has Ulysses protecting himself with a wand of mullein against the cagey Circe. Another name, hag taper, relates to saturating the dry seed head with tallow or other animal fats for use as a torch. It evolved etymologically speaking, from *high taper* to *hig taper* and then *hag*. *Haga* is the Anglo-Saxon term for "hedge." Native to Eurasia, it has been naturalized in North America for so long that it has been accepted into the materia medica of indigenous people. The origin of the word *mullein* has several variations. Some believe it derived from the Old English *moleyne*, in turn from the Old French *moleine*, a lung disease suffered by cattle. Other scholars think *mullein* derives from the French *malandre*, for boils on a horse's neck. This became *malen* and then to its current spelling. *Malanders* came to mean "lepers," and hence *malandrin*, an outlaw driven from society. Less likely is the explanation provided by the Oxford dictionary, that *mullein* is derived from the Old English *molegn*, meaning "curds." It may stem from the Latin *mollis* or Old French *moll* for "soft," as in *mollify* or *emollient*, in reference to the leaves, or from the English *wooleyn* for "woolen" due to the texture of the leaves.

Some authors believe it is the Holy Moly referred to in work authored by Homer. This also less likely, but who knows?

The soft leaves make handy disposable diapers, and sole inserts for worn shoes and slippers. Slip a fresh leaf into hiking boots for sore feet. The leaves contain rotenone, a natural insecticide. The leaf hairs, if examined closely, are a tangled web that discourages insect travel, but also act as a barrier to the intense sunlight that would damage delicate leaf cells. The hairs may protect against blowing dust associated with the dry soils on which it grows, helping the leaf stroma remain open for the uptake of carbon dioxide. I would not recommend using the leaf as toilet paper.

If you are hiking in dry areas and you run out of water, seek out the second-year stem. Snap it off at the point of least

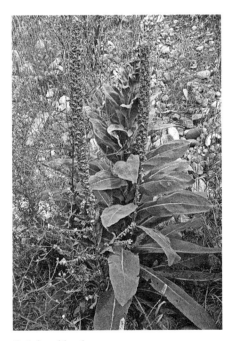

Dried seed heads

303

resistance, like asparagus, and peel. This interior pulp is edible and juicy, slightly sweet initially, and then has a bitter aftertaste. It will temporarily ease your thirst.

Traditional Uses

During the time of Charlemagne, mullein leaves were boiled and the decoction was poured into fishponds. The leaf saponins reduced the water surface tension and coated the gills of fish that literally drowned. Natives of Alberta used the seeds as a piscicide, to poison fish, by grinding them and putting them into bodies of water. Their narcotic activity stupefied the fish, making for easy harvest. The seeds of mullein are plentiful, with one plant capable of producing several hundred thousand seeds.

The dried seed heads and stems make excellent fire tinder. Natives across the prairies smoked the introduced plant leaves to alleviate lung congestion. The Hopi combined mullein and gromwell as a smoking mixture for "fits, witchcraft, and craziness." The Aniyunwiya (Cherokee) smoked the leaves to treat throat and lung problems and called it *ga lah la di,i ga di*. The name *Cherokee* is probably derived from a Muskogee word for "speakers of another language." The Apsaalooké (Crow) of southern Montana placed leaf poultices on the breasts of lactating mothers to increase milk production. *Apsaalooké* means "children of the large beaked bird," a term given to them by the Hidatsa, a neighboring tribe. The Dine'e (Navajo) call it "big tobacco." They combined the leaf with other herbs for coughing spasms. The name *Navajo* derived from a Tewa word for "planted fields." The Iswa, or Catawba, named it "gray leaf" and used leaf poultices for sprains and swellings. *Iswa* means "people of the river." The Anishinaabe name is *nookaadiziiganzh*.

> *Mullein has another major virtue to share with the Anishinaabeg. It has an oil [flower] that is effective against internal bleeding. It is healing to broken inner parts of the body, hemorrhoids, postoperative bleeding, bleeding ulcers, post-childbirth bleeding, etc. It will reach parts of the body one could not get at otherwise.... Float the flowers in a wide-mouthed glass jar of pure water. Put the top on the jar and place it in the window in the sun. The oil will accumulate on the top of the water. (Geniusz 2015, 188).*

Veterinarians feed freshly picked mullein leaves to cattle for coughs and tapeworms. Allison McCutcheon et al. (1995) found mullein extracts active against bovine herpes virus type I. In Italy, the roots are fed to pigs to fight intestinal afflictions. An older name was bullock's lungwort, due to the doctrine of signatures as related to the leaf shape. Today the powdered roots are mixed in feed to fatten poultry. In Germany, the plant is placed in granaries to drive away mice. The leaves were traditionally hung in hog barns to control lice. Mary Wuff and Gregory Tilford (2009) suggest mullein leaf may be used in treating canine herpes virus and feline viral rhinotracheitis. The leaf and seed are anthelmintic, but the seed is more powerful. Activity against roundworms (*Ascaridia galli*) and tapeworms (*Raillietina spiralis*) was noted in work by Niaz et al. (2012). Paralysis and death of *R. spiralis* suggests the extract is more wormicidal than the drug albendazole. Relaxation of intestinal tissue was noted in this study.

An extract of mullein is used today in Europe to produce a liqueur (Altvater Jägerndorfer). Flower extracts are used in preparations to tint blond hair, while the leaf fluid extract is added to hair restorative and tonic formulas. An insect associated with mullein, the mirid bug (*Campylomma verbasci*), has shown benefit to pear orchards. It is partially phytophagous and cannot complete its life cycle without feeding on mites and insects that attack the fruit, including the introduced European red mite. The beetle *Labidomera clivicollis* will curl up in mullein's warm, fuzzy leaves to hibernate for the winter.

The seed is long-lived. Seeds buried under a European church for 650 years germinated when exposed to light. In 1879, various "weed" seeds were bottled and reopened in 2000. In the case of mullein, 22 percent of the seeds germinated. Goldfinches love the ripe seeds.

Medicinal Uses

Constituents: *V. thapsus* leaves: various flavonoids, including hesperidin, verbascoside, and aucubin; an iridoid glycoside containing ajugol, verbascoside, a luteolin glycoside, and catalpol; caffeic acid, carotene, mucilage, rotenone, coumarin, gums, triterpene saponins, including songarosaponins D–F, bitter amaroid and essential oils, trace minerals, 10% protein. The fresh leaf contains 78% moisture. The fresh whole plant contains no less than 23 iridoids.

Flowers: glucose (8.35–11%), catechin tannins (15–22%), thapsic acid (0.2%), flavonoids including luteolin, apigenin, rutin, etc., and traces of essential oils (no alkaloids or carotenoids). They also contain 3% polysaccharides, comprising uronic

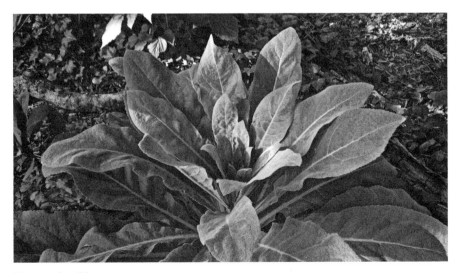

First year basal leaves

305

acids, 47% D-galactose, 1% L-fucose, and 25% arabinose; xyloglucan, glycoside esters, saponins, including thapsuins and hydroxythapsuins A and B; sterols, digiprolactone, iridoid monoterpenes, lignan glucosides, including 6f-0-apiosyl-verbascoside and eight phenylethanoid glycosides; as well as rotenone, and about 11% invert sugar.

Seeds: hemolytic aaponins, no alkaloids, beta-sitosterol; linolenic, stearic, palmitic, and oleic acids; 27% fats, mucilage, 18% protein.

Root: verbacose, octaose, nonaose, heptaose, aucubin, alpha-galactosidase.

Mullein leaf is cooling, restores dry and moist issues, is bitter, soothing, and a mildly demulcent herb with anti-inflammatory and antibacterial properties. That is, mullein promotes expectoration but also resolves excess phlegm and relieves chronic, unproductive coughs. Both lung phlegm dampness and dryness are relieved. This includes dry, hard coughs with sticky yet scanty mucus, but also thin white or viscous yellow mucus in cases of sub-acute bronchitis, spasmodic asthma, and whooping cough. For the latter, combine with sundew. For asthma, combine with coltsfoot root and balsam poplar bud tincture. For pneumonia, combine with coltsfoot and crampbark.

Research by Zhao et al. (2016) found verbascoside inhibits pneumolysin, a virulent factor of *Streptococcus pneumoniae*. It prevents lung damage via alveolar epithelial cell injury, preventing penetration of the bacterium into tissue. Hot infusions of mullein leaf induce sweating. It finds good use in the first stages of infection and fever. And although it acts principally on the lungs, it also soothes mucous membranes of the intestine and bladder. It relieves gastrointestinal inflammation in cases of gastritis, pancreatitis, and spasms. Use a milk decoction for intestinal distress accompanied by infections and/or bleeding.

Mullein is a most useful herb for strengthening the glandular systems, and the adrenal glands in particular. It combines well with licorice root for adrenal hypofunction and with burdock root for adrenal hyperfunction conditions. The leaf staunches bleeding in the lungs and intestinal tract. Smoking the fruity-scented leaf or drinking the leaf tea relieves acute asthma and bronchitis by relieving spasms and optimizing bronchial secretions. Be careful, as smoking mullein leaf can excessively dry out mucous membranes of the nasal passages, as will any smoke. Use a water pipe or vaporizer.

Mullein leaf is used when the cough is dry, irritating, and unproductive with a definite lack of mucus production. It is more for sub-acute or chronic coughs that persist to the point of an unproductive cough reflex. The leaf is salty with some mucilage that opens the lungs, reduces coughing, relaxes the larynx, and opens the sinuses. Matthew Wood notes the connection of mullein with lungs and kidneys. William Cook (1869) wrote the leaves possess "a peculiar and reliable power over the absorbent system, to which they seem a specific relaxant; and their power in promoting absorption in cellular dropsy … and similar accumulations of fluid, is truly remarkable." Keep in mind the rotenone in leaf is more toxic when inhaled than ingested, and it is used as an insecticide and fish poison in large concentrated doses.

In Ireland, fresh mullein leaf is renowned for the treatment of tuberculosis. In many texts you will find reference to the fresh leaf decocted in milk as a superior preparation for this disease. This suggests there are some as-yet unidentified constituents in the leaf that are fat soluble. Sore throats respond to well-strained hot leaf infusions. The leaves have small hairs that are particularly irritating, so straining the tea through a filter is very important. When combined with yarrow, the tea is taken internally for hemorrhoids, and cooled off for an effective retention enema to treat intestinal inflammation, peritonitis, fistula, and *E. coli* infections. In fact, the first mention of mullein for fistulas was recorded in the *Treatise of Fistula* by John Arderne in 1376.

Turker and Camper (2002) found the water extract of the leaf especially active against *Klebsiella pneumoniae, Staphylococcus aureus, S. epidermidis,* and *E. coli.* Lymphatic swellings, such as mumps and tonsillitis, are relieved by applying hot apple cider and mullein leaf poultices to the affected area. Glandular swellings, including swollen testes, can be relieved, using a hot fomentation of mullein leaf, snakeroot herb *(Sanicula marilandica),* and lobelia. Mastitis is relieved by placing a steamed fresh mullein leaf to the affected breast, combined with a cup or two of the infused leaf tea. Fresh wilted mullein leaves are placed in a jar and covered with a good vegetable oil and then sealed. For wounds or cuts, simply place a piece of leaf on the affected area and then bandage for 48 hours. Seldom will a scar develop. You can produce a 1:5 carrier oil with the freshly wilted leaves.

Varicose ulcers are washed with mild leaf infusions. Externally, the fresh leaf poultice relieves neuralgic pains and cramps, or can be applied for external hemorrhoid relief. If you make the above carrier oil with coconut, you can easily produce suppositories for rectal insertion. Combine with fireweed flower oil for a superior product. Matthew Wood (1997), in *The Book of Herbal Wisdom,* mentions mullein as an herb with "the intelligence to set bones." He has used it successfully in cases where it is difficult to set a bone properly, or make a chiropractic adjustment. Herniated disks, for example, sometimes respond to external application of mullein leaf or root tincture. In *The Earthwise Herbal,* he elaborates further.

It releases synovial fluid into the bursa and disperses internal fluids into the surrounding tissues, lubricating joints, muscles, bones, and ligaments. It is thus a remedy for complex fractures, where the bone needs to be lubricated, to be returned to its place. It is also indicated in spinal dryness, inflexibility, and pain, and nerve pain along pinched or irritated nerve tracts. (Wood 2009)

The basal rosette leaves or first year root are used for these spinal issues. Matthew shared the story of someone taping a fresh leaf over a broken rib, helping knit the break and reducing pain. Combine the herb with vervain for neck issues, or with horsetail for delicate bone issues of the hands and feet. Kiva Rose (2009) suggests using mullein leaf when the hips are painful, especially with rotation. It feels like you have a corkscrew instead of a lower back, especially when trying to sleep.

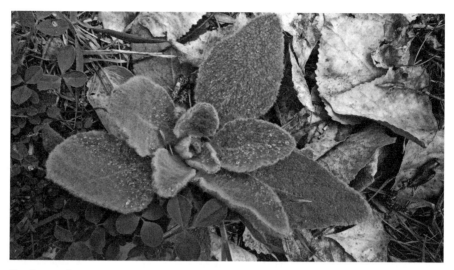

Basal rosette leaves

As mentioned in the introduction, I am an advocate of biochemic cell salts. Mullein contains both potassium and calcium phosphate, necessary for bone structure and the nervous system. I find a combination of mullein and comfrey leaves excellent for various respiratory conditions, including lung hemorrhage, and various gastrointestinal conditions and ulcerative states as well as kidney ailments with blood in the urine. Bone conditions, including osteomyelitis, benefit from a mullein-comfrey combination.

For gallstones, the whole plant is gathered after the first frost, when the ice crystals are still on the plant. This is stuffed into containers, mashed and bruised, allowed to ferment, and then drunk to dissolve stones. The French herbalist, Maurice Mességué, used mullein leaf decoction syrups for heart palpitations, tachycardia, bradycardia, and angina complaints. Trichomoniasis is a sexually transmitted disease caused by the organism *Trichomonas vaginalis*. Standard biomedical treatment is metronidazole, which has teratogenic and carcinogenic side effects. Work by Kashan et al. (2015) found mullein alcohol extracts induce apoptosis in the organism.

Verbascoside is one of the more interesting compounds in mullein. It is also found in lilac and scullcap, with more information in those sections in Chapters 7 and 8. Work by Sheng et al. (2002) suggests verbascoside may be useful in reducing stress-induced neurodegenerative diseases. Verbascoside may help to counteract muscle fatigue (Liao et al. 1999). Verbascoside significantly increases positive chronotropic and inotropic effects and the coronary perfusion rate in rat hearts (Pennacchio et al. 1996). Zheng et al. (1993) suggested verbascoside may have significant antioxidant, anti-inflammatory, and antitumor effect. Because verbascoside inhibits 5-lipooxygenase, the enzyme that catalyzes formation of inflammatory leukotrienes, it may play a key role in reducing inflammatory and allergenic conditions. Both verbascoside and luteolin decrease the oxidative stress associated with heroin use. Application in drug treatment is unknown, but is worth further investigation. The compound is anodyne (pain-relieving) and reduces peristaltic muscle activity. An in vitro study found verbascoside possesses cytotoxic effect on rat hepatoma and sarcoma cells, and cytostatic activity on human epithelial carcinoma cells (Saracoglu et al. 1995). Verbascoside shows activity against human gastric adenocarcinoma cells, and similar to DMSO, can reverse the cells' malignant nature and induce redifferentiation of these cells (Li et al. 1997). Zhang et al. (2002) found verbascoside affected telomerase activity and telomere length and induced apoptosis in gastric cancer cell lines. Telomere length on RNA strands is an important marker of longevity. Telomeres are like the small clip on the end of a shoelace. The fraying and shortening of telomeres is related to shortened life expectancy and increased risk of cellular malformations.

Tyrosine hydroxylase is a key enzyme in production of dopamine. Levels of this enzyme in the neurons in the substantia nigra of the brain are related to progression of Parkinson's disease. Verbascoside has been found to regenerate tyrosine hydroxylase-immunoreactive neurons in this region of brain (Liang et al. 2016). Work in 1980 found verbascoside decreases blood pressure and potentiates the antitremor effect of L-DOPA. Faba bean, scullcap, and mullein may be a great combination for Parkinson's disease. Verbascoside exerts corticosteroid-like inhibition of pro-inflammatory chemokines, suggesting benefit for inflamed skin conditions (Georgiev et al. 2012). Verbascoside (acteoside) stimulates lymphocyte-mediated interferon-gamma production, suggesting benefit in shortening the duration of viral infections (Song et al. 2016).

The compound is somewhat unstable and best preserved in an alcohol, or better yet, an oil base. Flower oil is better known, but the leaves contain higher levels of verbascoside and make a superior oil for external application to painful muscle, tendon, and joint pain. Use the similar 1:5 ratio as flower oil, noting that the fresh leaves are 80% water and require initial drying. Methanol extracts from leaves show activity against the influenza virus (Rajbhandari et al. 2009). Galanski et al. (1996) suggested mullein contains substances that inhibit protein biosynthesis (elongation factor eEF-2) and reduce tumor growth.

Catalpol, also found in scullcap species, enhances myeloid leukemia cell apoptosis when combined with imatinib mesylate (M. B. Kim et al. 2015). Catalpol combined with metformin, reduced blood sugar, cholesterol, and other markers in diabetic mice by increasing skeletal muscle function (Xia Li et al. 2014). It may help reduce adipose tissue inflammation and associated insulin resistance in type 2 diabetes. Catalpol may be protective against neurodegenerative conditions. A review of its potential therapeutic value was recently compiled by Jiang et al. (2015). Other studies suggest the potential to promote remyelination in MS and related conditions. The compounds luteolin and 3-O-fucopyranosyl-saikogenin F are antiproliferative and induce apoptosis in A549 lung cancer cells (Zhao et al. 2011).

All of the above properties regarding anticancer activity come with a caution by Henrietta A. Diers Rau (1968). She writes that mullein "should not be used in cancers and any other swellings where it would be injurious to have a deposit absorbed." Maybe, but this is highly doubtful. I believe she is simply copying a warning suggested by Cook regarding its use with carbuncles, buboes, and cancers. There is a certain logic to this, as mullein has some very useful properties with regard to reducing swelling and lymphatic congestion. Some herbal books suggest tannins found in mullein may be cancer-causing. The jury is still out, but mullein has considerably more anticancer activity than cancer-creating concerns. Chronic lymphatic congestion is, of course, a contributing factor in lymphoma, due to stagnation and possible mutation of abnormal cells.

Combine mullein leaf with alder bark and wild bergamot for acute lymphatic congestion and with cleavers and red root for more chronic conditions. Laura Avensaro recommends leaf infusions for mercury and chemical toxicity, kidney toxicity, and general environmental toxins in the body. I have found a combination of equal parts mullein leaf or root and goldenrod herb useful for enlarged prostate and night-time urination.

Combine in water mullein, garden sage, and rose bud or petal tincture for sore throats as a gargle, swished, and swallowed. Mullein root was decocted by the Catawba to treat croup in children. Various indigenous peoples took to smoking the leaves for pleasure, asthma, and coughs. The Menominee smoked the root for various pulmonary diseases. The bruised fall root can be applied to gout pain. The root is a diuretic and urinary tract astringent. It is warming or neutral, slightly bitter, drying, and mildly astringent.

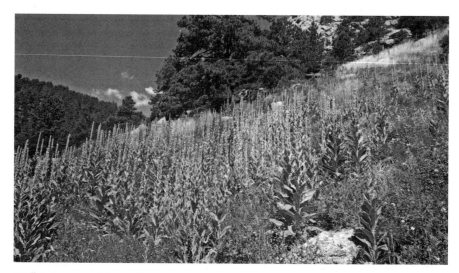

Mullein in a mountain meadow

Decoctions drunk before bedtime help bed-wetting and bladder incontinence caused by loss of tone following pregnancy or catheterization. It also works well for young children with weak bladders. It drains dampness of the lower burner, specifically the kidney and bladder. Children with enuresis after four years of age may be helped but only if due to bladder size structure and function. Equal parts of mullein root and corn silk are recommended. The root may be dried and powdered and put into 00 capsules. Mullein root strengthens sphincter control and tone, with great benefit to the elderly suffering incontinence and dribbling of urine. Stress incontinence is associated with aging or caused by a cystocele related to childbirth injury. Mullein root appears to restore tone to a prolapsed bladder. According to Charles Kane (2009, 152), "mullein root has a tonifying effect on the trigone muscle." This muscle, at the base of the bladder, is normally contracted, and for urine to enter the urethra, the trigone must relax. It combines well with stinging nettle root.

One day, a new client walked into my office. He was a well-known medicine man from a First Nation reservation south of Edmonton. After introductions, he told me his specific issue. He was suffering decreased urine flow that was painful when first coming forth, like a spasm of his bladder. A quick urine test revealed no infection, so we continued the consultation. I asked if he had ever used mullein, and he said he was not familiar with that herb. I told him it was found in British Columbia and he nodded. I suggested the root was specific for his issue, and that he ingest the tincture twenty drops three times daily in warm water for a few weeks. He returned about six weeks later with a big smile on his face. He sat down and looked at me and said, "You are a true healer. I will let my people know." That really made my day. And he did, over the years, refer many clients to my office.

Mullein root increases the volume of urination and decreases frequency. It can be used long term for urinary incontinence, recurring bladder infections, interstitial cystitis, and benign prostatic hypertrophy. For the latter, combine with fireweed leaf tea or tincture. For urinary incontinence, combine with wild strawberry root and cleavers. Combine with black cohosh with hypertension and licorice root with low blood pressure. Stinging nettle root and cleavers are good additions depending upon the picture pattern. It is a little known antispasmodic and sedative that combines well with cow parsnip seed in cases of Bell's palsy, trigeminal or facial neuralgia, as well as TMJ pain. For chronic arthritis of hands, hips, and other joints, use small doses of root tincture.

Mullein root is a little-known papaverine-like smooth-muscle relaxant and a digitalis-like cardiotonic, useful in cases of tachycardia and arrhythmia. The root may be useful for mild physical stress incontinence, or loss of urine associated with lifting weights, laughing, coughing, or running. It improves integrity of the tissue of the bladder and restores prolapsed tissue. It combines well with yellow pond lily, corn silk for the treatment of prolapsed bladder and cystocele, a bladder hernia protruding into the vagina usually due to injury caused during childbirth. It may be safely used during pregnancy for leakage and incontinence. For menopausal incontinence caused by urethral and vaginal membrane shrinkage, use the root in combination with black cohosh. If there is low adrenal function, combine with licorice root, as mentioned. Symptoms may include low blood pressure, night-time urination, frequent urination, light-colored urine, chronically dry skin and mucous membranes, and renal hypotension.

Mullein root combines well with the leaf for asthma and other spasmodic lung conditions. I like to blend it with sweet coltsfoot leaf and/or root in a smoking mixture. Use a water pipe or vaporizer to minimize smoke irritation. Ken Cohen, in his excellent book *Honoring the Medicine* (2003), mentions a Cherokee elder using mullein root for tobacco addiction. This is a fairly modern issue, as tobacco has long been a sacred herb used by various native people throughout North America.

Note: Mullein root should be harvested in the first fall or the early second spring. As the second-year plant begins to create a large columnar stem and then flowers and seeds, the root diminishes in size and energy.

Mullein flowers are a delight to pick in mid to late summer. They bloom in a random fashion on the long stalks and require hand-picking one at a time. It is very meditative.

The fresh flowers are jammed into a large glass jar and covered with a good-quality monosaturated oil. In a warm climate you can set this out in the sun for 10–14 days, shaking daily, and then strain and bottle in dark glass, labeled and stored in the fridge for later use. I like to put some in a 50 ml amber glass bottle with a dropper for ease of use. In cooler climates, use a ratio of 1 part flowers by weight to 5 parts oil by volume in a low-temperature crock pot for up to 4 hours. Cool and strain as above. If you have the time, a triple preparation is much more effective. After cooling, pressing, and straining the first batch, use the same oil for a second and then third batch of fresh flowers. You cannot purchase such a great product off the shelf.

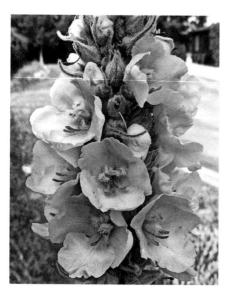

The flowers are relaxing, cool, neutral and sedative in nature, and are useful for hot, inflamed lung infections. They contain catechin tannins, flavonoids, mucilage, saponins, and traces of essential oil, but no carotenoids (despite their color) nor alkaloids. Taking ½ teaspoon of flower tincture in water before bedtime may improve your sleep. The flower tincture combines well with elderberry tincture for viral ear infections that have become chronic in nature. The flowers are heated in olive oil and then squashed and used to cure chilblains. Fresh crushed flowers are applied

Mullein flowers

to persistent warts. The flowers can be added to a bowl of hot water as a steam for respiratory weakness. Drape a towel over your head and the bowl and slowly inhale for up to five minutes. A hot fomentation of the fresh or dried flowers will help cramping of the large thigh muscles, when nothing else seems to help. Combine flower tincture with chokecherry bark for slipped discs that result in a sharp pain and burning sensation.

Ryan Drum, a west coast herbalist extraordinaire, mentions in his writings that when flowers or branches are removed, the plant exudes a black resinous gum that smells like vanilla. This resin can be gathered and made into an alcohol extract for baking. When tinctured, it is slightly psychotropic, so caution with dosage is advised. In Italy, the dried flowers are infused as tea for bronchial catarrh. The flowers possess antiviral activity against influenza A and B as well as herpes simplex (Zgórniak-Nowosielska et al. 1991). Apply flowers or prepared oil externally to affected areas for facial or genital herpes. Michael Moore (2003) noted the flower "seems most useful in women and children who have frequent outbreaks as often as monthly, triggered either by the sun, food allergies, or the estrogen surges before ovulation." I also noted the latter in my own clinical practice.

The flowers help reduce infection and pain associated with acute otitis media (Sarrell et al. 2001). The flowers in the form of a tea, oil or, tincture help relieve ear pain. Mullein flower oil combines well with garlic oil and Saint John wort carrier oil for ear pain in the young and old. Gently warm the combination before inserting a few drops. In the case of tinnitus, nerve deafness, and vertigo associated with the eighth auditory nerve, a few warm drops of mullein oil are inserted 3–4 times daily. This is combined with a tincture of equal parts yellow dock root, thuja leaf, cleavers, violet leaf, and echinacea root internally.

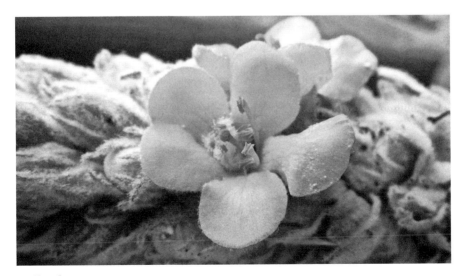

Mullein flower

A few drops of the oil soothe the most persistent cough and bring rapid relief to frost-bite when applied externally. Swollen glands and testicular pain are relieved. For hemorrhoids, itchy anus, or pain in the rectum, combine mullein flower and fireweed carrier oils as a suppository. It can be used for skin problems, including eczema, and difficult-to-heal hard and dry skin tumors. Combine it with other carrier and essential oils for external application to sprains, bruises, neuralgia, sore throat, swollen joints, and torn ligaments.

Internally, the oil is vermicidal, antiviral, and antibacterial. The flowers contain rotenone and insecticidal activity that help control and manage fleas in pets and farm animals. Mullein oil, 1 teaspoon taken internally 3–4 times daily, is an effective and safe vermifuge and anthelmintic. The flower oil helps alleviate infections in animals, especially dogs. Combine with St. John's wort oil for ear mites. Mullein flower oil relieves painful joints, cramps, arthritis, and rheumatic conditions. Dr. Cushing and Father Kneipp both suggested mullein oil for dribbling urine where the underwear is always slightly wet in children and older adults. Serkedjieva (2000) found the flowers are indeed antiviral and when combined with antanamine glucuronide (Symmetrel) produce an even more powerful antiviral synergy.

Even the seeds can be useful, with crushed seed infusions helping childhood asthma and convulsions. The seeds possess mild narcotic properties that easily pass through the

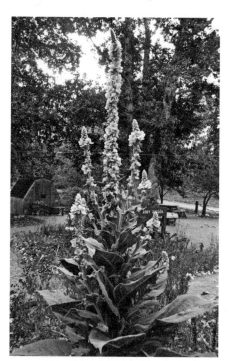

Mature second-year mullein

intestine to relieve obstructions and kill parasites. The seeds in small doses act as a kidney trophorestorative, like stinging nettle seed and goldenrod leaf. Caution is advised, as the seeds are semitoxic in moderate amounts.

Homeopathy

The homeopathic preparation is useful for excited fantasies, especially of a sensual nature. It is for excessive joyfulness with laughter. The client likes having people around and talking with them. Dreams of war and corpses are prevalent. They are affected by overpowering panic attacks and a fear of crowds and public places. There is a mania for cleanliness and washing. The left side of the body is more affected and ears feel stopped up. There is sensation of heavy weight in the legs going up and down stairs. Headaches are made worse by smoking tobacco. Lightning pain shoots over right side of face when talking, sneezing, biting hard, or even when touching teeth with tongue.

Dose: Mother tincture and low potencies. Proving by Hahnemann with five male provers using tincture in 1921. Also based on clinical observations by Hering and Mangialavori. For bed-wetting, use 5-drop doses of tincture morning and evening.

Essential Oil

An essential oil obtained by steam distilling the leaves and flowers is sometimes available. It is a light yellow oil with a vaguely nutmeg scent. It contains 14.3% of 6,10,14-trimethyl-2-pentadecanone and 9.3% of (E)-phytol. The oil has been found active against various bacteria, including *Bacillus subtilis, Staphylococcus aureus, Salmonella* Typhi, *Pseudomonas aeruginosa*, and the yeast *Aspergillus niger* (Morteza-Semnani et al. 2012). Work by Ghasemi et al. (2015) found no antibacterial or antifungal activity when he tested the essential oil. It may be useful in genital herpes and shingle pain, as well as cradle cap when diluted appropriately.

Doctrine of Signatures

Pallasdowney (2002) offers one of my favorite descriptions on this beautiful plant, based in part on the doctrine of signatures:

Mullein's stalk is stout, thick, and tall, and its base is especially strong. The entire plant is soft, fuzzy, hairy, and velvety. The plant's character of strength along with its softness represents its ability to cut through coughing and bronchial spasms that damage the soft hairs lining the mucous membranes. The velvety soft, hairy, downy leaves resemble the soft hairs of the mucous membranes.

The mullein's phallus-shaped terminal spike filled with flowers also represents strength with softness, promoting intimacy and gentleness. The densely packed lemon-yellow cuplike flowers, flower buds, and seeds are securely protected in the soft, woolly, phallic spike, demonstrating emotional openness yet a tightness offering security, protection, and personal space. This signature relates especially to men who are seeking true intimacy and security in expressing a soft, gentle, humble nature, or for women who want to strengthen yet soften their masculine nature.

Mullein's use as a torch is a signature of its ability to promote focus, purpose, and Light, thus guiding us toward our own inner selves. The woolly ear-like signature reminds us to listen to our inner selves and to others as they communicate with us.

The incredible absorbency of mullein leaves is a powerful signature. They act as a relaxant, and they promote absorption in cases of cellular dropsy, chronic disease, pleuritic effusions, and similar accumulations of fluid. Perhaps, on another level, this signature can be related to a person's process of assimilating emotional and mental states that no longer serve the individual.

The taste of the leaves is slightly bitter and their temperature is slightly cool. The leaves have a mucilaginous quality, and the roots and flowers give off a soothing aromatic scent. These qualities give a signature of the plant's physical ability to sooth irritated membranes, reduce fever, increase secretion, and clear the lungs.

Personality Traits

Matthew Wood (2008, 508) contributes to the discussion on mullein:

William LeSassier used to say that mullein was for "intellectuals and hot air people." I have confirmed this several times. It is for people who think too much and congest the mind, or suffer mental tightness and congestion following difficult projects. Mullein gives such a person a feeling like the mind is opened up to breezes on a fresh spring day—speaking from personal experience. William also emphasizes that the voice box is often affected. The voice can be too high or too low.

Kiva Rose (2009) offers a unique perspective:

I have also seen mullein flower tincture work very well in guiding and providing focus to those who feel they have lost their way or can't see their path. They often feel in the dark and disjointed, and the confusion leaves them tense and with a deep sense of abandonment. Consider it the perfect plant for those "hiding their light under a bushel" instead of letting it shine, usually from fear of rejection or out of confusion of how to shine.

Botanica Poetica

MULLEIN

Is Junior coughing hard at night?
His trachea is all inflamed
He's got you up, no sleep in sight
Well here's an herb, his cough to tame
Spasmodic cough it can improve
Help him to expectorate
Mucous membranes it can soothe
Lymphatic drainage facilitate
And if the ear is aching so
Use the oil as in a balm

Apply directly, 'cause you know
Ear pains it can gently calm
Mullein flowers shown to slay
Virus strains like the flu
If you're sick do not delay
Here's a tea designed for you
Verbascum thapsus, leaf and flower
Irritation you can soothe
For bronchitis you've got power
To fight catarrh and thus improve.

—Sylvia Chatroux (2004)

Astrology

Kranich (1984) writes:

Because the synodial rhythm is fifty days longer than two years, the conjunctions and oppositions of Mars and the sun occur in ever-changing sections of the zodiac. There are years, then, during which Mars enhances, and others during which it obstructs, the sun's influence. During some years, we may, for example, see more mulleins and thistles than during others.

RECIPES

Infusion: 1 tablespoon of dried leaves to 1 pint of boiling water. Let steep 20 minutes. Strain well in paper filter as the tiny hairs can be very irritating. Take 1–3 cups daily. The dried plant must be protected from light and particularly from moisture. Otherwise the plant changes color to brown or dark brown due to the iridoid content.

Fresh leaf decoction: Simmer 1 handful of fresh leaves in 1 quart of fresh milk, strained and drunk several times daily, sweetened with honey. It soothes the lungs, increases weight, and restores vitality. Leaves are picked in late spring before flowering, or the previous summer.

Dose: 2–3 ounces up to 4 times daily. Decoctions should be low-heat to avoid destroying the minor mucilage properties.

Decoction syrup: Simmer 2 handfuls of leaf and flowers in 2 quarts of water for 1 hour. When reduced by half, add honey or blackstrap molasses. Take 1 tablespoon of syrup 2 times daily between meals for heart complaints.

Tincture: 1–4 ml taken 3 times daily. The mother tincture is made from the fresh plant in flower. The leaf tincture is best made from first-year leaf for lung and kidney problems. The flower tincture is much stronger and more nervine. Root tincture is made from first-year fall root. For either flower, root, or leaf tincture, use 1:3 for fresh material and 1:5 for dry at 60% alcohol.

Capsules: Root powder. Take two 00 capsules with each meal for 6 weeks. Children ages 6 to 12 would take half the dosage.

Caution: Due to the diuretic action of the leaf, mullein may interfere with anti-inflammatory drugs, interfere with diabetic or hypertension drugs, or increase the risk of hypokalemia when taken with corticosteroids. Maybe.

Flower oil: Cover 1 part by weight of flowers with 5 parts of canola or olive oil by volume in a glass jar, and set in the sun for up to 2 weeks. Allow venting on top to prevent moisture spoilage. Strain well and bottle in dark glass. Warm up and use for ear problems: 5–8 drops in the affected ear held in with cotton. Externally, rub into affected joints and glandular swellings. Internally, 1–3 drops three times daily for urinary dribbling and incontinence in children, especially associated with bedtime and when the urine is alkaline. How can you easily tell if urine is acidic or alkaline? You can use a pH strip, or simply tear off a small piece of red cabbage and add to the urine. If it is acidic, the color of vegetable will turn red, and if it is alkaline, it will turn blue-purple. Mullein leaf, aspen bark, and fireweed in equal dried parts by weight can be covered with coconut oil in a crockpot. Simmer at low temperature for 6 hours. Strain and pour into suppository molds for hemorrhoids.

Bronchial syrup: Take 1 cup each of red clover blossoms, pine needles, and mullein leaves. In saucepan cover with 4 cups of water, bring to a boil, lower the heat, and simmer for 20 minutes. Strain the juice through double cheesecloth and add 1 pint of honey. Bring this to a boil, and store it in fridge. Take 1 or 2 teaspoons as needed.

Calamus

Calamus • Rat Root • Sweet Flag • Fire Root—*Acorus americanus* (Raf.) Raf.

The flower is a long thing … of a greenish yellow color, curiously checkered, as if it were wrought with a needle with green and yellow silk intermixt.

—John Gerard

You are often more bitter than I can bear,
You burn and sting me,
Yet you are beautiful to me your faint tinged roots.

—Walt Whitman

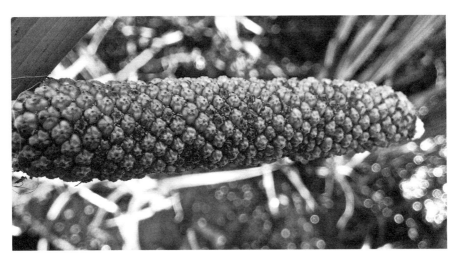

Calamus seed head

Calamus root is a universal panacea in the northern part of Canada. It is commonly known as rat root and is highly prized among indigenous peoples. It is an important herbal ally for a number of reasons, as you will soon find out.

Calamus may derive from the Greek *kalamos* or Arabic *kalon*, meaning "pen" or "reed," and probably from the Sanskrit *kalamas*. Kalamos was the son of the river god Meander, and he loved Karpos (Carpus), the son of Zephyrus and Chloris. When Karpos drowned, Kalamos was transformed into a reed, whose rustling song is a sigh of lamentation. Carpus became the "fruit of the fields" that die and are reborn each year. *Vacha* is the Sanskrit name for this plant, meaning "power of the voice." In Ayurvedic medicine, the related *Acorus calamus* is said to restore memory, communication, and self-expression and is widely used after a stroke, for shock, or for coma. Related words include *calamari*, meaning "squid," from the Latin *calamarium*, "ink horn" or "pen case"; *calumet*, another name for a native peace pipe made from the hollow reed; and *chalumeau*, the lower notes of a clarinet's range. *Acorus* derives from the Greek or Arabic *akoron*, and in turn from *kore* or *coreon*, meaning "the pupil of the eye." *Kore* is a Greek word for "girl" and is the original name of the goddess Persephone. Andrzej Szczeklik et al. (2012, 58–59) write:

> *Kore is the Ancient Greek word for a girl, and also for the pupil of the eye. The Greeks said that the soul was invisible in the form of a little girl, through the pupil. How could they have known that the pupil is the one and only tiny window that gives a view of the brain and of the ocular nerves?*

The last weekend of August, for the past fifteen years, has been reserved on my calendar for Rat Root Rendezvous. The location is south of Chip Lake, a long shallow body of water that is home to millions of calamus plants. Lori and Randy Breeuwsma are the generous hosts. Survivalists, wild-crafters, herbalists, wilderness guides and a host of veterans and newbies gather to reconnect, share skills, and listen to the stories of Mors Kochanski. Mors is a world-renowned author and teacher of the art of northern bushcraft, elucidated in his 1987 book. His knowledge of survival skills is second to none.

Randy, Mors, and I traveled together many years ago making plant videos of the boreal and aspen parkland forests of Alberta. We have kept in touch and enjoy each other's company whenever the opportunity arises. The highlight of the weekend is a hike down to the lake to gather rat root, named after the favorite food of muskrats. In fact, its flesh is so rich in the unusual flavor that some people find them difficult to eat. Personally I enjoy the spicy, peppery taste of the meat as well as the root, which is really a large rhizome. Collecting this medicinal plant requires getting wet, and although it is often found growing alongside the similar-looking cattail, it can be a struggle to collect the matted intertwined rhizomes. At first glance it appears like a cattail, but on closer inspection it's true nature is revealed. A flower–seed head at a 45-degree angle lets you know you have the correct plant, and the distinct scent of the rhizome.

Work by Albertazzi et al. (1998) suggests *Acorus* might be the most ancient surviving representative of the ancestral monocotyledonous plants. The plant has been prized and

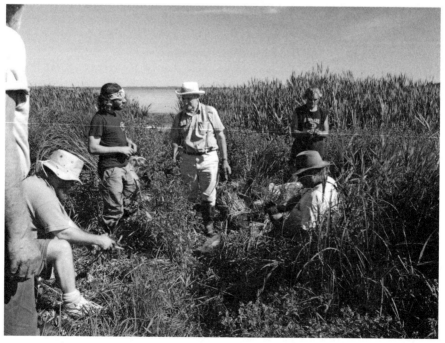

Mors (center) and friends harvesting rat root

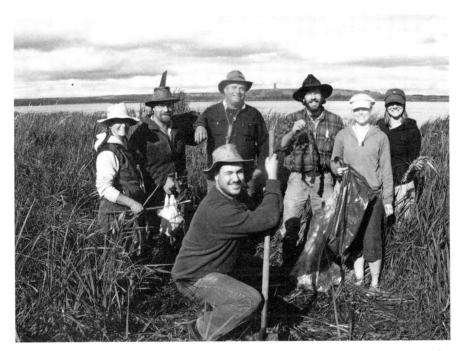

Note the prize-winning root dug by Al Wardale. To his right are noted survival instructors Randy Breeuwsma and Kelly Harlton.

praised throughout the world, and we are most fortunate that the safest variety is our western North American asarone-free diploid ($2n = 24$) type. This plant produces viable seed and was probably chosen tens of thousands of years ago for planting across western North America. It has two to six raised veins and a swollen center to the leaf in cross section. Frans Vermeulen and Linda Johnston (2011) contribute from their epic four-volume *Plants*:

> *There are various mythological and biological connections of the muskrat to Acoraceae. On a purely prosaic level, the muskrat enthusiastically dines on the plant's roots. It is an emblematic correlation that an animal, like the plant, living so happily in watery, muddy areas, is endowed with such enticing aromatic fragrances. Out of water rises earth and from earth rises the spiritual realm of heaven. The continuum between water, mud, earth, and heavenly bliss is traversed on the wings of intoxicating aromas.*

The rhizomes twist and bunch up in the swamp like thick mats, requiring strength, perseverance, and a sense of humor. An unofficial contest at our annual Rat Root Rendezvous involves digging up the longest intact rhizome, which can be eighteen inches or more.

The plant is both a panacea and sacred to the Cree of northern Alberta. I will often make a fresh root tincture after carefully washing and cutting it in small pieces after the harvest. But I also leave a lot in its whole dried form to give as gifts. There are many home-less people in Edmonton, with a high percentage of aboriginal descent. They may be found panhandling in my favorite part of town, and instead of money I reach into my pocket and give them a good-size piece. In some cases it will take a short while for a response, but in the end there is always a thank-you and a smile. In my mind, I am hoping that a spark of spiritual connection is taking place. But in any case, the gift of calamus makes me feel good.

It is much mentioned in the Bible, and was immortalized by the mystic Walt Whit-man, in his famous *Leaves of Grass*. Initially, twelve poems in the calamus chapter of *Leaves of Grass* (1855) were symbolic of the love of male comrades, adhesiveness, and personal attachment. The seventh edition, published in 1881, contains thirty-nine calamus poems. The gay liberation movement of the 1970s, still going strong, praised the calamus poems as a homosexual manifesto. Calamus has long symbolized male love, perhaps in part due to its symbolic penis-like spathe.

Traditional Uses

The Cree of Northern Alberta make great use of this muskrat food, or *wachaskomechiwin*. It is known as "rat root" or "muskrat root," *wacaskwatapih*, or simply *wihkes* or *wiyikiyo*. The Eastern Ojibwe name is very similar, *wike*, or *wee-kees*. The Swamp Cree who live near Hudson Bay call it "fire root" or "bitter pepper root," or *pow e men artic*. The Dene (Chipewyan) call it "muskrat food," *dzen ni*. The root is slowly chewed and used to over-come fatigue on long journeys.

The Asian calamus root, due to its content of alpha- and beta-asarone, is considered sedative, but the North American diploid is stimulating to the mind and relaxing to the body. It cuts phlegm and is used in relieving asthma. For cramped arms and legs, paralyzed limbs, or rheumatic swellings, poultices or hot fomentations are applied to affected areas. It is often chewed for diabetes, or held in the throat for a long time to "get rid of the tonsils by burning them off," according to one Cree healer. For earache, a small piece of root is softened in water and gently inserted.

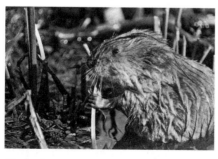

The Dene smudge dried rat root and inhale the smoke for headaches. The crushed root is boiled and cooled for stom-achache and to help pass pinworms. Some Thlingchadine (Dogrib) healers say rat root should not be taken within a few hours of modern medicines. The name *Thingchadine* means "dog flank people," based on a tradi-tional legend. Native drummers will often tie a string on the dried root and hang it around their necks. They can then chew

Muskrat

and suck on it to keep their singing voices strong hour after hour, hence the name "drummer's root" or "singer's root." The dried root definitely resembles the trachea in the doctrine of signatures.

The Kainai (Blood) of southern Alberta call it *pow-e-men-artic*, or fire root, and use the root to relieve coughs and treat liver ailments. The neighboring Blackfoot had to trade for the root and used it with tobacco as a smoking mixture, or alone as an abortifacient. The English settlers called the Kainai band "Bloods" due to their use of ocher for red face "paint." The Teton Dakota chewed calamus root and rubbed the paste on their faces to prevent excitement and fear. The Anishinaabe combined the root tea, with chokecherry bark for coughs. The Ojibwe used the root medicinally and call it *powemenarctic*, or "muskrat root." Note the extreme similarity to the Kainai name.

The Tsitsistis (Cheyenne) know it as "bitter medicine," *wi'ukh is e'evo*, and traded with their Dakota (Sioux) neighbors for the root. They tied a small piece on their children's necklace for both protection from night spirits and to numb teething pain. *Cheyenne* is a Sioux word meaning "relatives of the Cree." *Sioux* is from the Ojibwe word meaning "little snakes" and is today considered a derogatory term. They tossed pieces of the root on glowing rocks in the sweat lodge for cleansing purposes. The powdered root was combined with bark of red osier dogwood in smoking mixtures. It was known as a "ghost medicine," with the power to ward off evil. The leaves were braided or added to baby bundles for good luck and as an aromatic insecticide. The innermost tender leaf is edible, as is the flower bud before flowering. It is not really that tasty. The Pawnee name is *kahtsha itu*, meaning "medicine lying in water." The young green blades were traditionally braided into fragrant neck garlands. The Lakota name, *sinke tawote*, means "muskrat food." The specific name *sunkace*, meaning "dog penis," refers to the phallic shape of the seed head, which is found halfway up the stem of some plants at a 45-degree angle.

Tis Mal Crow (2001), a Native American root doctor, uses calamus root as an activator or accelerator that increases the potency of other herbs. He believes it should only be added in 1 part to 32 parts of other herbs, or the mixture may be dangerously strong. Calamus is used specifically with white-flowered medicines for this purpose; and violet leaves are used to activate green medicines. He notes the plant follows the doctrine of signatures:

> Calamus is another good doctrine of signatures plant. It grows in the swamp or bog in really smelly and sulfurous places, the coldest, dankest part of the swamp. The root also looks like a larynx. This shows us that it is good for colds and congestion, breaks up phlegm, and is good for the throat and voice.

Medicinal Uses

Constituents: *A. americanus* rhizome: 243 components, including mainly sesquiterpene and monoterpenes ketones, aconic and acoric acid, mucilage, bitters, tannins, choline, essential oils, acorin, acoretin, galangin, furfural, shyobunone, and iso-shyobunone (8.62%). Also found are 6-epishyobunone, elemicin, 2,6-di-epi-shyobunone, dehydroxy-isocalamendiol (22.81%), acorafuran, acorone, acoragermacrone, isoacoranone, acorenone, geranylacetate, and small amounts of calamendiols. Up to 26% acorone may be present in dried roots. Beta-asarone (cis-isoasarone) may or may not be present in diploid type, and if so, at an extremely low percentage. Alpha-asarone may be present in low amounts, if at all, and amines, such as dimethylamine, methylamine, and trimethylamine are also present.

Aerial leaves: tropone, beta-curcumene, acolamone, acoragermacrone, acoric acid, acorine, ascorbic acid, borneol, calarene, delta-guazulene, dimethylamine, mycrene, saponins, tannins, trans anethole, trimethylamine.

The rhizome is warm, pungent, bitter, and aromatic. I personally use the root tea or tincture for sore throat or for that feeling of an impending cold with flu-like symptoms. Calamus root is used, as a cold infusion, for all manner of digestive complaints, including hyperacidity. It stimulates the salivary glands and yet counteracts acidity and reduces heartburn and gas, combining well with meadowsweet (*Filipendula ulmaria*). Flatulence due to poor digestion is eased and appetite increased.

Cold infusions of the root promote pancreatic function, one sip before and one sip after meals three times daily in cases of mild late-onset diabetes. It is highly prized for its specific action on stomach cancer, working in a manner similar to *condurango* vine from South America. In Europe our calamus root is much prized for this purpose and warrants further investigation.

Small pieces can be chewed for kicking addictions to nicotine. When chewed, the juices combine with the taste of tobacco, causing nausea and working as aversion therapy. In small amounts it is stimulating and euphoric. It also affects the brain during withdrawal from cocaine, marijuana, heroin, and morphine. During this time, addicts experience intense craving, nausea, and vomiting, which calamus root can help modify. Later, when the brain can be stimulated by wheat, meat, and milk, *Acorus* seems to enable the process by which the brain recognizes these nondrug opiates. The herbalist 7Song suggests chewing the root is good for a pot hangover. I am not sure how he came upon this information.

Matthew Wood (2009, 58) writes of a case where it appeared palliative in Alzheimer's disease or related brain trauma:

> A woman in her fifties fell down a mountainside and sustained a head injury. She was extremely debilitated, to the point where she would get lost for hours two blocks from home. We tried peony root without success and then calamus. She said the effect was immediate, profound, and highly beneficial. Each time she took the tincture, the plant seemed to say to her, "Concentrate." It taught her a new and different way of thinking and rescued her from an almost helpless state.

Galangin, present in American calamus rhizome, inhibits acetylcholinesterase activity, an approach widely used in the search for the treatment of Alzheimer's disease (Guo et al. 2010).

324

The compound is a potent inhibitor of BACE1, a key enzyme for beta-amyloid production. This suggests possible neuroprotective benefit, including prevention or treatment of Alzheimer's (Zeng et al. 2015). Elemicin, also found in nutmeg oil, is psychoactive. The wonderful herbalist Jim McDonald (2016) contributes greatly to the conversation.

> *Calamus is best understood as a plant whose spirit teaches those who make relationship with it how to live in a good way upon the Earth; to live gently, lucidly, perceptively. She is subtle, and teaches a subtlety of perception, a subtlety of awareness.... Those who do not perceive such subtleties will likely find little in her of merit (though they could most benefit from such teachings). But make no mistakes: the plant is incredibly wise and quite sentient. If perhaps you cannot feel what she is putting out, she can certainly feel what you are. It is impossible to really describe what my relationship with this plant is like. How would you describe an orange to someone who had never tasted one? The best that can be done, I suppose, is to offer such descriptions as strike near the mark. There's something about Calamus I've always likened to the song of crickets. If I were to describe her using the idea of resonance, of sound, I would think of the long, slow undulating rhythm of crickets, and the way you come to feel if you sit out in the evening and just let that music wash over you ... the way your tension dissipates, the way your mind slowly lets go of its many errant simultaneous thoughts, one by one, till you're just there, right where you're at, and perfectly contented to be there. Tibetan "singing" bowls create a similar effect in me, if they continue for a long enough time ... but they don't quite compare to crickets, or the rustling of leaves in the wind, or the running of water over stones.*

Small pieces of dried root relieve toothache and teething pain in young children and adults. A tincture of the fresh root is a good parasiticide applied to the skin and hair for lice, scabies, and crabs. The root can be powdered and rubbed into affected areas as well. A hot poultice of the mashed or powdered root is applied to injured extremities where circulation is impaired and tissue damage severe. It is most useful in metabolic sluggishness where there is an accumulation of toxins. Like bogbean (*Menyanthes*), it is a gentle, cleansing, digestive herb. Calamus root is good for digestive stagnation associated with gas, bloating, belching, and congestion. A body-temperature enema can be helpful for rectal pain associated with hemorrhoids without bleeding. Be careful with irritable bowel issues, as the root is not demulcent.

Individuals with low-grade annoying fevers and poor vital energy will enjoy this herb. Sweet flag, especially the fresh root, promotes menses delayed by chilled or exhausted dispositions. Decoctions are useful in muscle spasms, restlessness, and insomnia and are most sedative to the central nervous system. Acoric acid is a sesquiterpene with hypotensive properties. Some authors have speculated high levels of organic potassium in the rhizome help relieve asthma, hay fever, hiccups, and muscular dystrophy. This is too simple an explanation, in my opinion.

The asarone-free genotype calamus shows antispasmodic properties (Keller et al. 1985). Other calamus genotypes do not share this property. Work by Gilani et al. (2006) confirmed this antispasmodic nature and suggested the activity was calcium channel–like in action. The rhizome exhibits antifungal and antibacterial activity but is not antiviral in nature. The rhizome extract shows significant activity against *Mycobacterium tuberculosis*, with less toxicity to three human cell lines than the DMSO positive control (Webster et al. 2010). Scientists have identified additional compounds in *Acorus* acting on the body chemicals other than from a strictly histaminic perspective in stopping bronchial constriction during asthmatic attacks. Methyl isoeugenol, for example, is an expectorant, antispasmodic, antihistaminic, and antibacterial. Shah and Gilani (2010) determined the bronchodilating activity is mediated through multiple pathways.

It makes a stimulating morning bath, showing the different effects gained by external versus internal application. Baths are very useful for general exhaustion during convalescence, anemia, and diabetic conditions. Gary Raven, a traditional healer from Manitoba, recommends calamus, wild licorice (*Glycyrrhiza lepidota*), and white water lily root be grated and used as a tea for diabetes. Small slices can be chewed to treat high cholesterol. Choline counteracts excessive cholesterol and assists the manner in which it prevents its potential buildup on arterial walls.

Calamus root is very active on the human peroxisome proliferator–activated receptor associated with fat and blood sugar regulation (Rau et al. 2006). Other herbs showing similar activity include corn silk, cayenne, water plantain, and stinging nettle. Work by Acuna et al. (2002) on American calamus found high antioxidant activity in ethanol extracts of the rhizome. A substance other than beta-asarone in calamus root, extracted by ethyl acetate, enhances adipocyte differentiation and may have a benefit in the treatment of type 2 diabetic conditions. It appears to have rosiglitazone-like activity (Hao-Shu Wu et al. 2007). Calamus root appears to decrease serum glucose and triglycerides and increase insulin sensitivity in genetically obese mice (Wu et al. 2009). Calamus root protects brain tissue from free radicals produced by excessive oxygen. This can occur in various brain-related disorders, including stroke, where a restored flow of oxygen to previously deprived cells can cause brain-tissue damage. A formula of calamus root and Oriental cedar seed (*Thuja orientalis*) as well as figwort, *Lycium* fruit, and licorice root is used in TCM for ADD, depression, and Alzheimer's disease.

Beta-asarone, found in European and Asian-type calamus, may be of benefit in cognitive impairment including Alzheimer's disease (Geng et al. 2010; Chang and Teng 2015) and may help prevent epileptic activity (Hazra et al. 2007). American calamus contains shyobunone, iso-shyobunone, and acorenone. The former compound shows GABA(A) modulation and the latter two only weak modulating properties (Zaugg et al. 2011). *Acorus* root lectins have been identified and studied by Bains et al. (2005). They significantly inhibit growth of J774, a murine macrophage cancer cell line, and to a lesser extent, B cell lymphoma tissue. The leaves of *A. calamus* inhibit pro-inflammatory cytokine release and may be useful for treating skin disease (Kim et al. 2009).

TMA-2, a controlled drug in the United States, is a hallucinogen with at least ten times the potency of mescaline. Asarone is naturally converted to TMA-2 in the body by amination shortly after ingestion. This only occurs, however, when either alpha- or beta-asarone are present. In chemical structure, alpha-asarone is similar to mescaline from the peyote cactus, while beta-asarone is more chemically like myristicin, found in nutmeg and kava-kava. The wild western North American root contains little if any asarone. Alexander Shulgin (1991), the great psychedelic chemist, manufactured TMA-2 and took amounts ranging from 10 to 40 milligrams. At 40 milligrams, the drug was "benign and peaceful and lovely … some visuals but not intrusive. Moderate good-mannered kaleidoscopic imagery against dark. Music superb. Clear thinking. Calmly cosmic. This is a seminal, or archetypal psychoactive material."

It appears that European roots have been planted and are taking hold in the northeastern United States. This triploid cytotype does contain asarone derivatives and produces sterile seeds. There is considerable confusion over the viability of *A. americanus* seeds. I have personally germinated fresh seeds from northern Alberta. The original *Acorus calamus* toxicity studies fed rats a diet containing 500 parts per million of Asian calamus essential oil until they formed malignant intestinal tumors. So what? This is science? A similar piece of nonsensical toxicology testing was performed on sassafras a number of years ago, suggesting safrole was toxic when injected into mice. Many herbalists, including myself, believe the European variety is safe for use. The asarone-free variety is abundant in northwestern North America, and that is the root I harvest and use.

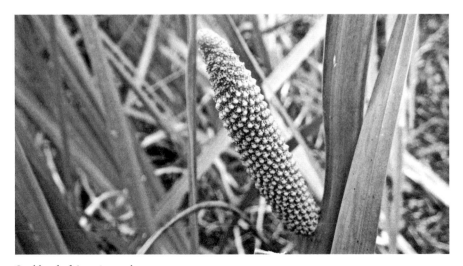

Seed head of American calamus

Essential Oils

I have steam-distilled both the rhizome and leaves of *Acorus americanus*. The rhizome contains some unusual constituents, including shyobunones (13–45%), isoshyobunone (8–13%), beta-farnesene, methyl eugenol, calamenen (4%), beta-sesquiphellandrene (3%), preisocalamenediol (7–12%), calamenol (5%), alpha-cadinol, linalool, calamone, azulene, camphor, acolamone, pinene, acorone, and isocorone (11%), acorenone (9–18%), asaralde-hyde, and cineole, among 243 recorded volatile components. The aldehyde with the characteristic odor is (Z,Z)-4,7-decadienal ($C_{10}H_{16}O$). Its concentration in the oil is 500 parts per million, and the odor threshold value 4.2 parts per billion. The concentration is about 100,000 times its odor threshold, indicating the importance of this compound to overall odor composition.

Steam distillation of the fresh root yields a yellow and then reddish volatile oil (up to 6%) that is heavy, earthy, and slightly sweet with bitter undertones. It is described by some writers as resembling dried milk and sweet leather, and has been compared to the fragrance of a milk truck or a shoe repair shop.

The essential oil produced from fresh rhizomes is finer and more soluble in weak alcohol. In my own distillations, at 40% moisture, the yield is about 0.7%. The fresh rhizome oil is very difficult to obtain and definitely has a worldwide demand. The outer rhizome peel contains the most essential oil and should not be peeled before distillation.

Oil from the leaves is a straw-yellow camphor-rich product containing butyric and oenanthylic acids as esters. Yield is about 0.5–1.0%. Work by Radusiene et al. (2007) looked at the essential oil composition of various *Acorus calamus* leaves and found 84 constituents representing at least 86% of the essential oil. *Acorus calamus* oil was used by the Egyptians as part of an ointment given to Moses that contained myrrh, cinnamon, and cassia infused in olive oil. Its mind-altering effects are used for meditation and psychic development and in perfume blends for its smooth middle notes. The North American fragrance market presently uses about $30 million of imported oils annually.

Beta-asarone is low or undetectable in the diploid cytotype North American root essential oil (Keller and Stahl 1983). It can be used for congested kidneys and bladder infections. Bronchitis and asthmatic complaints, with a need for antibacterial and antispasmodic properties, suggest using calamus essential oil. Isoasarone-free calamus essential oil exhibits an antispasmodic effect, while oils from Asian *Acorus calamus*, containing up to 96% isoasarone, possesses no spasmolytic effect. Alpha-cadinol is active against human colon cancer cell line HT-29 (He et al. 1997). Calamenene induces dendritic cell maturation, with a strong Th1 direction. This may have an application as an adjuvant in cancer vaccines.

Either steam with or rub 5% diluted in carrier oil onto the chest to achieve the calming effect. Massages relax tense and sore muscles; tired feet and varicose veins feel rejuvenated and toned. For a footbath, use calamus oil and a dispersant in hot water, or a few drops of oil in a cool bath to help relieve menopausal hot flashes. Steam with calamus root essential oil for rhinitis and sinusitis. Place a few drops of oil into a bowl of hot boiled water and inhale, placing a towel over the head to trap the aromatic vapors more efficiently. The scent prolongs sleeping time in a dose-dependent manner. Calamus oil can be mixed as a 5% dilution in silverweed root tincture and water as a mouthwash for gingivitis. It is a digestive and biliary stimulant, useful in anorexia, gas pains, and digestive spasms. The oil clears phlegm in the gastrointestinal tract and calms nervous problems such as vertigo and tension headaches. The oil will assist those suffering intermittent fevers and is mildly vermifuge in action.

It has been noted that considerable amounts of heat are given off at the time of flowering. The temperature near the early spring flower head is often 45 degrees warmer than the surrounding air. This helps attract insects that assist in cross-pollination. Skunk cabbage, another great respiratory herb, utilizes the same strategy. The flowers could be steam distilled and investigated further. I may have to do this one day. Shyobunone and isoshyobunone are strongly insecticidal, suggesting the essential oil may be a useful addition to insect repellants (H. P. Chen et al. 2015).

Studies in the Czech Republic found the essential oil content was higher in the spring (0.8–2.6%) than fall (1.0–1.8%). Although it may not be relevant to North America, the same researchers found a close negative relationship between essential oil content, the concentration of calcium in the water, and the pH of the substrate. Work in Russia found rhizomes and roots dried in the sun yield 10% and 30% less essential oil, respectively, than plant material dried in the shade. Calamus root oil is often combined with catnip oil and beaver castor as a muskrat lure in the boreal forest lakes and swamps.

Hydrosol

The hydrosol of dried Canadian calamus root is masculine and earthy, while the fresh root is similar but even greener. I like both, but many people find it too intense. The pH is 4.6. Suzanne Catty (2001) writes, "The hydrosol makes a gently astringent aftershave on its own, or combined with sandalwood, cedar wood, or bay laurel. It probably has some benefit in various digestive problems concerning the liver, stomach, and pancreas, and is worthy of further research." I agree.

Flower Essence

Years ago I created an *Acorus americanus* flower essence and trialed it for possible clinical application. It is a research essence of the Prairie Deva flower essence line. Calamus flower essence appears helpful to those individuals who have difficulty with temperature regulation. Cold or hot night sweats, menopausal flushes, or individuals who experience one-sided heat or cold in body would benefit. Individuals who have noticeable heat loss from the head, or who are Sulphur types homeopathically, may find this flower essence especially useful for skin conditions.

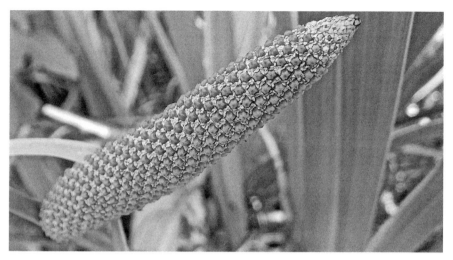

Calamus flower head

Myths and Legends

Ranco (2007) recorded the following legend:

> It is said that in the old days, the Penobscot people were suffering from a great plague. Many were ill, many had died. One of the leaders, severely troubled about the illness sweeping his people, prayed to the Creator for help. That night, the Muskrat appeared to him in his dreams.
>
> "You have prayed for help for your people", said the Muskrat, "and I have come to help you. Look carefully and remember."
>
> The man looked closely and saw the Muskrat turn himself into a plant. He examined the plant closely until he knew it well. He looked deeper and saw that the spirit and power of the Muskrat was contained within the root of the plant and thus knew that this was the part of the plant he was to use.
>
> When he awoke, he dressed and traveled to the place where he had been shown the plant would be found. There he dug it up and made medicine for his people. In this way the Penobscot people were healed and sweet flag, muskrat root, came to the people.

Note: The Penobscot people now refer to themselves as Panawahpskek, meaning "rocks spread out," the geographic location of their homeland.

Botanica Poetica

Calamus to calm you down
A GI tonic quite renown
If colic is the situation
Spasm or nervous tension
Relax and sooth, it's known to do
A GI cramp it will undo
Volatile oils there are within
Reducing flatulence therein
Ulcer, gastritis, a poor appetite
Sweet flag helps to set things right
A demulcent to coat and soothe
Dyspepsia you could improve
It's a spice that clears the mind
Better focus you will find
To quit tobacco, ease the hype
For the excited nervous type
But here's a piece of sound advice
Don't abuse this bitter spice
Not high dose, not continuous
Otherwise it's dangerous
So when you think of calamus
Think aromatic bitter, par excellence!

—Sylvia Chatroux (2004)

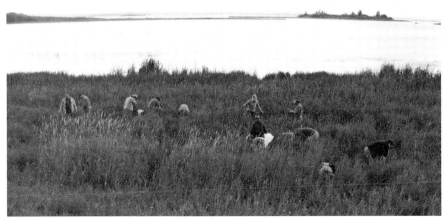

Harvesting calamus root

RECIPES

Cold infusion: This is necessary, as heat and boiling destroy some vital properties. Soak 1 ounce of chopped fresh or dried root in 1 quart of water overnight. Gently warm in the morning and drink ½ cup before meals.

Tincture: 20–30 drops up to 3 times daily. Small amounts reduce stomach acidity, while larger doses increase acid production. Make a fresh rhizome tincture at 70% at 1:3, or from the dried rhizome at 1:5, and 40% alcohol. Cut the root into thin slices when fresh, as the dry root becomes hard like a rock.

Essential oil: 2–3 drops twice daily. If used externally, dilute with carrier oil. It works like arnica for relieving deep pain.

Decoction: For bath: Bring 1 ounce of root to simmer in 1 quart of water for 20 minutes. Strain and add to a hot bath for nervous exhaustion. For enema, use only 2 teaspoons of dried root to 5 ounces of water. Strain and cool to body temperature. C. Chen et al. (2009) found a 1-hour decoction reduced beta-asarone content in European roots by 85%. Note the above indication for cold infusion of the North American variety, helping retain valuable volatiles.

Caution: Avoid during pregnancy. It is worthy of note that the European calamus contains up to 15% beta-asarone and is considered free of side effects or health hazards by the *PDR for Herbal Medicines* when taken in therapeutic doses. *Acorus calamus* from India may contain up to 70% beta-asarone. This variety could be a health concern if taken for any period of time.

10

Rutting Moon Herbal Allies

Rhodiola

Roseroot—*Rhodiola rosea* L.

Every herbalist has their favorite plant. Mine is Rhodiola rosea.

—Chris Kilham

Mine as well! I have a very close and personal connection with my herbal ally *Rhodiola*. In 2002 I identified roseroot in a report commissioned by the province as the number-one medicinal herb of choice for commercial production in Alberta. Later, as chairman of The Alberta Natural Health Agricultural Network, I helped initiate the Rhodiola Project, which began the cultivation of several million plants in 2004 to 2007. This selection was based on several market factors, including hardiness, commercial demand, and other variables. Siberian *Rhodiola rosea* is widely wild-crafted and will soon be on the endangered species list. Government support helped fund and build a processing facility to assist small-acreage farmers benefit from this new potential agricultural opportunity.

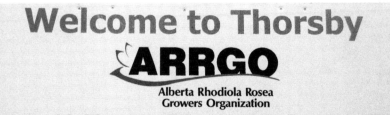

Rhodiola *facility*

Roseroot requires fourteen hours of daylight to come out of its dormant state and begin to photosynthesize and grow. It is hardy to −76°F, is drought resistant, and will grow on poor, even gravelly soil. Yields of 5,520 pounds per acre were found in central Alberta based on five-year growth.

The rhizome has a mild roselike scent when cut or bruised as well as a beautiful pink color. *Rhodiola rosea* was the binomial chosen by Linnaeus for the rose- or geranium-like scent of the dry root. He reported use of the plant as an astringent to treat hernia, leucor-rhea, headache, and hysteria.

There are three species of *Rhodiola* in North America. Roseroot is found from the mountains of North Carolina to the arctic circle. *Rhodiola rhodantha* is native to the Rocky Mountains from New Mexico up to the Canadian border. *Rhodiola integrifolia* may be a hybrid of the two, found widely in the Rocky Mountains with some isolated populations in Minnesota and New York.

When researching the species to grow, a group of Alberta agriculturist ventured into the nearby Rockies and found several species, but none contained the rosavins and salidro-sides desired by the herb industry. Bertalan Galambosi, a research scientist from Finland, helped our organization with a large donation of viable seeds to start our project. I was fortunate enough to spend a few days with this esteemed senior scientist when he visited my hometown of Edmonton. He retired in 2011.

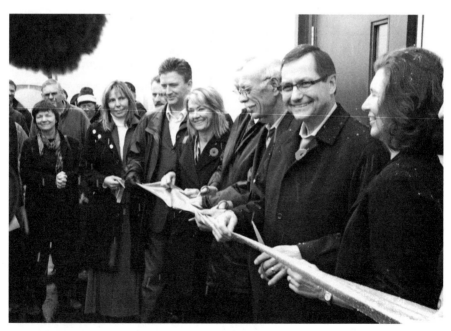

Alberta premier Ed Stelmach at the grand opening of the plant

Traditional Uses

According to the Eclectic physician John King, the Cree chewed the leaves of roseroot for wounds and drank a tea. Although edible, the leaves should be eaten in moderation due to several constituents that cause emetic and cathartic response. Roseroot was traditionally boiled with other plants by the Inuit for stomach and intestinal discomfort. The raw flowers were eaten as a treatment for tuberculosis. The root was eaten raw or cooked as a potherb by natives of Alaska. The boiled root was prized by Inuit and combined with various animal fats and blubbers. They placed the leaves and roots into a sealskin poke with water and allowed this to ferment. It was then frozen for winter use and served as mentioned above.

Roseroot was prepared as a poultice for hemorrhoids by the Nlaka'pamux (Thompson), while native peoples in western Yukon chewed the roots and spit the mixture into others suffering from sore mouth. The Haida used the plant medicinally and as a mouth freshener after taking a fish-grease laxative. The plant is known as *k'aa gaananang*. Roseroot and lousewort *(Pedicularis lanata)* shoots were often combined fresh or with other summer greens in a raw salad. The Athapaskans chew or decoct the roseroot for sore throats, colds, and as an eyewash. The Dena'ina of Alaska call the plant *diqus nula*, possibly meaning "light's sleep." Their uses are similar to the Athapaskans, as well as treating athlete's foot with a soak. The tea was given to expectant mothers to facilitate childbirth.

It is said the Vikings consumed roseroot to give them the extra strength needed for their long, arduous journeys. Maybe. In fact, the first recorded mention of roseroot was by Dioscorides in *De Materia Medica*, dating from the first century CE:

> *Rhodia radix grows in Macedonia, being like to Costus, but lighter, and uneven, making a scent in the bruising, like that of Roses. It is of good use for the aggrieved with headache, being bruised and layered on with a little Rosaceum, and applied moist to the forehead and the temples.*

The fresh root has some scent, but when dried, the root smells like rose. It was added to skin tonics and at one time called poor man's rose water and sprinkled on clothes. Roseroot was grown in many English cottage gardens and on old walls and cliffs for its scented root. The whole plant, when hung in a house, is said to deter insects for several weeks. The cultivated plants are not as strongly scented, but the dried roots have a distinct rose scent. The plant is dioecious, with male and female flowers on different stems. The female flowers are a dark yellow to red, with very distinctive domed clusters of unisexual flowers. They develop plump follicles or seed heads shaped like tiny wineskins. The male flowers are a yellow to gold tint.

In 2014 I had the great pleasure of visiting Iceland. Anna Rósa Róbertsdóttir kindly hosted me. She is the foremost herbalist in the country and author of *Icelandic Herbs and Their Medicinal Uses*. I was amazed to see roseroot growing everywhere—in the wild, in people's front yards, and even in graveyards. The legendary thirteenth-century Ukrainian prince Daniel of Galicia had a reputation that rivaled Casanova's. He used roseroot, apparently quite successfully, as an aphrodisiac. It may cause mild euphoria and hangovers if taken in excess. In Russia, a bouquet of *Rhodiola* is presented to married couples, helping ensure good fertility and healthy offspring. In Scotland it was known as priest's *pintel*, meaning "priest's penis." The herb was placed in the first *Pharmacopoeia* of Sweden in 1775.

Medicinal Uses

Constituents: *S. roseum:* flavonoids, tannins, gallic acid derivatives, organic acids, salidroside/rhodioloside (hydroxy-phenethyl glycoside), sedamine, parathirosol (aglycone), cinnamic alcohols, p-tyrosol, vimalin; rosin, rosarin, and rosavin-cinnamyl glycosides; sachaliside, picein, rhodionin, rhodiolgin, rhodiolgidin, (-)rosiridol, rhodoflavonoside, gallic acid, lotasutralin, rhodalidin, mongrhoside, flavonoid glycosides, such as gossypetin-7-o-l-rhamnopyranoside and rhodioflavonoside; various caffeic and coumaric acids, triandrin, and lariciresinol 4-glucoside, trans-p-hydroxycinnamic acid, gossypetin-7-O-l-rhamnopyranoside, tricin (4f,5,7-trihydroxy-3,5f-dimeth-oxyflavone) and its 7- and 5-O-glucosides; 17 amino acids, trace minerals, and vitamins.

In Ukraine, roseroot is known as golden root (*R. rosea*). It has been studied extensively for its medicinal properties by Ukrainian and Russian scientists. In 1961 the Russian botanist G. V. Krylov went to Siberia to begin study on the root, and by 1975 the Ministry of Health approved *Rhodiola* extract as a medicine and tonic. Today in Ukraine a medicinal alcoholic drink called *nastojka* is prepared by mixing vodka and roseroot in equal parts by weight.

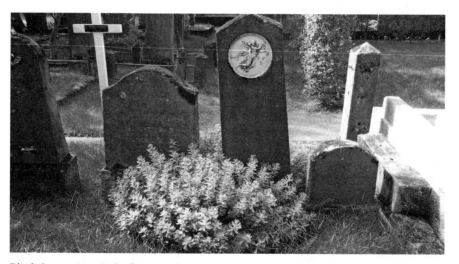

Rhodiola rosea *in an Icelandic cemetery*

Roseroot is an adaptogen, like ginseng, wild sarsaparilla, eleutherococcus, schisandra berry, and *reishi* mushroom: a substance that is "innocuous, causing minimal physiological disorder; nonspecific in action; and increasing resistance and normalizing function in the body, irrespective of the direction of the pathological change" (Brekhman and Dardymov 1969). These plants influence the hypothalamic-pituitary-adrenal axis (HPAA) and in turn, our digestion, immune system, moods, emotions, energy storage, and expenditure. They influence and regulate our hormones and endocrine glands, bringing balance and adaptation to stress. Cortisol is a major stress hormone of a chronic nature. Adrenaline increases when we are presented with an immediate danger, but cortisol is the hormone of long-term stress. A deficiency of cortisol is linked to chronic fatigue syndrome, insomnia, and general burnout. Elevated levels include autoimmune conditions as well as increased risk of cardiovascular events and cancer.

Fintelmann and Gruenwald (2007) rated *Rhodiola* good or very good in clinical trials with 80% of physicians and patients subjectively approving of its performance. It showed very few side effects, with a 99% safety rating. Studies in Russia suggest the chemically active compounds can improve learning and memory and reduce stress. In one study of mental fatigue in 128 students, the placebo group had an increase in errors of 13% after 1 hour, a 37% increase after 4 hours, and an 88% increase after 6 hours. Those students taking *Rhodiola* had a 56% decrease in errors after 4 hours. A randomized controlled trial of 40 male medical students ages 17 to 19 followed them during stressful examination times and gave them either roseroot or placebo. Significant improvement in physical fitness, mental fatigue, and self-assessment of general well-being were found in the herb group compared to placebo after 20 days (Spasov et al. 2000). A study by Bystritsky et al. (2008) looked at reduction of generalized anxiety disorder (GAD) in 10 patients ages 34 to 55. They took 340 mg of roseroot daily for 10 weeks, and a reduction in Hamilton Anxiety Rating Scale (HAM-A) scores similar to clinical trials was noted.

David Winston, professional member of the American Herbalist Guild, suggests that "this cooling adaptogen is perfect for excess constitutions with hypertension, liver-fire rising headaches (red face, ears, and eyes and sharp pain behind the eyes), and excessive anger." I have found this as well. Goldenroot tincture has proven efficient in treating chronic gum disease such as peridontosis when gargled three times daily with water.

Studies show it naturally stimulates the level of dopamine in the brain, improves brain cell activity, and helps the body use oxygen more efficiently. Roseroot is useful in treating depression by enhancing the transport of tryptophan and 5HTP to the brain and inhibiting both MAO and catechol-O-methyltransferase (COMT). Serotonin is destroyed by COMT, and rosavin can decrease COMT by 60% and raise serotonin levels by 30%. COMT inhibitors are a new class of drugs being developed for treating Parkinson's disease. They are used with L-DOPA, reducing its breakdown before it enters the brain, and thereby increasing availability to the brain. Faba bean and roseroot sound like a great combination to me. Work by Daphne van Dierman et al. (2009) found *Rhodiola* is a potent antidepressant that inhibits MAO-A and may be useful in senile dementia due to inhibition of MAO-B. A double-blind randomized placebo-controlled study of 89 subjects has found roseroot of benefit in mild to moderate depression (Darbinyan et al. 2007). Dosage was 340–680 mg daily for six weeks, with little difference found in the higher dosage group. A study on 57 subjects with major depression was conducted by Mao et al. (2015). The results were modest, with no significant difference between groups taking *Rhodiola* or sertraline. However, *Rhodiola* reported significantly less adverse events and was better tolerated. Therefore, it may have a more favorable risk-to-benefit ratio for mild to moderate depression.

Roseroot appears to target various levels on the regulation of cell response to stress, affecting various components of neuroendocrine and neurotransmitter receptor sites. Amsterdam and Panossian (2016) conducted a thorough review of two randomized double-blind placebo-controlled trials of 146 patients with major depressive disorder and seven open-label studies of 714 individuals with stress-induced mild depression. The conclusions were positive. The plant requires fourteen hours of sunlight or better to grow. This suggests, of course, winter daylight hours are often eight hours or less. I have found in clinical practice that it works well for seasonal affective disorder (SAD), a significant health concern in higher latitudes, where it grows more rapidly.

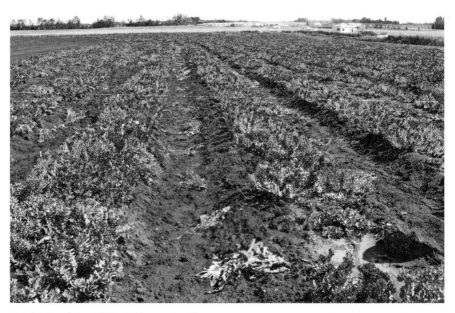

A field of commercial Rhodiola rosea *in Alberta*

In a recent study of 35 men with erectile dysfunction or premature ejaculation, 26 showed substantial improvement after taking 150–200 mg daily for three months. Levels of 17-ketosteroids in the seminal fluid showed an increase in production of sex hormones. In a placebo-controlled study of the herb's ability to mobilize fatty acids from adipose tissue, 120 patients were given roseroot or placebo. Serum lipid levels were tested at rest and one hour after exercise. The *Rhodiola* group showed 6% greater serum fatty acid levels at rest, and 44% after one hour of exercise, due in large part to the herb activating adipose lipase, which helps break down body fat for energy. Another clinical study at the Georgian State Hospital treated 130 obese patients for 90 days; 92% of those taking *Rhodiola* lost an average of 20 pounds, while the control group on the same diet lost an average of only 8 pounds. Korean scientists screened 93 plants against HIV-1 protease, and roseroot rated the most potent; with 70.4% inhibition at a concentration of 100 mcg/ml (Min et al. 1999). *Rhodiola* extract (600 mg daily) or placebo was given to 48 male and female marathon runners for thirty days prior, the day of, and seven days after running. Results found protective effects against virus replication following this prolonged and intense exercise (Ahmed et al. 2015).

Extracts inhibit division of HL-60 cells. The mild action of the extract, as well as its cytostatic and antiproliferative activity, raise hopes for its use in anticancer therapy by enhancing the effectiveness of existing cancer drugs (Majewska et al. 2005). T. S. Chen et al. (2008) found roseroot a more powerful antioxidant than Siberian ginseng (*Eleutherococcus*) or *amla* (Indian gooseberry). Work by De Sanctis et al. (2004) found roseroot to significantly protect human red blood cells from glutathione depletion, suggesting antioxidative protection. A study involving 24 young athletes showed 200 mg daily, before exercise, statistically improved performance and lowered lactate levels (De Bock et al. 2004). This Belgian study suggests acute herb intake can improve endurance-exercise capacity. In another study of 112 subjects, 89% of those taking roseroot showed rapid improvement in various sports, including track and field, swimming, speed skating, and skiing competitions. A four-week study on fourteen trained male athletes found significant reduction of plasma fatty acids and lower blood lactate and plasma creatine kinase (Parasi et al. 2010). A small study of only 12 patients found the herb useful in superficial bladder carcinoma, improved their urothelial tissue integration, parameters of leukocyte integrins, and T cell immunity (Bocharova et al. 1995). Work by Ming et al. (2005), identified a rhodioflavonoside cytotoxic to human prostate cancer cell lines.

Women's health may benefit from roseroot as well. In a study of 40 women with secondary amenorrhea (lack of menstruation), a dose of 100–150 mg per day resulted in normalized periods for 25 women, and 11 women eventually became pregnant. A randomized double-blind placebo-controlled parallel study of 60 men and women ages 20 to 55 with chronic fatigue was conducted by Olsson et al. (2009). Half took four capsules (576 mg) daily and the control half took placebo. After twenty-eight days, mental performance improved, ability to concentration increased, and cortisol response to awakening stress decreased. According to the authors, this is the first study to show a proprietary *Rhodiola* extract benefits patients with chronic stress-induced fatigue. A parallel-group randomized double-blind placebo-controlled trial of students ages 18 to 55 in the Faculty of Nursing at the University of Alberta was conducted in 2011. A forty-two day course of 364 mg of *Rhodiola* found fatigue worsened compared to placebo. This was very disappointing, as I encouraged the government to conduct a trial on Alberta-grown *Rhodiola*. The authors say the results should be interpreted with caution, but something went wrong (Punja et al. 2014).

Modulation of cortisol levels is a key mechanism of adaptogenic activity. Herbert et al. (2006) suggest corticosteroids damage the brain and cognitive function. My father-in-law was a personal case I observed firsthand. Cortisone cream for pustular psoriasis on the bottom of his feet helped alleviate the pain of walking, but the rapid decrease in mental concentration and memory was significant. "Roid rage" is commonly associated with chronic use of cortisone. As *Rhodiola rosea* becomes scarcer from wild-crafted source, the introduction of less-studied species can be expected to reach the market.

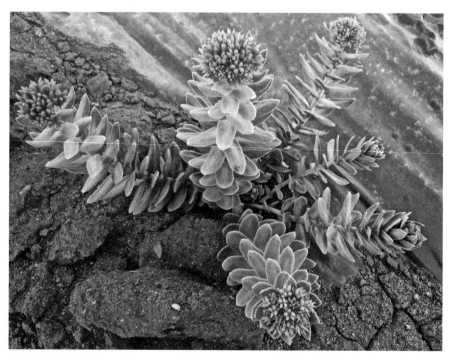

Young Rhodiola *plants*

Salidroside is a marker in *Rhodiola rosea*, along with a group of rosavins. Salidroside, from roseroot, shows activity against coxsackie virus B3, associated with viral myocarditis. It may combine well with astragalus root for this condition (Wang et al. 2009). I had three cases of viral myocarditis associated with coxsackie in my years of clinical practice, and all cases resulted in successful outcomes. Salidroside inhibits high glucose-

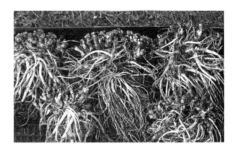

Four-year old Rhodiola rosea *roots*

induced mesangial cell proliferation associated with diabetic nephropathy, suggestive of a protective mechanism (Yin et al. 2009). Salidroside inhibits human breast cancer cell line MCF-7 both in vitro and in vivo by inducing apoptosis (Zhao et al. 2015). Other studies suggest the compound inhibits cancer of the lungs, colon, glioma, bladder, and adenoids as well as fibrosarcoma.

The herb shows good tyrosine inhibition and the highest xanthine oxidase inhibition among herbs tested (C. H. Chen et al. 2009). This suggests benefit in treating uric acid excess or gouty and rheumatic conditions. It may combine well with tamarack needles for gout. *Rhodiola* may be a short-term support for hypothyroid issues induced by hormonal withdrawal and related to TSH levels (Zubeldia et al. 2010). More work is needed to unravel the whole picture, as the herb is quite safe on its own. Mouse studies suggest possible success in treating opioid addiction and smoking cessation (Mattioli and Perfumi 2011). Roseroot may be useful in treating drug-resistant strains of the bacterium responsible for gonorrhea *(Neisseria gonorrhoeae)*. Both salidroside and rosavin exhibit significant inhibition (Cybulska et al. 2011). Bearberry *(Arctostaphylos uva-ursi)* and black cherry *(Prunus serotina)* also inhibited growth of this bacterium in the same study.

A word of warning about adulterated products. Patov et al. (2006) identified a way to synthesize rosavin in a one-step glycosylation of cinnamyl alcohol with a disaccharide. Is adulteration far behind, or already here? You can purchase *Rhodiola rosea* from China at 1%, 2%, 3%, 4%, and higher upon request. Adulteration with *R. crenulata* is another issue, again topping up this herb with rosavin from other sources. In a study by Booker et al. (2016), forty commercial products were sourced from different suppliers. Approximately one-fifth

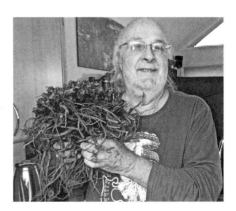

The author with a five-year-old root

of products claiming to be *R. rosea* contained no rosavin, and others contained no salidroside. Around 80% of the remaining commercial products were lower in rosavin and appeared to be adulterated with other *Rhodiola* species. Buyer beware—or do what I did and grow your own. Or encourage your farming friends to grow it for you as long as they have sufficient fourteen-hour days of sunlight.

Essential Oil

Roseroot has a lovely roselike fragrance that can be captured in carrier oils and may be amenable to steam distillation. Terpenes and aroma volatiles from rhizomes of *R. rosea* from Norway have been isolated by both steam distillation (SD) and headspace solid-phase microextraction (HS-SPME) coupled with gas chromatography and mass spectrometry analysis. The dried rhizomes contained 0.05% essential oil with the main chemical classes: monoterpene hydrocarbons (25.40%), monoterpene alcohols (23.61%), and straight-chain aliphatic alcohols (37.54%). The most abundant volatiles detected in the essential oil were *n*-decanol (30.38%), geraniol (12.49%), and 1,4-p-menthadien-7-ol (5.10%), and a total of 86 compounds were identified in both the SD and HS-SPME samples. Geraniol was identified as the most important roselike odor compound besides geranyl formate, geranyl acetate, benzyl alcohol, and phenylethyl alcohol. Floral notes such as linalool and its oxides, nonanal, decanol, nerol, and cinnamyl alcohol highlight the flowery scent of roseroot rhizomes.

Work in Finland found up to 36% myrtenol, 16% trans pinocarvol, and 12% geraniol as well as up to 12% dihydrocumin alcohol. Work by Evstatieva et al. (2010) found a 48–57% variation of geraniol, and a yield of 0.1–2.5% of a pale yellow oil.

Flower Essence

Rhodiola rosea flower essence is for issues surrounding ego, forgiveness, and acceptance. It helps one depersonalize perceived injustice or acknowledgment of an indifference as opposed to deliberate betrayal. The essence may be helpful in softening emotional armor that has hardened from years of criticism. If you do anything important, there will always be critics. If you don't like criticism, don't do anything important. This is a research essence of Prairie Deva flower essences.

Personality Traits

Vermeulen and Johnston (2011) offer insight into the family:

> There is a distinct polarity in this family [Crassulaceae], from boost to bust. On one hand, there is a boost to endurance, stamina, liveliness, and prolonged lifespan. These "life plants" and "live-long" plants are well named. Equally, on the other side is a bust with death-like stupe-faction, depression, anesthesia, shrinking, feeling lost, collapse and paralysis of mind and body.

The proficiency and longevity can be credited to their ability to adapt and survive in harsh environments, including severe family life or profound grief. Enduring harsh, stark, and extreme environments necessitates preparing for the worst. Having a hardened exterior as protection from their surroundings is reflected physically with corns, skin indurations, and hardness. With steadfast determination, calm courage, strength, and resistance, they can hang onto the very cliff of existence, finding a small crack in which to anchor and prosper.

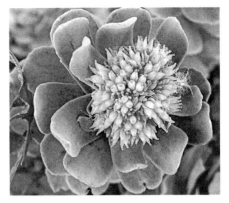

Rhodiola rosea *flower*

RECIPES

Tincture: 5 to 20 drops of fresh plant tincture daily. Tincture is made at 1:3 and 70% alcohol; dried root 1:5 at 45–50% alcohol. Add up to 10% glycerin due to high tannin content. This will avoid precipitation of tannins and reduce the puckering effect in the mouth due to astringency. Work by Hellum et al. (2010) suggests potent inhibition of CYP3A4 enzyme system, although this is highly theoretical at this point. The metabolic capacity of CYP2C9 in humans is modest but may interfere with phenytoin and warfarin (Thu et al. 2016). This is possible, but highly unlikely. Kucinskaite et al. (2007) found 70% ethanol extracts yield the highest rosavin content, but lower salidrosides. At 40% alcohol there are considerably less rosavins extracted. Ultrasonic extraction with 50% alcohol for one hour at 77°F shows promise (Staneva et al. 2009).

Roseroot: Standardized extracts with a minimum of 3–4% rosavin, 1% salidroside, and 40% polyphenols appear to be the new standard. Take 100 mg capsules 2 to 3 times, 30 minutes before meals. Roots dried at 160–175°F suffer no damage to active ingredients.

Infusion or decoction: 1 teaspoon of dry root to 1 cup water. Use up to 1 cup daily. Dosages over 10 grams of juice or 3.5 grams of the dried plant are said to bring on diarrhea, vomiting, and queasiness. No cases of poisoning have been recorded in recent times. Do not use in cases of inflammatory conditions of the gastrointestinal or urinary tract.

Caution: Individuals prone to anxiety may feel jittery or agitated. Many herbal students believe roseroot is stimulating; it is not. The herb is contraindicated in patients with bipolar spectrum disorders taking antidepressants. Activity of doxorubicin on metastatic cancer was unimpaired, and hepatotoxicity greatly reduced, when combined with *Rhodiola* extract (Brinker 2010).

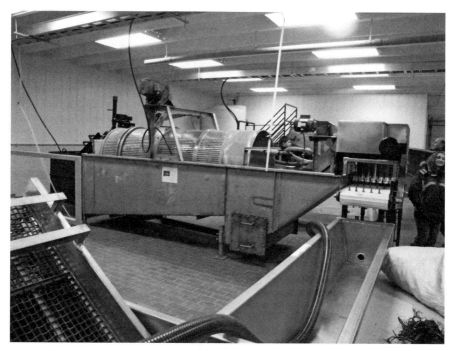

A dryer in the Thorsby, Alberta, Rhodiola *plant*

Cultivation

Roseroot seeds, both fresh and stored for eight months, have the highest germination rate after forty-five days of stratification, reaching 90% and 82.6%, respectively. The quickest method of clonal micropropagation of roseroot is activation of the axillary meristems of growing shoots. The explants used are seeds or buds of mixed type, since vegetative buds give rise only to assimilation shoots, which cannot form roots.

The best time for isolating buds is June–July or September–October. They are sterilized for 1 minute in 70% ethanol, 5 minutes in 3% hydrogen peroxide, then propagated in a medium containing, per liter, 0.2 mg BAP plus 0.1 mg IAA. They are then transplanted into vermiculite for two weeks at 85–90% relative humidity and then into a mixture of equal parts soil, humus, and vermiculite. Root cuttings in fall have a 96% success rate. Some agriculturalists use zeatin and other compounds for micro-propagation and in vitro cultures. Research conducted in Estonia found good success when seeds were stratified for sixty to ninety days in September, grown in a greenhouse, and planted at the end of May. Roots harvested at the end of the third year yielded 60 tons per acre.

Rhodiola rosea has been introduced as a potential economic crop in Bulgaria. Research found propagation by rhizome cutting a successful strategy, with planting to harvesting taking only three years. From seed takes four to five years, and biomass production from rhizome cutting is higher than seed-propagated plants. The male possesses higher medicinal value than the female on the basis of total amount of rosavins and salidroside.

Wild Sarsaparilla

Wild Sarsaparilla • Rabbit Root—*Aralia nudicaulis* L.

> *I call for wild sarsaparilla, a soft prayer, deep within self.*
> *Autumn, vivid colors on a hillside, leaves strewn on granite rocks,*
> *I see you, wild sarsaparilla.*
> *Stalks, a gold ocher, dance in evening wind, one last greeting before winter.*
>
> —Laurie Lacey

> *The Moon Rabbit is lying against the bunker, dreaming and thinking about life and dreaming the impossible possible and creating its own true stories.*
>
> —Florentijn Hofman

> *Say, friend—you got any more of that good sarsaparilla?*
>
> —*The Big Lebowski,* 1998

Wild sarsaparilla is one of my favorite plants of the northern forest. It was one of my first plant allies with which I became well-acquainted. There are millions of acres of wild sarsaparilla found throughout the northern prairies and far into the boreal forest. This is what initially piqued my interest. I finished a science degree in botany at the University of Alberta in 1971, and I had had my fill of academia. Shortly thereafter I hitchhiked with my friend Peter Johnson throughout the Caribbean and South America. That we survived the adventure is a novel or a movie in itself. I later found myself with six friends living on a hippie commune situated on the south shore of Lesser Slave Lake in northern Alberta. I was twenty-three years old.

The single house had four bedrooms, no electricity or running water, and was heated by woodstoves. For a city kid, this was a new adventure, and I soon began to look at the local wild plants in this unique environment. But before going any further, I should give you a bit more background information. Our communal property was at the top of a hill that quickly became known by the locals as Hippie Hill. On one side was a reserve called Driftpile, now the Driftpile First Nation, and to the west was Sucker Creek First Nation. It was a local joke that Driftpile was where all the drifters piled up, including me, I guess.

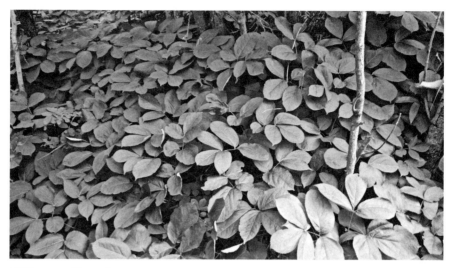

Wild sarsaparilla patch

Rose Auger was a well-known medicine woman on the former reserve and had a well-deserved reputation as a generous person and a healer. Russell Willier lived on the reserve to the west, and he had just taken on the honor and burden of a medicine bundle handed down for ten generations through his grandfather. Rose was always smiling and laughing, and when I would visit she would offer me some muskeg tea (Labrador tea) simmering on the back of her woodstove. Her Cree name, *oh-soh-ka-pow-skoa*, meant "Woman Who Stands Strong."

One day I asked her if she would teach me about local plant medicine. She looked at me with her kind, dark eyes and said, "Maybe." I rose to leave and said I would be back the next day. She did not reply. Bright and early on a beautiful July morning I showed up at her place. She came outside and told me to go into the forest, find the first plant to which I was attracted, spend time with it, and return the next day with what it told me. I was surprised and did not know what to say. I was a university-trained botanist and had never heard of plants conversing with humans. But off I went.

I immediately spotted this beautiful wild sarsaparilla. I only knew its name because I had looked it up in a book the previous summer. I knew from my botanical Latin that the name *sarsaparilla* derived from the Spanish *sarza*, meaning "bramble," and *parilla*, for "vine." And I knew that *nudicaulis* meant "bare stem" or "naked stem," from the Latin *nudus* and Greek *kaulos*. I noted immediately that the flower and leaf stems separated just above the root. I was feeling good. I sat down cross-legged in the quiet forest and began to await a revelation about the plant. My left brain was searching for clues that would somehow guide my intuition. Did I mention that I was twenty-three years old? An hour passed, and except for noting the emerging flower buds and the distinct three stems, each with three to five leaves, I was stumped.

The next morning I went to Rose and told her it had something to do with the third and fifth chakras. She looked at me puzzled and replied, "No." I knew I had not tried very hard, so the next morning I went back to my original site. I decided to dig up a neighboring plant and noted the stem extended into the ground and soon traveled off in opposite directions. At first I thought this may be a geographic clue, but I soon found other wild sarsaparilla that put out stolons in opposite directions but not distinctly north, south, east or west.

I pulled a leaf and tasted. It was mildly bitter, sweet, and balsamic, but somewhat salty as well. Again I noted that some stems had three leaves and others five. I cleaned a piece of rhizome (underground stem), chewed on it, and swallowed the pleasant-tasting earthy juice. It would make a nice tea, I thought. At this point I decided to take a few tokes of another herbal medicine and lay down for a nap. I awoke to the cracking of branches and a building storm. Time to head home.

The next morning I went to see Rose and told her what I had found out. She looked at me with a slight roll of the eyes and said, "No." That evening I went home and thought about this turn of events. I decided this was not for me, and I would look at the local library for books on native plants and medicine. I went through all the stages of denial, anger, and resignation before heading to bed. But my sleep was restless, and in the morning I decided to give it one more try. Would the plant talk to me?

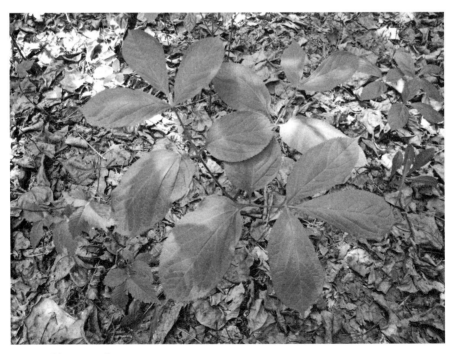

Young wild sarsaparilla

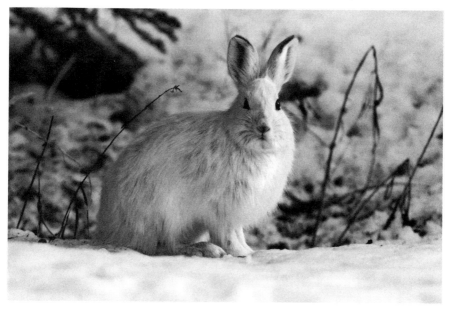

Rabbit

The next morning I was sitting with the plant and put myself into a meditative state. Pretty soon I was sitting with my eyes closed when I heard a rustle. I opened them to see on my far right a large snowshoe hare. It perked up its large ears and then looked directly at me. It slowly loped over to the wild sarsaparilla plant, only a few feet away. The rabbit looked directly at me, took a nibble of a leaf, looked right at me, and slowly trundled off. I sat there, not sure of what had happened, and then smiled.

The next morning I went to see Rose. I told her I believed the plant had something to do with rabbits. At that, her eyes lit up and a big smile came across her face. "I will teach you," she said. Only later did I find out the Cree name for the plant translates as "rabbit root."

Of course, it was over many more years that I learned additional secrets from this amazing plant. Rose passed away in August 2006 after healing herself of lymphatic cancer in the 1990s. I have another amazing story to share about Rose. One long, cold winter night in 1979, my good friend and best man Terry Anderson, an original resident of Hippie Hill, and I envisioned a public celebration of music on the summer solstice weekend. Our larger community already celebrated the longest day of the year with a feast and party, but we wanted to create something larger. It was born that summer and named the North Country Fair (NCF), after a Bob Dylan song. The sun barely skims under the horizon at that time of year, so the festivities continued day and night. The community built a school that was financially supported in part by the NCF. I remember taking the young elementary students for plant walks in the surrounding forest. One youngster later went on and received his PhD from Duke University on the study of lichens. The fair in 2016 celebrated its 38th anniversary.

Shortly after year four of the fair (1983), our northern community suffered the tragic loss of four friends in a single traffic accident. A long story short, I volunteered to make sure the fair continued the next year, and among the duties I assigned myself was to feed all the volunteers and performers. On the second morning, preparing for breakfast, I went to light the large propane stove. The explosion blew me right across the floor into the wall. I lay there, stunned, and looked at my bare arms, now angry red and swollen. My face was hot, and I thanked goodness I was wearing glasses. People helped set me down on a picnic table outside. My brother David was there, and he observed, and later shared with me, what happened next.

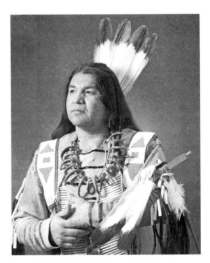

Rose heard the explosion and was moving her cherubic body as fast as possible to where I was seated. David watched in disbelief as Rose put her hands close to my burned body and threw "flames" off me, twenty feet into the air. She continued this for over five minutes, until no more were seen. I don't remember any of this as I was in shock. The next morning I awoke without any sign of redness or burn on my face or arms. It was amazing. She was a true medicine woman.

I knew her son Dr. Dale Auger as well. He was an amazing, talented man who sadly died at only fifty years of age. He was an incredibly gifted artist. His legacy of oil paintings can be found in the book *Medicine Paint*, published in 2009.

Dale Auger

Traditional Uses

The Cree of northern Alberta call the plant *waposociyipîyk*, meaning "rabbit root." The Dene (Chipewyan) further north, call it *gajie*, "rabbit berry." The Plains Cree also call it rabbit root, or *wâ-pus-wo-tcha*. I quickly learned compresses of the root could be applied to cuts and wounds. The root was given to children to chew while teething or to treat gum infections. The root was decocted with Labrador tea to improve appetite and taken with calamus root for respiratory conditions such as pneumonia and bronchitis. The latter decoction was used to soak fishing nets, often made with dogbane fiber, to help mask human scent and give good luck with the catch. The fruiting stalk was decocted and given to new mothers to stimulate breast milk production. The leaf tea is diaphoretic and helps promote sweating.

Cree runners would chew on the roots as a source of energy while traveling as quickly as possible to neighboring tribes. I later heard various Cree healers call it natural Viagra due to its ability to help impotence and erectile dysfunction. I was told this at a community healing ceremony and heard it mentioned several times, in a joking manner, from a number of sources. At this particular gathering and feast, I was honored and treated to moose nose, a delicacy of the boreal forest. Knowledgeable midwives encourage sips of the root infusion to help relax a hard cervix before delivery. The root exhibits antiandrogenic activity and may be useful in conditions as varied as polycystic ovarian syndrome and pubescent acne. Some herbalists suggest the tea or tincture of root helps reduce the Herxheimer reaction associated with spirochete die-off and the unpleasant effects of Lyme's disease. Combine equal parts of teasel and wild sarsaparilla root as one possible combination.

Forty years later I coauthored a book with David Young and Russell Willier called *A Cree Healer and His Medicine Bundle* (2015). In this book, Russell reveals the seventy-some plants in a tenth-generation medicine bundle and how he uses various plant parts for healing. Russell lived west of my home near Joussard. He calls the plant *waposociyipiyk* and uses the root for heart, lung, liver, and kidney ailments. He calls the larger, older "male" version bear root and the smaller, darker-leaved versions "female" or rabbit root. He used both sizes of roots in combinations for a variety of medicines. But what does "rabbit root" really mean? And where does it come from? My good friend and an amazing herbalist Matthew Wood shared this in *The Earthwise Herbal: A Complete Guide to New World Medicinal Plants*:

> The Cree name for Aralia nudicaulis *translates as "rabbit root," according to Rogers. This indicates their conception of the therapeutic direction of the medicine. In the Far North, on the Canadian Shield where the Cree live, the rabbit is associated with starvation and emaciation. When the snow is high, only the rabbits can get out on top of the snow, so the deer population dies out and the people have to rely on the rabbit. However, the latter does not provide a complete diet because it lacks good-quality oils. Thus, rabbit medicines are used to antidote the ill-effects of emaciation and atrophy. They are largely nutritive and support the bones and muscles.* (Wood 2009)

Matthew notes the root of the related spikenard (*Aralia racemosa*) is a "bear medicine" due to its hairy tuft rising from the ground. It is oilier in nature than rabbit root.

I have observed over the years that the three stems, when young, will hold two, three, or four leaves. A mature plant of five to seven years old will exhibit three stems, each with five leaves. The older plants are the ones I personally prefer to harvest. I later learned the root was widely harvested in the late nineteenth-century for inclusion in root beer. These regional beverages varied throughout North America, but often contained alterative herbs that would help cleanse and invigorate individuals who suffered a long winter of salted and dried meats. I believe the root would make a great commercial product as an energy and tonic drink. Carbonated for the market, of course.

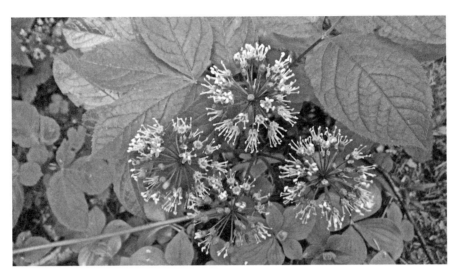

Wild sarsaparilla in early flower

Medicinal Uses

Constituents: *A. nudicaulis* root: campesterol, stigmasterol, beta-sitosterol, alpha- and beta-amyrin, (3R) falcarinol, (3R, 9R, 10S) panaxydol, salseparin, potassium chloride, basserin, albumen, pectin, acetic acid, essential oils, and various minerals. 100 grams of fresh root contain 97 mg Calcium, 30 mg phosphorus, 225 mg potassium, 34 mg magnesium, 0.1 mg copper, 0.4 mg zinc, 1.5 mg iron oxide, 6 mg manganese, and 2.4 mg chloride. Protein leaf studies conducted at Purdue in 1993 indicate that *A. nudicaulis* is a morphologically distinct species but is closely related to *A. racemosa*. A test for unknown alkaloids was positive.

Endophytes on rhizomes include palitantin, botrallin, craterellin C, mycosporulone, spiromassaritone and massarigenin D. Various Eclectic physicians, such as John King, recommended the root either be decocted or made into syrup as a substitute for sarsaparilla (*Smilax* species). King writes that it

> possesses alterative properties and is used in decoction or syrup as a substitute for sarsaparilla in all cases where an alternative is required. It is likewise used in pulmonary diseases. Externally, a decoction of it has been found beneficial as a wash in zona [shingles] and in indolent ulcers. (Felter and Lloyd 1898)

The root was official in the U.S. *Pharmacopoeia* from 1820 to 1882. William Buchan, a medical doctor, published the first edition of *Domestic Medicine* in 1769, an influential and popular book in its time. He mentions a pint of root decoction may be drunk daily as a cancer cure. My friend Gerry Ivanochko lived for a number of years in Lac La Ronge, Saskatchewan. We ran into each other at various wild-crafting and medicinal plant conferences over the decades. He participated in a study by Wang et al. (2006) looking at extracts of the rhizome, stem, leaf, and fruit. Extracts of the rhizome showed in vitro activity against human colon and leukemia cancer cell lines, while the fruit showed activity against human cervical cancer cell lines.

The dark purple drupes, containing one seed, can be made into syrups, cordials, and wines with a flavor similar to elderberry. I made wine one fall that was unremarkable but drinkable. Work at the University of Guelph in 1994 found the energy value of the berries is higher than blueberry, pin cherry, or saskatoon berry.

In 1996 I spoke at a Medicinal and Aromatic Plant of the Prairies Conference in Olds, Alberta. My herbal friend Terry Willard was there, and he talked about the energetics of the ginseng family. Wild sarsaparilla and devil's club (*Oplopanax horridus* [Sm.] Miq.) are the only two members of this famous family growing in northern Alberta. He began by describing Chinese or Korean ginseng *(Panax ginseng)* as a sports car, like a hot, fast Lamborghini or Porsche. I could relate to the analogy, as the root of this precious medicine is warming and stimulating and works well for individuals with kidney yang deficiency. He then described American ginseng *(P. quinquefolius)* being like a Volvo. I related to this as well, as I had been a longtime Volvo owner. American ginseng root is cooler and more calming to the nervous system but still possesses good energetics. As I was listening, this thought came into my mind: "And wild sarsaparilla is like a Ford Tempo." That is, the root, taken over a period of time, has some of the same benefits as other members of the ginseng family, and it is milder, but it will get you there.

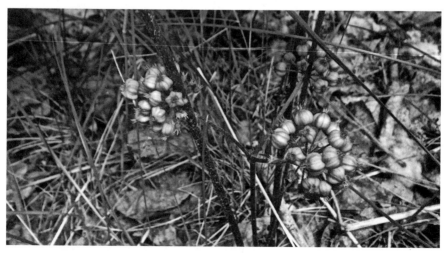

Immature berries

While the ginseng cousins have central roots that resemble human bodies complete with arms and legs, wild sarsaparilla has long, underground stems that spread out widely. This suggests less concentrated activity spread over a larger sphere of influence. Both ginseng species are in the class of herbs known as adaptogens. The mode of activity and strength is somewhat less in rabbit root but will help balance your hormonal and endocrine system, energetically speaking. Adaptogens increase the capacity of the body to "adapt" to stressful situations by reducing stress response. In order to be a true adaptogen, the herb must meet three defining criteria: an adaptogen must be innocuous and cause minimal disturbance of normal physiology; its action should be nonspecific and increase resistance to adverse influence; and it should normalize action irrespective of the direction of the preceding pathological changes. That is, an adaptogen will normalize glandular function, whether high or low, and will alter reactivity of the HPAA. Vermeulen and Johnston (2011) expand on this concept:

> *A spectrum of conditions may be associated with increased and prolonged activation of the HPA axis, including melancholic depression, anorexia nervosa with or without malnutrition, obsessive-compulsive disorder, panic anxiety, chronic active alcoholism, alcohol and narcotic withdrawal, excessive exercising, poorly controlled diabetes mellitus, childhood sexual abuse, and hyperthyroidism.*
>
> *Hypoactivation or depletion of the stress system, on the other hand, has been linked with post–traumatic stress disorder, atypical seasonal depression, chronic fatigue syndrome, fibromyalgia, hypothyroidism, poststress conditions, postpartum, menopause, and nicotine withdrawal.*

More study is required, but I believe wild sarsaparilla is adaptogenic and will prove so with further research. Michael Moore, noted herbalist, found cold infusions of the root help treat hypofunction of the adrenal cortex and reduce hyperlipidemia associated with liver stress. My good friend Martin Osis discovered a footbath of the decocted root relieves gout pain within the hour.

Alpha- and beta-amyrin, also found in crampbark, exhibit hepato-protective activity in animal research. Alpha-amyrin is a competitive inhibitor of porcine pancreatic elastase, suggesting anti-inflammatory properties. It targets chymotrypsin, trypsin, cyclic AMP–binding phosphatase, calium^{2+}-dependent protein kinase C, collagenase, and HIV-1 protease receptor, all indicative of antiarthritic benefit. Beta-amyrin inhibits oxidative stress, apoptosis, inflammation, and hepatic fibrosis (Thirupathi et al. 2016). Beta-amyrin palmitate, also found in the root, is an antidepressant through an increased release of epinephrine. More careful analysis of the root is needed. The fresh root may be more useful for medicine than the dried.

Many years ago, my brother and I were working on an American ginseng product to reduce symptoms of colds and flu. This later turned into a natural supplement, Ginse, to replace the use of antibiotics in livestock. I had access to lab equipment and we did an in vitro study on splenocytes showing activity from fresh sarsaparilla root extracts 40% more active than the prepared ginseng product. The dried root showed little activity.

Both alpha- and beta-amyrin possess anti-inflammatory activity potentiated by indomethacin, suggesting prostaglandin and TNF-alpha inhibition (Aragao et al. 2007). Work by Holanda et al. (2008) found alpha-, beta-amyrin is a pain reliever working through an opioid mechanism. The root and two of its compounds, (3R) falcarinol and (3R,9R,10S) panaxydol, have been found to exhibit strong activity against *Mycobacterium tuberculosis*. The compounds show an MIC of 25.6 μM and 36 μM, respectively, and IC_{50} of 15.3 μM and 23.5 μM, respectively (Li et al. 2012). Later work by Li et al. (2015) identified six endophytes in the rhizomes that show activity against the same destructive organism. This may explain in part the traditional success of the root in various respiratory conditions, including tuberculosis.

One compound, mycosporulone, shows activity against penicillin-resistant *Staphylococcus aureus* and *Pseudomonas aeruginosa*. The compound is not toxic to normal human cells but is cytotoxic against human tumor cell lines MDA-MB 231 and PC(3), and the murine L-1210 leukemia cell line (Guiraud et al. 1999). Panaxydol induces apoptosis in cancer cells (Kim et al. 2011). Later work by Kim et al. (2016) demonstrated in vivo anticancer activity associated with panaxydol. Panaxydol may help reduce amyloid beta neurodegeneration associated with Alzheimer's disease (Nie et al. 2008).

Mary Barnes, noted herbalist, writes, "*Aralia nudicaulis* has softer energetics than *Oplopanax horridus* while still having adaptogenic and lung supportive properties." I agree. And it is less nasty thorn-wise and a lot easier to collect. The Araliaceae family contains a number of interesting medicinal plants. Frans Vermeulen and Linda Johnston produced a four-volume *Plants: Homeopathic and Medicinal Uses from a Botanical Family Perspective*. They wrote:

> Araliaceae won't accept the natural decline wherein youthful vigor and well-being are replaced by aging debility. Aralia is noted for the "constant dread of disease." They seek indestructible, enduring, eternal, everlasting life. Clinging to the dream of longevity, all their energy goes to rejuvenation, where it is possible to postpone or prevent the natural wane of functions.... The dilemma for the Araliaceae is how to stay flexible and youthful while embracing all stages of life with open-minded enthusiasm and joy. The wisdom to do this is the true preserver of health and life. (Vermeulen and Johnston 2011, 493)

Flower Essence

I have to agree. Some twenty-five years ago I prepared a flower essence from the small green-white flowers, one of the research essences available from Prairie Deva flower essences. I wrote:

> Wild sarsaparilla flower essence is specifically for men reaching middle-age crises. It is useful for those seeking resolution with maturation of sexuality and even diminished sex drive. Negative aspects include unhealthy relationships and "conquest" issue with younger females, or the need for artificial stimulation through strip clubs, peep shows, magazines, or porn.

On the positive side, the flower essence helps individuals get in touch with the spiritual side of sexuality and learn how to truly receive pleasure from their partners.

WILD SARSAPARILLA

(Aralia nudicaulis)
The northern woods are far too cold
To grow ginseng of any sort,
But one wild cousin, truth be told
Is a handy, dandy medicinal wort.
The Cree they call it rabbit root
It helped them thrive in winter snow,
It gave them fat and energy to boot
This is an adaptogen so you know.
Widely used to make root beer
The species name means "bare stem"
Herb Viagra you have here
T'is a phytochemical gem!
Best of all its free for all
Tons just waiting for those who know,
Leaves turn yellow, pick root in fall,
It'll keep you healthy when cold winds blow.

—RDR

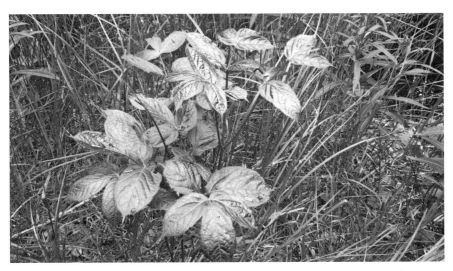

Mature plant

RECIPES

Tincture: For reasons cited above, I prefer a fresh root tincture, prepared optimally at 1 part fresh finely cut root to 3 parts of a menstruum containing 60% alcohol. Dry root tincture is prepared 1:5 and 40% alcohol. Take 1–2 teaspoons as desired.

Decoction: If you desire a decoction, be sure to cut the roots diagonally after washing and place on a nylon screen to thoroughly dry. Use 1 heaping teaspoon of dried root per pint of water and gently simmer for 15 minutes. Strain and enjoy a cup or two daily.

Caution: Avoid in pregnancy (speculative), especially early pregnancy, due to its empirical emmenagogue effect (Brinker 2010).

Harvesting

I prefer to harvest the roots in the fall, just as the leaves are turning yellow. Don't wait too long, however, as once the leaves have fallen, it can be very difficult to find the roots. Wild sarsaparilla is a woodland plant, and does not like direct sunlight. When forests are clear-cut, an abhorrent and unsustainable practice, the plant leaves turn bright red or purple in an attempt to reduce solar radiation. After a few years, the herbs die off from this environmental assault.

As mentioned, the roots travel in opposite directions, so I generally will follow one stolon for as long as possible, usually to another plant in the area. I have pulled some over ten feet long, so it does not take long to harvest your year's supply. It is important to slice the freshly harvested roots soon after washing. Otherwise the whole roots will dry rock-hard and be very difficult to prepare into medicines.

Bear Root

Alpine Bear Root ♦ Alpine Sweet Vetch ♦ Utah Sweet Vetch ♦ Northern Chainpod—*Hedysarum alpinum* L.

Northern Hedysarum ♦ Boreal Sweet Vetch—*Hedysarum boreale* Nutt. ♦ *H. boreale* var. *mackenzii* (Richardson) S. L. Welsh

> And through the night, behind the wheel, the mileage clicking west
> I think upon Mackenzie, David Thompson and the rest
> Who cracked the mountain ramparts and did show a path for me
> To race the roaring Fraser to the sea.

> —Stan Rogers

Never sell the bear's skin before one has killed the beast.

—Jean de la Fontaine

Hedysarum derives from the Greek root *hedys*, meaning "sweet," and *arum* for "smell." *Alpinum* means "of the alpine." *Boreale* means "northern." *Mackenzii* is named in honor of Alexander Mackenzie, the Scottish explorer and fur trader of the late-eighteenth century. He was the first European to cross North America, exiting the Fraser River to the west. An American edition of his book *Voyages from Montreal to the Frozen and Pacific Oceans* (1801) was presented to Meriwether Lewis, by Thomas Jefferson. He carried it with him on his famed 1804–1806 expedition with William Clark to the Pacific Ocean.

The bear is considered ancestral and a symbol of resurrection by various native peoples. It is the alchemical symbol for the primary state of matter. Living in the boreal forest for a better part of my adult life has given me a unique perspective on bears. Every summer I come upon a number of black bears, and if I mind my own business, they are no problem. If you ever find yourself between a mama bear and her cubs, well, that is a different story, and is best handled by backing away, quietly and quickly.

Grizzly bears, on the other hand, are somewhat unpredictable. I was walking with Timba, my faithful Samoyed dog, south of my cabin one early fall, picking raspberries. I came around a sharp bend in the path and there was a silver-tip grizzly with his back to

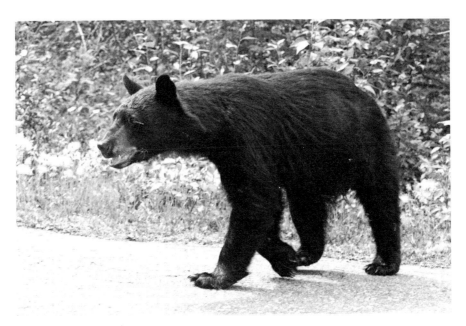

Black bear crossing road

us. I was worried Timba would bark, but fortunately, we were able to back out and run down the trail. But not before the grizzly stood up and turned around, sniffing the air. We were downwind, but when he put his giant paws in the air, he was over sixteen feet tall. The silver-tip is the last of the plains grizzlies, driven into the mountains by human encroachment.

Bear root, or alpine sweet vetch, is an important food plant for both grizzly bears and humans in survival settings. The root is optimally balanced in protein and nonprotein energy. A side dish of ants adds a good source of lipids. I often joke, but with a serious note, that when you come upon a hillside of bear root decimated by bear claws, you do not linger, and you do not pitch your tent anywhere near the site.

The root has been eaten by native people in a variety of ways: raw, boiled, baked, or fried. The young roots have a mild anise-like taste, a mix of coconut and pea flavor. The peeled cooked roots are more like carrots or parsnips, while the roasted root can be compared to potato chips.

Traditional Uses

The Dene Tha name for bear root is "slave carrot," *dene thae.* Alaskan natives will always eat bear root with fat or oil, claiming the root alone will cause constipation. Bear grease is

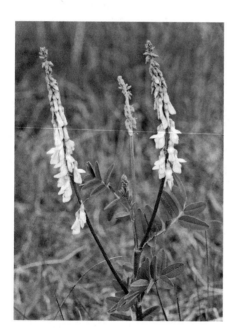

Bear root (courtesy of Glen and Maureen Lee, Regina, Saskatchewan)

often used for this purpose. At many ceremonies I was honored to attend, a bucket of bear grease was passed around to smear on the already deep-fried bannock. Bear grease is a remedy for *witiko,* a creature that eats human flesh raw or half roasted. The Cree believe that grease from the bear, the fattest of big game animals, is an ideal *witiko* cure. This is based on several factors. Bears resemble humans, and are given the honorary name *apitawiõiniw,* meaning "half human." They are spiritual animals with certain body parts, including intestinal fat, concentrating their power. And the bear is the one animal in the boreal forest that will hunt, kill, and eat people. It is believed that bears haunt the graves of executed *witiko.*

The Inuit call the plant *masu* or *masru.* As well as utilizing the root for food, they dried, powdered, and boiled it as a diuretic. The word *Inuit* means "the people." They were previously referred to as Eskimos, a derogatory Cree term meaning "raw-meat eaters." Some authors suggest the name means "snowshoe lacers"; this is less likely. Herbalists of Tibet know bear root as red sweet vetch, or *srad-marbo*. The aerial parts are used for heart and kidney issues. The Gwich'in of the Mackenzie Delta (also named for Alexander Mackenzie) prefer to eat the cooked roots with duck or fish oil. When boiled, the juice is also drunk. Elders say the raw root relieves diarrhea, while the cooked root will increase a sick person's appetite. The Dene Tha sun-dried the roots and cut them into small pieces. For sore eyes, the patient was covered with a blanket and a small piece of root was burned on a fire to create healing smoke. Treatment was about a half hour in length.

Alpine bear root is easily distinguished from northern or *mackenzii* species by its smaller, straggly pink-purplish flowers and conspicuous, dark, regular veins on the lower side of the leaf. The latter plant was blamed for the death of a young man named Chris McCandless. His life story on survival in Alaska was the inspiration for the book *Into the Wild* (1997), written by Jon Krakauer. In his diary, he writes "extremely weak. Fault of seed. Much trouble just to stand up. Starving. Great jeopardy." The movie, by Sean Penn, is well done. Work by Edward Treadwell, a graduate student at the University of Alaska, found no evidence of toxins in *H. mackenzii*. The much larger root probably explains why *H. alpinum* is preferred, rather than any poisonous content. Or is it the seeds that are toxic?

Apparently not, according to Treadwell and Clausen (2008). Recent work, suggests the presence of L-canavanine (1.2%) in the seed. The authors conclude the consumption of the seeds likely contributed to the death of Chris McCandless (Krakauer et al. 2015). I highly doubt it. At least not in a few days. Alfalfa seed, for example, contains L-canavanine. Ingestion by monkeys of alfalfa seeds (up to 40% of diet for seven months) induced lupus erythematosus–like symptoms. This is likely due to L-canavanine, a nonprotein amino acid with the structural analogue of arginine. It may block absorption of B_6 and enzyme cofactors. Monkeys, rodents, and rabbits were fed food made from alfalfa seed as well as alfalfa hay and tablets containing high doses of L-canavanine sulfate. The sprouts only played a marginal role in the two studies, and the connection between

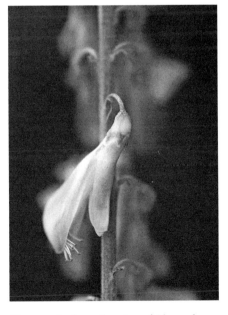

Close-up of a flower (courtesy of Glen and Maureen Lee, Regina, Saskatchewan)

sprouts, as humans consume them, and lupus has never been proven. Supermarket alfalfa sprouts are one week old, whereas the study was one- to three-day-old nongreen oven-dried seedlings. In fact, when sprouts mature, there is no trace of canavanine at all (Bell 1960). I am amused and dismayed when I read in herbal books written by pharmacists that alfalfa sprouts should be avoided by patients with lupus. The sprouts contain no trace of this amino acid.

Other important medicinal herbs containing canavanine are *Baptisia australis, Cytisus scoparius, Genista tinctoria,* soy (*Glycine soja*), white sweet clover (*Melilotus albus*), red clover, Russian olive, and sea buckthorn. Although bear root is a valuable survival food, it should be tested carefully for allergenic response, especially by those individuals already sensitive to strawberries. The roots are enjoyed by grizzly bears, and you can avoid their territory by observing the bank-side digging of this delicacy. Both grizzly and black bears suppress appetite during hibernation under control of leptin. This satiety hormone is secreted by fat cells into the blood stream, affecting appetite centers of the brain.

In western North America, at least in the north, bears begin the transitions to hibernation in September or October. This follows a period of hyperphagia. Black bears will consume 15,000 to 20,000 kilocalories per day and consume excessive amounts of water. During hibernation their heart rate will drop to 8 to 21 beats per minute and oxygen uptake is cut in half. They are not "true" hibernators like ground squirrels, as they can be aroused from sleep. Scientists now call this "winter lethargy" or "winter sleep." Bear root is the major food of grizzly bears posthibernation, along with deer and elk. By July their diet may switch to cow parsnip, horsetail, and other vegetation along with animal protein.

The Dena'ina of Alaska call it wild potato or Alaska carrot, as well as *k'tl'ila,* meaning "rope." This refers to the use of long roots for quick bundling. It is probably their most important wild food other than fruit. It is boiled and the water given to babies when a mother's milk is not available. Like many roots, they are best in spring or fall, becoming dry and tough in summer. The related *H. mackenzii* is known as "brown bear's wild potato."

Both species are recommended for land reclamation. The seed yield for bear root is 100,000 seeds per pound from wild plants and slightly higher numbers from nursery harvest. Considering the potential of bear root over the other two species (see "Medicinal Uses" below), it is the most valuable for dual-purpose plantation. In Russia bear root is highly valued for its medicinal properties, with ongoing research into improving production and cultivation. Mature bear root plants live for up to twenty years (Treshow and Harper 1974), unless bears get them first. In 2004, my company, Earth Medicine Consulting, was asked by the Alberta government to identify ten medicinal plants for commercialization. *Rhodiola rosea* was the number one pick, and it has proven to be a good choice. My other choices were *echinacea pallida* var. *angustifolia, Urtica dioica, Silybum marianum, Trigonella foenum-graecum, Actaea racemosa, Astragalus membranaceus,* and *Hedysarum alpinum.* Our team received a Bronze Premier's Award of Excellence for this contribution to agriculture.

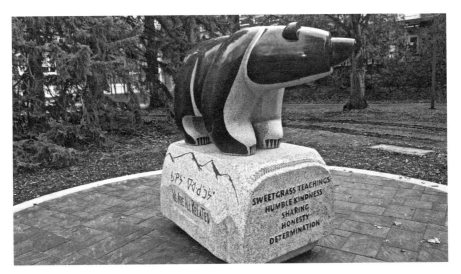

Sweetgrass bear on the University of Alberta campus

Medicinal Uses

Constituents: *H. alpinum* root: mangiferin (C-glucosylxanthone 1.0% of dry weight), iso-mangiferin, alpizirin, quercetin, and hyperoside.

Leaf: polystachoside (guaiaverin), hyperoside, hedisaride, and hedisaride-I; alpizarin $C_{19}H_{18}O_{11}$ (2-beta-C-D-glucopyranosyl-1,3,6,7-tetrahydroxyxanthone); mangiferin content of leaves and flowers varies from 1.19–3.43% in 1–3-year-old plants. Total sum of xanthones 4.3%; flavonoids (0.108%), including quercetin, quercitrin, and hyperoside.

Seeds: galactomannans, L-canavanine.

H. boreale root: saponins and tannins.

Mangiferin inhibits herpes simplex 2 while iso-mangiferin is more effective than acyclovir and other traditional controls (Zheng and Lu 1989). There is one French patent on bear root as a potential source of mangiferin. Alpizarin has been isolated from the aerial parts of *H. alpinum*. In addition to antiviral (antiherpetic) activity, alpizarin possesses cardiac stimulating activity, strengthens capillaries, and reduces inflammation. It helps repair various inflamed conditions of the gastric mucosa. In studies by Sokolov et al. (1988), the plant showed no significant action on the central nervous system, the tone of peripheral vessels, or the smooth musculature of the intestine. It failed to influence carbohydrate metabolism or blood coagulation.

Mangiferin has been shown in mouse studies to increase insulin sensitivity and anti-diabetic activity (Miura et al. 2001). Mangiferin helps decrease insulin resistance with no effect on normal blood glucose levels. It dissolves well in water so is easily extracted. It is an iron chelator and has a number of other useful medicinal benefits, including inhibition of cancer (Matkowski et al. 2013). It enhances tumor cell cytotoxicity in normal and tumor-bearing mouse macrophages and antagonizes in vitro the cytopathic effect of HIV (Guha et al. 1996). Yoshimi et al. (2001) found mangiferin at levels of 0.1% reduced intestinal neoplasms, suggesting chemopreventive activity. In North America colon cancer is presently the second-highest cause of death among both sexes and is increasingly found in young adults. Mangiferin induces apoptosis and cell cycle arrest in A549 human lung carcinoma cells (Shi et al. 2016). Colitis may be ameliorated by mangiferin (Lim et al. 2016). This is not surprising considering its anti-inflammatory influence on intestinal membranes. Hikino et al. (1976) correlated the content of gamma-aminobutyric acid (GABA) in the root with its hypotensive effect. Mangiferin and hyperoside are found in the aerial parts of St. John's wort.

Mangiferin appears to perform antioxidant activity at different levels of the oxidation sequence. It acts by decreasing localized oxygen concentration and thereby generating mangiferin phenoxy radicals, binds metal ions ($Fe^{2+/3+}$) in forms that will not allow the generation of tissue-damaging species such as hydroxyl and highly reactive oxo-ferryl radicals, regulates polymer chain lengthening (membrane lipids) by interacting with the reactive oxygen species, scavenges intermediate radicals such as lipid peroxy and alkoxy radicals to prevent continued H abstraction from cellular lipid molecules, and maintains cellular oxidant-antioxidant balance.

Mangiferin, as mentioned above, has a number of roles to play in blood sugar dysregulation. It inhibits aldose reductase, helping protect eye health associated with hyperglycemia. Mangiferin protects against nephropathy in diabetic-induced rats (Li et al. 2010). Progressive renal failure is common in diabetics and leads to severe complications and organ failure. Mangiferin significantly reduces diabetic symptoms, including antilipidemic and antiatherogenic activity (Muruganandan et al. 2005). Mangiferin decreases inflammation and preserves lysosomal integrity, indicative of cardiac protection (Prabhu et al. 2009). Newer studies suggest mangiferin is both anti-inflammatory and anticancer in nature (Vyas et al. 2012). Mangiferin improved serum lipids in overweight patients with high blood cholesterol (Na et al. 2015). This double-blind randomized trial of 97 men was conducted for 12 weeks with one group receiving 150 mg of mangiferin daily and the other a placebo. The aglycone of mangiferin, norathryiol, reverses obesity and high fat diet–induced insulin resistance (Ding et al. 2014). Mangiferin enhances the sensitivity of human myeloma cells to anticancer drugs by suppression of the NF-kappa-B pathway. This malignancy has a five-year survival rate of about 35%. When used in combination with anticancer drugs the expression of p53 increased and induced apoptosis, activation of caspase-3 and the accumulation of the cells in the sub-G1 phase of the cell cycle (Takeda et al. 2016).

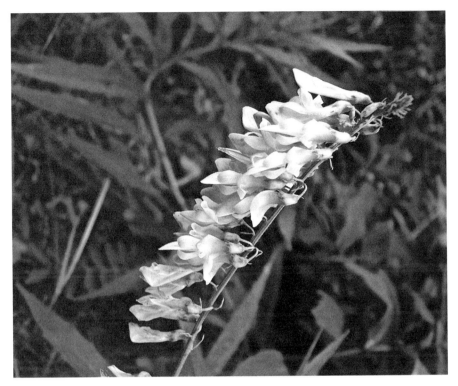

Bear root in full flower

Guaiaverin is a flavonoid also found in fireweed. Bear root should be more thoroughly investigated, due both to its potential medicinal applications and widespread availability of the plant.

Myths and Legends

Teit (1912, 218–21) recorded a Nlaka'pamux narrative:

> *"The Four Black Bears," in which a hunter living near the famous root-digging ground of Botanie (Beta'ni) Valley had two wives, Grizzly Bear and Black Bear. Grizzly became jealous of the man's attention to his Black Bear wife. One day she said to her husband, "I am going to dig roots. Come along with me, so I may not feel lonely! You can do shooting at the same time." She wanted to kill Black Bear's children, so she told her own children to entice the young Black Bears by saying, "Let us play at feasting!" and then setting a basketful of nqá ux, a "pudding" of roots and berries in front of them and inducing them to eat heavily so that they would lose their strength.*

Personality Traits

Jack Tressider (2000) offers this insight into bear symbolism:

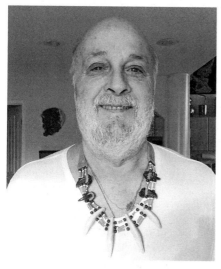

Bear claw necklace given to author

As a symbol of primeval force, the bear was an incarnation of the god Odin in Scandinavia, where the fierce Berserkers wore bearskins into battle. It is linked with many other warlike divinities, including the Greek mother goddess Artemis (whose cultic maidens were "bears"), the Germanic Thor and the Celtic Artio, whose worshippers included the people of Berne (Swiss city of "the bear"). The bear is also an emblem of masculine courage in China, where dreams of a bear presaged the birth of sons. As a symbol of strength, the bear is an ancestral figure to the Ainu of northern Japan, and plays a similar role in mythology of the Algonquin tribe of Native Americans. Elsewhere it is sometimes linked with lunar and resurrection symbolism, perhaps because of its hibernation.

Shamans wear bear-masks to communicate with forest spirits. Although she-bears appear widely as symbols of maternal strength, care, and warmth, Jung linked them with dangerous aspects of the unconscious. In Christian and Islamic traditions, the bear is cruel, lustful, and vengeful, and it can represent gluttony in Western art.

Ed McGaa (2004, 28) explains:

Bear medicine encourages all upon the planet to discern and expose false ego and false superiority, which persuade some people that they can cover up or distort the truth because they are "better," "wiser," "more intellectually blessed," or "more important" than the rest of the world's citizens.

According to Robert A. Brightman (2002, 32):

Crees experience and act both ceremonially and productively on the boreal fauna not as objective qualities but as entities mediated by social meanings.... Bears are understood, by many Cree, as exceptional animals, possessing intelligence equaling or exceeding that of humans. It is said that bears, for example, understand spoken Cree, a competence not conventionally generalized to other animals.

RECIPES

Root: It can be boiled, baked, or roasted. I know this will sound pathetic to survivalists, but if you have a solar-powered food processor, you will get a less fibrous meal.

Infusion: The leaves can be infused: 1 ounce dried plant to 1 pint of water, for various viral conditions. Water extractions produce a clear yellow extract with a sweet, tea-like smell.

Tincture: Tincture the entire plant fresh, including the root chopped finely. Use 50 % alcohol at 1:4 ratio. Take 20–30 drops up to 3 times daily for inflammation, blood sugar dysregulation, and antiviral benefit. Ethanol yields a light-green extract with solids that is strong and sweet but black and sticky. The water or alcohol tincture is light green.

Note: There is no literature suggesting bear root was traditionally used for chronic conditions, only as a diuretic or for treating diarrhea. It deserves to be more widely studied.

Several *Hedysarum* species are used in traditional Chinese medicine (Dong et al. 2013), and more research could provide herbalists with a useful and plentiful addition to the boreal forest materia medica.

Epilogue

THE TWENTY HERBAL ALLIES presented above are by no means the complete story of my learnings of plant medicine over the past four decades. In fact, I was hard-pressed to narrow down my favorites for this book. As I was writing each chapter, I would catch myself thinking about other herbal allies of the boreal forest. Perhaps, in time, I will be able to share some further plant adventures.

References

Acuna, U. M., D. E. Atha, J. Ma, M. H. Nee, and E. J. Kennelly. 2002. "Antioxidant Capacities of Ten Edible North American Plants." *Phytotherapy Research* 16(1): 63–65.

Adachi, Y., Y. Kanbayashi, I. Harata, et al. 2014. "Petasin Activates AMP-Activated Protein Kinase and Modulates Glucose Metabolism." *Journal of Natural Products* 77(6): 1262–69.

Agra, L. C., M. P. Lins, P. da Silva Marques, et al. 2016. "Uvaol Attenuates Pleuritis and Eosinophilic Inflammation in Ovalbumin-Induced Allergy in Mice." *European Journal of Pharmacology* 780: 232–42. doi:10.1016/j.ejphar.2016.03.056.

Ahmad, M., and K. Aftab. 1995. "Hypotensive Action of Syringin from *Syringa vulgaris*." *Phytotherapy Research* 9(6): 452–54.

Ahmad, M., A. H. Gilani, K. Aftab, and V. U. Ahmad. 1993. "Effects of Kaempferol-3-O-Rutinoside on Rat Blood Pressure." *Phytotherapy Research* 7: 314–16.

Ahmad, M., G. H. Rizwani, K. Aftab, V. U. Ahmad, A. H. Gilani, and S. P. Ahmad. 1995. "Acteoside: A New Antihypertensive Drug." *Phytotherapy Research* 9: 525–27.

Ahmed, M., D. A. Henson, M. C. Sanderson, D. C. Nieman, J. M. Zubeldia, and R. A. Shanely. 2015. "*Rhodiola rosea* Exerts Antiviral Activity in Athletes Following a Competitive Marathon Race." *Frontiers in Nutrition* 2(24).

Ahmed-Belkacem, A., A. Pozza, F. Munoz-Martinez, et al. 2005. "Flavonoid Structure-Activity Studies Identify 6-Prenylchrysin and Tectochrysin as Potent and Specific Inhibitors of Breast Cancer Resistance Protein ABCG2." *Cancer Research* 65(11): 4852–60.

Akao, T., K. Kawabata, E. Yanagisawa, et al. 2000. "Baicalin, the Predominant Flavone Glycuronide of *Scutellariae* Radix, Is Absorbed from the Rat Gastrointestinal Tract as the Aglycone and Restored to Its Original Form." *Journal of Pharmacy and Pharmacology* 52(12): 1563–68.

Akhavan-Karbassi, M. H., M. F. Yazdi, H. Ahadian, and M. J. Sadr-Abad. 2016. "Randomized Double-Blind Placebo-Controlled Trial of Propolis for Oral Mucositis in Patients Receiving Chemotherapy for Head and Neck Cancer." *Asian Pacific Journal of Cancer Prevention* 17(7): 3611–14.

Akyol, Sumeyya, Mehmet Akif Gulec, Haci Kemal Erdemli, and Omer Akyol. 2016. "Can Propolis and Caffeic Acid Phenethyl Ester (CAPE) Be Promising Agents against Cyclophosphamide Toxicity?" *Journal of Intercultural Ethnopharmacology* 5(1): 105–7. doi:10.5455/jice.20160127024542.

Albertazzi, F., J. Kudla, and R. Bock. 1998. "The Cox2 Locus of the Primitive Angiosperm Plant *Acorus calamus*: Molecular Structure, Transcript Processing, and RNA Editing." *Molecular and General Genetics* 259(6): 591–600.

Al-Salem, H. S., R. S. Bhat, L. Al-Ayadhi, and A. El-Ansary. 2016. "Therapeutic Potency of Bee Pollen against Biochemical Autistic Features Induced Through Acute and Sub-Acute Neurotoxicity of Orally Administered Propionic Acid." *BioMed Central Complementary and Alternative Medicine* 16(120). doi:10.1186/s12906-016-1099-8.

Al-Waili, N. S. 2001. "Therapeutic and Prophylactic Effects of Crude Honey on Chronic Seborrheic Dermatitis and Dandruff." *European Journal of Medical Research* 6(7): 306–8.

———. 2004. "Natural Honey Lowers Plasma Glucose, C-Reactive Protein, Homocysteine, and Blood Lipids in Healthy, Diabetic, and Hyperlipidemic Subjects: Comparison with Dextrose and Sucrose." *Journal of Medicinal Food* 7(1): 100–7.

Al-Waili, N. S., and A. Haq. 2004. "Effect of Honey on Antibody Production against Thymus-Dependent and Thymus-Independent Antigens in Primary and Secondary Immune Responses." *Journal of Medicinal Food* 7(4): 491–94.

Amoros, M., E. Lurton, J. Boustie, L. Girre, F. Sauvager, and M. Cormier. 1994. "Comparison of the Anti-Herpes Simplex Virus Activities of Propolis and 3-Methylbut-2-Enyl Caffeate." *Journal of Natural Products* 57: 644–47.

Amsterdam, J. D., and A. G. Panossian. 2016. "*Rhodiola rosea* L. as a Putative Botanical Antidepressant." *Phytomedicine* 23(7): 770–83. doi:10.1016/j.phymed.2016.02.009.

An, J., Z. Li, Y. Gong, J. Ren, and J. Huo. 2016. "Amentoflavone Protects against Psoriasis-Like Skin Lesion through Suppression of NF-kappa-B Mediated Inflammation and Keratinocyte Proliferation." *Molecular Cell Biochemistry* 13(1–2): 87–95.

Andrews, Tamra. 2000. *Nectar and Ambrosia*. Santa Barbara, CA: ABC-CLIO.

Aragao, Gisiei Frota, Marta Cristhiany Cunha Pinheiro, Paulo Nogueira Bandeira, Telma Leda Gomes Lemos, and Glauce S. de Barros Viana. 2008. "Analgesic and Anti-Inflammatory Activities of the Isomeric Mixture of alpha- and beta-Amyrin from *Protium heptaphyllum* (Aubl.)." *Journal of Herbal Pharmacotherapy* 7(2): 31–47.

Atteya, R., M. E. Ashour, E. E. Ibrahim, M. A. Farag, and S. E. El-Khamisy. 2016. "Chemical Screening Identifies the B-Carboline Alkaloid Harmine to Be Synergistically Lethal with Doxorubicin." *Mechanisms of Ageing and Development* 60(4–5):381–89. doi:10.1016/j.mad.2016.04.012.

Auger, Dale, and Mary-Beth Laviolette. 2009. *Medicine Paint: The Art of Dale Auger*. Vancouver: Heritage House.

Aversano, Laura. 2002. *The Divine Nature of Plants*. Columbus, NC: Swan·Raven and Co.

Awad, R., J. T. Arnason, V. Trudeau, et al. 2003. "Phytochemical and Biological Analysis of Scullcap (*Scutellaria lateriflora* L.): A Medicinal Plant with Anxiolytic Properties." *Phytomedicine* 10(8): 640–49.

Baananou, S., E. Bagdonaite, B. Marongui, et al. 2015. "Supercritical CO_2 Extract and Essential Oil of Aerial Part of *Ledum Palustre* L.—Chemical Composition and Anti-Inflammatory Activity." *Natural Products Research* 29(11): 999–1005.

Baba, M., Y. Jin, A. Mizuno, et al. 2002. "Studies on Cancer Chemoprevention by Traditional Folk Medicines XXIV. Inhibitory Effect of a Coumarin Derivative, 7-Isopentenyloxycoumarin, against Tumor-Promotion." *Biological and Pharmacology Bulletin* 25(2): 244–46.

Bains, J. S., V. Dhuna, J. Singh, S. S. Kamboj, K. K. Nijjar, and J. N. Agrewala. 2005. "Novel Lectins from Rhizomes of Two *Acorus* Species with Mitogenic Activity and Inhibitory Potential towards Murine Cancer Cell Lines." *International Immunopharmacology* 5(9): 1470–78.

Baldea, N. L., A. Martineau, A.Benhaddou-Andaloussi, J. T. Arnason, É. Lévy, and P. S. Haddad. 2010. "Inhibition of Intestinal Glucose Absorption by Antidiabetic Medicinal Plants Derived from the James Bay Cree Traditional Pharmacopeia." *Journal of Ethnopharmacology* 132(2): 473–82.

Baldwin, I. T., and J. C. Schultz. 1983. "Rapid Changes in Tree Leaf Chemistry Induced by Damage: Evidence for Communication between Plants." *Science* 221(4607): 277–79.

Bankova, V., A. S. Galabov, D. Antonova, N. Vilhelmova, and B. Di Perri. 2014. "Chemical Composition of Propolis Extract ACF and Activity against Herpes Simplex Virus." *Phytomedicine* 21(11): 1432–38. doi:10.1016/j.phymed.2014.04.026.

Barberan, F. A. T. 1986. "The Flavonoid Compounds from Labiatae." *Fitoterapia* 57: 67–95.

Barnes, Burton V. 1966. "The Clonal Growth Habit of American Aspens."*Ecology* 47: 439–47.

Bartfay, W. J., E. Bartfay, and J. G. Johnson. 2012. "Gram-Negative and Gram-Positive Antibacterial Properties of the Whole Plant Extract of Willow Herb (*Epilobium angustifolium*)." *Biological Research for Nursing* 14(1): 85–89.

Batchelor, John. 1892. *The Ainu and Their Folklore.* London: Religious Tract Society.

Battinelli L., B. Tita, M. G. Evandri, and G. Mazzanti. 2001. "Antimicrobial Activity of *Epilobium* spp. Extracts." *Il Farmaco* (Societa chimica italica) 56(5–7): 345–48.

Baureithel, K. H., K. B. Büter, A. Engesser, W. Burkard, and W. Schaffner. 1997. "Inhibition of Benzodiazepine Binding In Vitro by Amentoflavone, a Constituent of Various Species of *Hypericum*." *Pharmaceutica Acta Helvetiae* 72(3): 153–57.

Beattie, K. D., P. G. Waterman, P. I. Forster, D. R. Thompson, and D. N. Leach. 2011. "Chemical Composition and Cytotoxicity of Oils and Eremophilanes Derived from Various Parts of *Eremophilia mitchellii* Benth. (Myoporaceae)." *Phytochemistry* 72(4–5): 400–8.

Bell, E. A. 1960. "Canavanine in the Leguminosae." *Biochemical Journal* 75(3): 618–20.

Beresford-Kroeger, Diana. 2010. *Arboretum Borealis*. Ann Arbor, MI: University of Michigan Press.

Beretz, A., F. Briançon-Scheid, A. Stierlé, G. Corre, R. Anton, and J. P. Cazenave. 1986. "Inhibition of Human Platelet Cyclic AMP Phosphodiesterase and of Platelet Aggregation by a Hemisynthetic Flavonoid, Amentoflavone Hexacetate." *Biochemical Pharmacology* 35(2): 257–62.

Bickel, D., T. Röder, H. J. Bestmann, and K. Brune. 1994. "Identification and Characterization of Inhibitors of Peptio-Leukotriene-Syntheses from *Petasiteshybridus*."*Planta Medica* 60(4): 318–22.

Bidartondo, M. I., and T. D. Bruns. 2001. "Extreme Specificity in Epiparasitic Monotropoideae (Ericaceae): Widespread Phylogenetic and Geographical Structure." *Molecular Ecology* 10: 2285–95.

Birket-Smith, K. 1931. "The Roles of Men and Women in Eskimo Culture." *American Anthropologist* 33(4): 635.

Björkman, Erik. 1960. "*Monotropa hypopitys* L.: An Epiparasite on Tree Roots."*Physiologia Plantarum* 13: 308–27.

Black, P., A. Saleem, A. Dunford, et al. 2011. "Seasonal Variation of Phenolic Constituents and Medicinal Activities of Northern Labrador Tea, *Rhododendron tomentosum* ssp. *subarcticum*, an Inuit and Cree First Nations Traditional Medicine." *Planta Medica* 77(14): 1655–62.

Blanchan, Neltje. 1917. *Wild Flowers Worth Knowing*. Self-published. Reprinted Charleston, SC: BiblioBazaar, 2007.

Bocharova, O. A., B. P. Matveev, A. Baryshnikov, K. M. Figurin, R. V. Serebriakova, and N. B. Bodrova. 1995. "The Effect of a *Rhodiola rosea* Extract on the Incidence of Recurrences of a Superficial Bladder Cancer (Experimental Clinical Research)." *Urologiia i Nefrologiia* (Moscow) 2: 46–47.

Bol'shakova, I. V., E. L. Lozovskaia, and I. I. Sapezhinshii. 1998. ["Antioxidant Properties of Plant Extracts"]. *Biofizika* (Moscow) 43(2): 186–88.

Booker, A., B. Jalil, D. Frommenwiler, et al. 2016. "The Authenticity and Quality of *Rhodiola rosea* Products." *Phytomedicine* 23(7): 754–62.

Borchardt, J. R., D. L. Wyse, C. C. Sheaffer, et al. 2008. "Antimicrobial Activity of Native and Naturalized Plants of Minnesota and Wisconsin." *Journal of Medicinal Plants Research* 2(5): 98–110.

Brattström, A., A. Schapowai, I. Maillet, B. Schnyder, B. Ryffel, and R. Moser. 2010. "*Petasites* Extract Ze 339 (PET) Inhibits Allergen-Induced Th2 Responses, Airway Inflammation and Airway Hyperreactivity in Mice." *Phytotherapy Research* 24(5): 680–85.

Brekhman, I. I., and I. V.Dardymov. 1969. "New Substances of Plant Origin which Increase Non-specific Resistance." *Annual Review of Pharmacology and Toxicology* 9: 419–30.

Bretz, W. A., N. Paulino, J. E. Nör, and A. Moreira. 2014. "The Effectiveness of Propolis on Gingivitis: A Randomized Controlled Trial." *Journal of Alternative and Complementary Medicine* 20(12): 943–48.

Brightman, Robert A. 2002. *Grateful Prey: Rock Cree Human-Animal Relationships*. Regina, Canada: Canadian Plains Research Center, University of Regina.

Brinker, Francis N. D. 2010. *Herbal Contraindications and Drug Interactions Plus Herbal Adjuncts with Medicines*. 4th Edition. Sandy, OR: Eclectic Medical Publications.

Brock, C., J. Whitehorse, I. Tewfik, and T. Towell. 2014. "American Scullcap (*Scutellaria lateriflora*): A Randomized, Double-Blind Placebo-Controlled Crossover Study of Its Effects on Mood in Healthy Volunteers." *Phytotherapy Research* 28(5): 692–98.

Brown, Annora. 1970. *Old Man's Garden*. Sidney, BC, Canada: Gray's.

Bruchac, J., and J. London. 1992. *Thirteen Moons on Turtle's Back: A Native American Year of Moons*. New York: Putnam & Grosset.

Budzynska, B., K. Skalicka-Wozniak, M. Kruk-Slomka, M. Wydrzynska-Kuzma, and G. Biala. 2016. "In Vivo Modulation of the Behavioral Effects of Nicotine by the Coumarins, Xanthotoxin, Bergapten, and Umbelliferone." *Psychopharmacology* (Berlin) 233(12):2289–300. doi:10.1007/s00213-016-4279-9.

Buhner, Stephen Harrod. 1998. *Sacred and Herbal Healing Beers*. Boulder, CO: Brewer's.

———. 2002. *The Lost Language of Plants: The Ecological Importance of Plant Medicine to Life on Earth*. White River Junction, VT: Chelsea Green.

———. 2013. *Healing Lyme Disease Coinfections*. Rochester, VT: Healing Arts.

Burdock, G. A. 1998. "Review of the Biological Properties and Toxicity of Bee Propolis (Propolis)." *Food and Chemical Toxicology* 36(4): 347–63.

Burgalassi, S., N. Nicosia, D. Monti, G. Falcone, E. Boldrini, and P. Chetoni. 2007. "Larch Arabinogalactan for Dry Eye Protection and Treatment of Corneal Lesions: Investigation in Rabbits." *Journal of Ocular Pharmacology Therapy* 23(6): 541–50.

Burns Kraft, T. F., M. Dey, R. B. Rogers, et al. 2008. "Phytochemical Composition and Metabolic Performance Enhancing Activity of Dietary Berries Traditionally Used by Native North Americans." *Journal of Agricultural and Food Chemistry* 56(3): 654–60.

Bystritsky, A., L. Kerwin, and J. D. Feusner. 2008. "A Pilot Study of *Rhodiola rosea* (Rhodax) for Generalized Anxiety Disorder (GAD)." *Journal of Alternative and Complementary Medicine* 14(2): 175–80.

Calderón, Eduardo. 1982. *Eduardo el Curandero: The Words of a Peruvian Healer.* Berkeley, CA: North Atlantic Books.

Campbell, Joseph. 1991. *Primitive Mythology: The Masks of God.* Book 1. New York: Penguin.

Card, David R. 2005. *Facial Diagnosis of Cell Salt Deficiency.* Prescott, AZ: Hohm Press.

Carr, Emily, and Emily Henrietta Woods. 2006. *Wild Flowers.* Victoria, Canada: Royal BC Museum.

Casteels, P., C. Ampe, L. Riviere, et al. 1990. "Isolation and Characterization of Abaecin, a Major Antibacterial Response Peptide in the Honeybee *(Apis mellifera)*." *European Journal of Biochemistry* 187(2): 381–86.

Catty, Suzanne. 2001. *Hydrosols: The Next Aromatherapy.* Rochester, VT: Healing Arts.

Causey, J., R. Robinson, J. Feirtag, R. Fulcher, and J. Slavin. 1999. "Effects of Larch Arabinogalactan on Human Peripheral Blood Mononuclear Cells: Results from In Vivo and In Vitro Human Trials." *Federation of American Societies for Experimental Biology Journal* 13(A589).

Cavanagh, D., J. Beazley, and F. Ostapowicz. 1970. "Radical Operation for Carcinoma of the Vulva: A New Approach to Wound Healing." *Journal of Obstetrics and Gynaecology of the British Commonwealth* 77(11): 1037–40.

Chan, F. L., H. L. Choi, P. S. Chen, and Y. Huang. 2000. "Induction of Apoptosis in Cancer Cell Lines by a Flavonoid, Baicalin." *Cancer Letters* 160(2): 219–28.

Chang, W., and J. Teng. 2015. "Beta-Asarone Prevents A-beta$_{(25-35)}$–Induced Inflammatory Responses and Autophagy in SH-SY5Y Cells: Down Expression Beclin-1, LC3B, and Up Expression Bci-2." *International Journal of Clinical Experimental Medicine* 8(11): 20658–63.

Chappell, Peter. 2003. *Emotional Healing with Homeopathy: Treating the Effects of Trauma.* Berkeley, CA: North Atlantic Books.

Chase, Pamela, and Jonathan Pawlik. 1991. *Newcastle Trees for Healing.* Van Nuys, CA: Newcastle.

Chatroux, Sylvia Seroussi. 1998. *Materia Poetica: Homeopathy in Verse.* Ashland, OR: Poetica.

———. 2004. *Botanica Poetica: Herbs in Verse.* Ashland, OR: Poetica.

Chen, C., D. Spriano, and B. Meier. 2009. "Reduction of beta-Asarone in Acori Rhizoma by Decoction." *Plant Medica* 75(13): 1448–52.

Chen, C. H., H. C. Chan, Y. T. Chu, et al. 2009. "Antioxidant Activity of Some Plant Extracts towards Xanthine Oxidase, Lipoxygenase, and Tyrosinase." *Molecules* 14(8): 2947–58.

Chen, H. P., K. Yang, L. S. Zheng, C. X. You, Q. Cai, and C. F. Wang. 2015. "Repellant and Insecticidal Activities of Shyobunone and Isoshyobunone Derived from the Essential Oil of *Acorus calamus* Rhizomes." *Pharmacogosy Magazine* 11(44): 675–81.

Chen, J. H., W. L. Chen, and Y. C. Liu. 2015. "Amentoflavone Induces Antiangiogenic and Anti-Metastatic Effects through Suppression of NF-kappa-B Activation in MCF-7 Cells." *Anticancer Research* 35(12): 6685–93.

Chen, Q., L. Yang, G. Zhang, and F. Wang. 2013. "Bioactivity-Guided Isolation of Antiosteoporotic Compounds from *Ligustrum lucidum*." *Phytotherapy Research* 27(7): 973–79.

Chen, S., J. Gao, D. Halicka, F. Traganos, and Z. Darzynkiewicz. 2008. "Down-Regulation of Androgen-Receptor and PSA by Phytochemicals." *International Journal of Oncology* 32(2): 405–11.

Chen, T. S., S. Y. Liou, and Y. L. Chang. 2008. "Antioxidant Evaluation of Three Adaptogen Extracts." *American Journal of Chinese Medicine* 36(6): 1209–17.

Cheng, L., F. Li, R. Ma, and X. Hu. 2015. "Forsythiaside Inhibits Cigarette Smoke-Induced Lung Inflammation by Activation of Nrf2 and Inhibition of NF-kappa-B." *International Immunopharmacology* 28(1): 494–99.

Cho, H. J., S. G. Jeong, J. E. Park, et al. 2013. "Antiviral Activity of Angelicin against Gammaherpes Viruses." *Antiviral Research* 100(1): 75–83.

Christopher, John R. 1976. *School of Natural Healing.* Provo, UT: BiWorld.

Chung, H., Y. M. Jung, D. H. Shin, et al. 2008. "Anticancer Effects of Wogonin in Both Estrogen Receptor Positive and Negative Human Breast Cancer Cell Lines In Vitro and in Nude Mice Xenografts." *International Journal of Cancer* 122(4): 816–22.

Chung, K. S., H. J. An, S. Y. Cheon, K. R. Kwon, and K. H. Lee. 2015. "Bee Venom Suppresses Testosterone-Induced Benign Prostatic Hyperplasia by Regulating the Inflammatory Response and Apoptosis." *Experimental Biology and Medicine* (Maywood, NJ) 240(12):1656–63. doi:10.1177/1535370215590823.

Cieniak, C., R. Liu, A. Fottinger, et al. 2013. "In Vitro Inhibition of Metabolism but Not Transport of Gliclazide and Repaglinide by Cree Medicinal Plant Extracts." *Journal of Ethnopharmacology* 150(3): 1087–95. doi.org/10.1016/jep.2013.10.029.

Clark, T. N., K. T. Ellsworth, S. Jean, et al. 2015. "Isolation of Phomopsolide A and 6(E)-Phomopsolide A as Antimycobacterial Natural Products from an Unidentified Endophyte of the Canadian Medicinal Plant *Heracleum maximum*." *Natural Product Communication* 10(10): 1647–48.

Cohen, Ken. 2003. *Honoring the Medicine: The Essential Guide to Native American Healing.* New York: Ballantine.

Cole, I. B., J. Cao, A. R. Alan, P. K. Saxena, and S. J. Murch. 2008. "Comparisons of *Scutellaria baicalensis*, *Scutellaria lateriflora*, and *Scutellaria racemosa*: Genome Size, Antioxidant Potential, and Phytochemistry." *Planta Medica* 74(4): 474–81.

Coles, William. 1656. *The Art of Simpling.* Reprinted Pomeroy, WA: Health Research, 1986.

Cooper, R. A., P. Wigley, and N. F. Burton. 2000. "Susceptibility of Multiresistant Strains of *Burkholderia cepacia* to Honey." *Letters in Applied Microbiology* 31(1): 20–24.

Coulson, S., A. Rao, S. L. Beck, E. Steels, H. Gramotnev, and L. Vitetta. 2013. "A Phase II Randomized Double-Blind Placebo-Controlled Trial Investigating the Efficacy and Safety of ProstateEZE Max: A Herbal Medicine Preparation for the Management of Symptoms of Benign Prostatic Hypertrophy." *Complementary Medical Research* 21(3): 172–79. doi:10.1016/j.ctim.2013.01.007.

Crow, Tis Mal. 2001. *Native Plants, Native Healing: Traditional Muskogee Way.* Summertown, TN: Native Voices.

Culpepper, N. 1652. *The English Physician: Culpepper's Complete Herbal.* Reprinted London: Arcturus, 2009.

Cuny, G. D., N. P. Ulyanova, D. Patnaik, et al. 2012. "Structure-Activity Relationship Study of beta-Carboline Derivatives as Haspin Kinase Inhibitors." *Bioorganic and Medicinal Chemistry Letters* 22(5): 2015–19.

Cybulska, P., S. D. Thakur, B. C. Foster, et al. 2011. "Extracts of Canadian First Nations Medicinal Plants, Used as Natural Products, Inhibit *Neisseria gonorrhoeae* Isolates with Different Antibiotic Resistance Profiles." *Sexually Transmitted Diseases* 38(7): 667–71.

Dalben-Dota, K. F., M. G. Faria, M. L. Bruschi, S. M. Pelloso, M. E. Lopes-Consolaro, and T. I. Svidzinski. 2010. "Antifungal Activity of Propolis Extract against Yeasts Isolated from Vaginal Exudates." *Journal of Alternative and Complementary Medicine* 16(3): 285–90. doi:10.1089/acm.2009.0281.

Dampc, A., and M. Luczkiewicz. 2015. "Labrador Tea—the Aromatic Beverage and Spice: A Review of Origin, Processing, and Safety." *Journal of Science Food and Agriculture* 95(8): 1577–83.

Darbinyan, V., G. Asianyan, E. Amroyan, E. Gabrielyan, C. Malmström, and A. Panossian. 2007. "Clinical Trial of *Rhodiola rosea* L. Extract SHR-5 in the Treatment of Mild to Moderate Depression." *Nordic Journal of Psychiatry* 61(5): 343–48.

De Bock, K., B. O. Eijnde, M. Ramaekers, and P. Hespel. 2004. "Acute *Rhodiola rosea* Intake Can Improve Endurance Exercise Performance." *International Journal of Sports Nutrition and Exercise Metabolism* 14(3): 298–307.

De Bock, Martin, Jose G. B. Derraik, Christine M. Brennan, et al. 2013. "Olive (*Olea europaea* L.) Leaf Polyphenols Improve Insulin Sensitivity in Middle-Aged Overweight Men: A Randomized, Placebo-Controlled, Crossover Trial." *PLOS One* 8(3): e57622. doi:10.1371/journal.pone.0057622.

De Sanctis, R., R. De Bellis, C. Scesa, U. Mancini, L. Cucchiarini, and M. Dacha. 2004. "In Vitro Protective Effect of *Rhodiola rosea* Extract against Hypochlorous Acid-Induced Oxidative Damage in Human Erythrocytes." *Biofactors* 20(3): 147–59.

Dewey, Laurel. 2001. *Plant Power.* Revised Edition. Markham, Canada: Safe Goods/New Century.

Dhawan, K., S. Kumar, and A. Sharma. 2004. "Beneficial Effects of Chrysin and Benzoflavone on Virility in 2-Year-Old Male Rats." *Journal of Medicinal Food* 5(1): 43–48.

Ding, H., Y. Zhang, C. Xu, et al. 2014. "Norathyriol Reverses Obesity- and High-Fat-Diet–Induced Insulin Resistance in Mice through Inhibition of PTP1B." *Diabetologia* 57(10): 2145–54.

Dion, C., E. Chappuis, and C. Ripoll. 2016. "Does Larch Arabinogalactan Enhance Immune Function? A Review of Mechanistic and Clinical Trials." *Nutrition Metabolism* 13(28).

Dong, P., Y. Zhang, J. Gu, et al. 2011. "Wogonin, an Active Ingredient of Chinese Herb Medicine *Scutellaria baicalensis*, Inhibits the Mobility and Invasion of Human Gall Bladder Carcinoma GBC-SD Cells by Inducing the Expression of Maspin." *Journal of Ethnopharmacology* 137(3): 1373–80.

Dong, Y. M., D. Y. Tang, N. Zhang, Y. Li, C. H. Zhang, and M. H. Li. 2013. "Phytochemicals and Biological Studies of Plants in Genus *Hedysarum*." *Chemistry Central Journal* 7(124). doi:10.1186/1752-153X-7-124.

Drag, M., P. Surowiak, M. Drag-Zalesinska, M. Dietel, H. Lage, and J. Oleksyszyn. 2009. "Comparison of the Cytotoxic Effects of Birch Bark Extract, Betulin, and Betulinic Acid towards Human Gastric Carcinoma and Pancreatic Carcinoma Drug-Sensitive and Drug-Resistant Cell Lines." *Molecules* 14(4): 1639–51.

Ducrey, B., A. Marston, S. Goehring, R. W. Hartmann, and K. Hostellman. 1997. "Inhibition of 5-Alpha-Reductase and Aromatase by the Ellagitannins Oenothein A and Oenothein B from Epilobium Species." *Planta Medica* 63: 111–14.

Dufour, D., A. Pichette, V. Mshvlidadze, M. E. Bradette-Hebert, and S. Lavoie. 2007. "Antioxidant, Anti-Inflammatory, and Anticancer Activities of Methanolic Extracts from *Ledum groenlandicum* Retzius." *Journal of Ethnopharmacology* 111(1): 22–28.

Duke, James A. 1983. *Handbook of Energy Crops*. Unpublished.

———. 1985. *Handbook of Medicinal Herbs*. Boca Raton, FL: CRC.

Durzan, Don J. 2009. "Arginine, Scurvy, and Cartier's 'Tree of Life.'" *Journal of Ethnobiology and Ethnomedicine* 5(5). doi:101186/1746-4269-5-5.

Eason, Cassandra. 2008. *Fabulous Creatures, Mythical Monsters, and Animal Power Symbols: A Handbook*. Westport, CT: Greenwood Press.

Ebeling, S., K. Naumann, S. Pollok, et al. 2014. "From a Traditional Medicinal Plant to a Rational Drug: Understanding the Clinically Proven Wound Healing Efficacy of Birch Bark Extract." *PLOS One* 9(1): e86147.

Eiden, M., F. Leidel, B. Strohmmeier, C. Fast, and M. H. Groschup. 2012. "A Medicinal Herb *Scutellaria lateriflora* Inhibits PrP Replication In Vitro and Delays the Onset of Prion Disease in Mice." *Front Psychiatry* 3(9).

Ellingwood, F. 1915. *American Materia Medica, Therapeutics and Pharmacognosy*. Reprinted Whitefish MT: Kissinger, 2010.

El Sayed, A. M., S. M. Ezzat, and O. M. Sabry. 2016. "A New Antibacterial Lupane Ester from the Seeds of *Acokanthera oppositifolia* Lam." *Natural Product Research* 4(April): 1–6.

Eltaher, S., G. F. Mohammed, S. Younes, and A. Elakhras. 2015. "Efficacy of the Apitherapy in the Treatment of Recalcitrant Localized Plaque Psoriasis and Evaluation of Tumor Necrosis Factor-alpha (TNF-alpha) Serum Level: A Double-Blind Randomized Clinical Trial." *Journal of Dermatological Treatment* 26(5): 335–39.

Enomoto, R., C. Koshiba, C. Suzuki, and E. Lee. 2011. "Wogonin Potentiates the Antitumor Action of Etoposide and Ameliorates Its Adverse Effects." *Cancer Chemotherapy Pharmacology* 67(5): 1063–72.

Evstatieva, Ljuba, Milka Todorova, Daniela Antonova, and Jordanka Staneva. 2010. "Chemical Composition of the Essential Oils of *Rhodiola rosea* L. of Three Different Origins." *Pharmacognosy Magazine* 6(24): 256–58. doi:10.4103/0973-1296.71782.

Felter, H. W., and J. U. Lloyd. 1898. *King's American Dispensatory*. Cincinnati: Ohio Valley Co.

Ferguson, Diane. 2001. *Native American Myths*. London: Collins and Brown.

Fintelmann, V., and J. Gruenwald. 2007. "Efficacy and Tolerability of a *Rhodiola rosea* Extract in Adults with Physical and Cognitive Deficiencies." *Advances in Therapy* 24(4): 929–39.

Flint, Margi. 2005. *The Practicing Herbalist: Thoughts for Meeting with Clients*. Marblehead, MA: EarthSong.

Fokina, G. I., T. V. Frolova, V. M. Roĭkhel, and V. V. Pogodina. 1991. ["Experimental Phytotherapy of Tick-Borne Encephalitis"]. *Voprosy virusologii* [Problems of Virology]. 36(1): 18–21.

Fong, Y. K., C. R. Li, S. K. Wo, et al. 2012. "In Vitro and In Situ Evaluation of Herb-Drug Interactions during Intestinal Metabolism and Absorption of Baicalein." *Journal of Ethnopharmacology* 141(2): 742–53.

Fraser, M. H., A. Cuerrier, P. S. Haddad, J. T. Arnason, P. L. Owen, and T. Johns. 2007. "Medicinal Plants of Cree Communities (Quebec, Canada): Antioxidant Activity of Plants Used to Treat Type 2 Diabetes Symptoms." *Canadian Journal of Physiology and Pharmacology* 85(11): 1200–14.

Frédérich, M., A. Marcowycz, E. Cieckiewicz, V. Mégalizzi, L. Angenot, and R. Kiss. 2009. "In Vitro Anticancer Potential of Tree Extracts from the Walloon Region Forest." *Planta Medica* 75: 1–4.

Freitas, S. F., L. Shinohara, J. M. Sforcin, and S. Guimarães. 2006. "In Vitro Effects of Propolis on *Giardia duodenalis* Trophozoites." *Phytomedicine* 13(3): 170–75.

French Pharmacopoeia. 10th ed. Paris: French Ministry of Health, 1988.

Freysdottir, J., M. B. Sigurpaisson, S. Omarsdottir, E. S.Olafsdottir, A. Vikingsson, and I. Hardardottir. 2011. "Ethanol Extract from Birch Bark *(Betula pubescens)* Suppresses Human Dendritic Cell–Mediated Th1 Responses and Directs It towards a Th17 Regulatory Response In Vitro." *Immunology Letters* 136(1): 90–96.

Fulda, S., C. Friesen, M. Los, et al. 1997. "Betulinic Acid Triggers CD95 (APO-1/Fas) and P53-Independent Apoptosis via Activation of Caspases in Neuroectodermal Tumors." *Cancer Research* 57(21): 4956–64.

Fulda, S., I. Jeremias, H. H. Steiner, T. Pietsch, and K. M. Debatin. 1999. "Betulinic Acid: A New Cytotoxic Agent against Malignant Brain-Tumor Cells." *International Journal of Cancer* 82(3): 435–41.

Fulda, S., and G. Kroemer. 2009. "Targeting Mitochondrial Apoptosis by Betulinic Acid in Human Cancer." *Drug Discovery Today* 14(17–18): 885–90.

Gafner, S., C. Bergeron, L. L. Batcha, et al. 2003. "Inhibition of [3H]-LSD Binding to 5-HT7 Receptors by Flavonoids from *Scutellaria lateriflora*." *Journal of Natural Products* 66(4): 535–37.

Galanski, W., J. Ghiabicz, A. Paszkiewicz-Gadek, C. Marcinkiewicz, and A. Gindzienski. 1996. "The Substances of Plant Origin That Inhibit Protein Biosynthesis." *Acta PoloniaePharmaceutica* 53(5): 311–18.

Galochkina, A. V., V. B. Anikin, V. A. Babkin, L. A. Ostrouhova, and V. V. Zarubaev. 2016. "Virus-Inhibiting Activity of Dihydroquercetin, a Flavonoid from *Larix sibirica*, against Coxsackievirus B4 in a Model of Viral Pancreatitis." *Archives of Virology* 161(4): 929–38.

Gao, Jiayu, Alberto Sanchez-Medina, Barbara A. Pendry, Michael J. Hughes, Geoffrey P. Webb, and Olivia Corcoran. 2008. "Validation of a HPLC Method for Flavonoid Biomarkers in Scullcap *(Scutellaria)* and Its Use to Illustrate Wide Variability in the Quality of Commercial Tinctures." *Journal of Pharmacy and Pharmaceutical Sciences* 11(1): 77–87.

Gao, Rong, Bang-Hao Zhu, Shi-Bo Tang, Jiang-Feng Wang, and Jun Ren. 2008. "Scutellarein Inhibits Hypoxia- and Moderately High Glucose–Induced Proliferation and VEGF Expression in Human Retinal Endothelial Cells." *Acta Pharmacologica Sinica* 29(6): 707–12.

García-Pérez, M. E., M. Royer, A. Duque-Fernandez, P. N. Diouf, T. Stevanovic, and R. Pouliot. 2010. "Antioxidant, Toxicological, and Antiproliferative Properties of Canadian Polyphenolic Extracts on Normal and Psoriatic Keratinocytes." *Journal of Ethnopharmacology* 132(1): 251–58.

Geng, Y., C. Li, J. Liu, et al. 2010. "Beta-Asarone Improves Cognitive Function by Suppressing Neuronal Apoptosis in the beta-Amyloid Hippocampus Injection Rats." *Biological and Pharmaceutical Bulletin* 33(5): 836–43.

Geniusz, Mary Siisip. 2015. *Plants Have So Much to Give Us, All We Have to Do Is Ask: Anishinaabe Botanical Teachings.* Minneapolis: University of Minnesota Press.

Georgiev, M., S. Pastore, D. Lulli, et al. 2012. "*Verbascum xanthphoeniceum*–Derived Phenylethanoid Glycosides Are Potent Inhibitors of Inflammatory Cytokines in Dormant and Interferon-gamma–Stimulated Human Keratinocytes." *Journal of Ethnopharmacology* 144(3): 754–60.

Gerard, John. 1633. *The Herbal or General History of Plants.* Revised English Edition by Thomas Johnson, Mineola, NY: Dover, 2015.

Ghasemi, F., F. Rezaei, A. Araghi, and M. A. Tabari. 2015. "Antimicrobial Activity of Aqueous-Alcoholic Extracts and the Essential Oil of *Verbascum thapsus* L." *Jundishapur Journal of Natural Pharmaceutical Products* 10(3).

Gheldof, N., X. H. Wang, and N. J. Engeseth. 2003. "Buckwheat Honey Increases Serum Antioxidant Capacity in Humans." *Journal of Agriculture Food Chemistry* 51(5): 1500–5.

Gilani, A., A. J. Shah, M. Ahmad, and E. Shaheen. 2006. "Antispasmodic Effect of *Acorus calamus* L. Is Mediated through Calcium Channel Blockade." *Phytotherapy Research* 20(6): 1080–84.

Glinski, Z. 2000. "Immuno-Suppressive and Immuno-Toxic Action of Contaminated Honeybee Products on Consumers." *Medycyna Weterynary Journal* 56(10): 634–38.

Godfrey, A., and P. R. Saunders. 2010. *Principles and Practices of Naturopathic Botanical Medicine.* Volume I. Toronto: CCNM.

Goun, E. A., V. M. Petrichenko, S. U. Solodnikov, T. V. Suhinina, and M. A. Kline. 2002. "Anticancer and Antithrombin Activity of Russian Plants." *Journal of Ethnopharmacology* 81(3).

Grinnell, G. B. 1905. "Some Cheyenne Plant Medicines." *American Anthropologists* 7: 37–43.

Grohmann, Gerbert. 1989. *The Plant.* Volume 2. Kimberton, PA: Bio-Dynamic Farming and Gardening Association.

Grossmann, M., and H. Schmidramsl. 2000. "An Extract of *Petasites hybridus* Is Effective in the Prophylaxis of Migraine." *International Journal of Clinical Pharmacology and Therapeutics.* 38(9): 430–35.

Grzegorczyk-Karolak, I., K. Golab, J. Gburek, H. Wysokinska, and A. Matkowski. 2016. "Inhibition of Advanced Glycation End-Product Formation and Antioxidant Activity by Extracts and Polyphenols from *Scutellaria alpina* L. and *S. altissima* L." *Molecules* 21(6).

Guan, T., Y. S. Qian, L. F. Huang, Y. Li, and H. B. Sun. 2011. "Maslinic Acid, a Natural Inhibitor of Glycogen Phosphorylase, Reduces Cerebral Ischemic Injury in Hyperglycemic Rats by GLT-1 Up-Regulation." *Journal of Neuroscience Research* 89(11): 1829–39.

Guha, S., S. Ghosal, and U. Chattopadhay. 1996. "Antitumor, Immunomodulatory and Anti-HIV Effect of Mangiferin, a Naturally Occurring Glucosylxanthone." *Chemotherapy* 42: 443–51. doi:10.1159/000239478.

Guillet, Alma. 1962. *Make Friends of Trees and Shrubs*. New York: Doubleday.

Guiraud, P., R. Steiman, F. Seigle-Murandi, and N. Buarque De Gusmao. 1999. "Antimicrobial and Antitumor Activities of Mycosporulone." *Journal of Natural Products* 62(9): 1222–24.

Guo, A. J., H. Q. Xie, R. C. Choi, et al. 2010. "Galangin, a Flavonol Derived from Rhizoma *Alpiniae officinarum*, Inhibits Acetylcholinesterase Activity In Vitro." *Chemico-Biological Interactions* 187(1–3): 246–48. doi:10.1016/j.cbi.2010.05.002.

Guseinova, V. E., V. I. Golyshevskaya, L. P. Cherednichenko, and E. A. Fomina. 1992. "Examining the Antimicrobial Properties of Medicinal Plant Species." *Farmatsiya* (Moscow) 41 (1992): 21–24.

Habib, F. K., M. Ross, A. Lewenstein, X. Zhang, and J. C. Jaton. 1995. "Identification of a Prostate Inhibitory Substance in a Pollen Extract." *The Prostate* 26(3): 133–39.

Hageneder, Fred. 2005. *The Spirit of Trees: Science, Symbiosis, and Inspiration*. New York: Continuum.

Haghighi, F., M. M. Matin, A. R. Bahrimi, M. Iranshahi, F. B. Rassouli, and A. Haghighitalab. 2014. "The Cytotoxic Activities of 7-Isopentenyloxycoumarin on 5637 Cells via Induction of Apoptosis and Cell Cycle Arrest in G2/M Stage." *DARU Journal of Pharmaceutical Sciences* 22(1): 3.

Hall, Dorothy. 1988. *Creating Your Herbal Profile*. New Canaan, CT:Keats.

Hamel, Paul B., and Mary U. Chiltoskey. 1975. *Cherokee Plants*. Sylva, NC: Herald.

Hanchuk, Rena Jeanne, and Andriy Nahachewsky. 1999. *The Word and Wax: A Medical Folk Ritual among Ukrainians in Alberta*. Edmonton, Canada: Canadian Institute of Ukrainian Study.

Hanrahan, J. R., M. Chebib, N. L. Davucheron, B. J. Hall, and G. A. Johnston. 2003. "Semisynthetic Preparation of Amentoflavone: A Negative Modulator at GABA(A) Receptors." *Bioorganic and Medicinal Chemistry Letters* 13(14): 2281–84.

Hao, H., Y. Aixia, L. Dan, F. Lei, Y. Nancai, and S. Wen. 2009. "Baicalin Suppresses Expression of Chlamydia Protease-Like Activity Factor in Hep-2 Cells Infected by *Chlamydia trachomatis*." *Fitoterapia* 80(7): 448–52.

Harbilas, Despina, Louis C. Martineau, Cory S. Harris, et al. 2009. "Evaluation of the Antidiabetic Potential of Selected Medicinal Plant Extracts from the Canadian Boreal Forest Used to Treat Symptoms of Diabetes. Part II." *Canadian Journal of Physiology and Pharmacology* 87(6): 479–92.

Harbilas, Despina, Diane Vallerand, Antoine Brault, et al. 2012. "*Larix laricina*, an Antidiabetic Alternative Treatment from the Cree of Northern Quebec Pharmacopoeia, Decreases Glycemia and Improves Insulin Sensitivity In Vivo." *Evidence-Based Complementary and Alternative Medicine* 2012. doi:10.1155/2012/296432.

Hata, K., K. Ishikawa, K. Hori, and T. Konishi. 2000. "Differentiation-Inducing Activity of Lupeol, a Lupane-Type Triterpene from Chinese Dandelion Root (*Hokouei-Kon*), on a Mouse Melanoma Cell Line." *Biological and Pharmacology Bulletin* 23(8): 962–67.

Hauer, J., and F. A. Anderer. 1993. "Mechanism of Stimulation of Human Natural Killer Cytotoxicity by Arabinogalactan from *Larix occidentalis.*" *Cancer Immunology and Immunotherapy* 36(4): 237–44.

Havlik, Jaroslav, Raquel Gonzalez de la Huebra, Katerina Hejtmankova, et al. 2010. "Xanthine Oxidase Inhibitory Properties of Czech Medicinal Plants."*Journal of Ethnopharmacology* 132(2): 461–65.

Hazra, R., K. Ray, and D. Guha. 2007. "Inhibitory Role of *Acorus calamus* in Ferric Chloride-Induced Epileptogenesis in Rat." *Human and Experimental Toxicology* 26(12): 947–53.

He, K., L. Zeng, G. Shi, G.-X. Zhao, J. F. Kozlowski, and J. L. McLaughlin. 1997. "Bioactive Compounds from *Taiwania cryptomerioides.*" *Journal of Natural Products* 60: 38–40.

He, Y. Q., G. Y. Ma, J. N. Peng, Z. Y. Ma, and M. T. Hamann. 2012. "Liver X Receptor and Peroxisome Proliferator–Activated Receptor Agonist from *Cornus alternifolia.*" *Biochimica et Biophysica Acta* 1820(7): 1021–26.

Hearne, Samuel. 2010. *A Journey from Prince of Wales's Fort in Hudson's Bay, to the Northern Ocean in the years 1769, 1770, 1771, 1772.* Gale Ecco Publishers.

Hellson, John C. 1974. *Ethnobotany of the Blackfoot Indians.* No. 19. Ottawa, Canada: National Museums of Canada.

Hellum, B. H., A. Tosse, K. Hoybakk, M. Thomsen, J.Rohloff, and O. Georg Nilsen. 2010. "Potent In Vitro Inhibition of CYP3A4 and P-Glycoprotein by *Rhodiola rosea.*" *Planta Medica* 76(4): 331–38.

Heo, J. H., D. O. Kim, S. J. Choi, D. H. Shin, and C. Y. Lee. 2004. "Potent Inhibitory Effect of Flavonoids in *Scutellaria baicalensis* on Amyloid-beta protein–Induced Neurotoxicity." *Journal of Agricultural and Food Chemistry.* 52(13): 4128–32.

Heo, J. H., H. J. Lee, Y. S. Kim, et al. 2007. "Effects of Baicalin and Wogonin on Mucin Release from Cultured Airway Epithelial Cells." *Phytotherapy Research* 21(12): 1130–34.

Herbert, J., I. M. Goodyer, A. B. Grossman, et al. 2006. "Do Corticosteroids Damage the Brain?" *Journal of Neuroendocrinology* 18(6): 393–411.

Herrendorff, R., M. T. Faleschini, A. Stiefvater, et al. 2016. "Identification of Plant-Derived Alkaloids with Therapeutic Potential for Myotonic Dystrophy Type I." *Journal ofBiological Chemistry* 291(33). doi:10.1074/jbc.M115.710616.

Hertrampf, Anke, C. Grundemann, S. Jager, M. Laszczyk, T. Giesemann, and R. Huber. 2012. "In Vitro Cytotoxicity of Cyclodextrin-Bonded Birch Bark Extract." *Planta Medica* 78(9): 881–89.

Hevesi, T. B., B. Blazics, and A. Kery. 2009. "Polyphenol Composition and Antioxidant Capacity of *Epilobium* Species." *Journal of Pharmaceutical and Biomedical Analysis* 49(1): 26–31.

Hidaka, Saburo, Yoshizo Okamoto, Satoshi Uchiyama, Akira Nakatsuma, Ken Hashimoto, S. Tsuyoshi Ohnishi, and Masayoshi Yamaguchi. 2006. "Royal Jelly Prevents Osteoporosis in Rats: Beneficial Effects in Ovariectomy Model and in Bone Tissue Culture Model." *Evidence-Based Complementary and Alternative Medicine* 3(3): 339–48. doi:10.1093/ecam/nel019.

Hiermann, A., H. Juan, and W. Sametz. 1986. "Influence of *Epilobium* Extracts on Prostaglandin Biosynthesis and Carrageenin-Induced Oedema of the Rat Paw." *Journal of Ethnopharmacology* 17: 161–69.

Hikino, H., S. Funayama, and K. Endo. 1976. "Hypotensive Principle of *Astragalus* and *Hedysarum* Roots." *Planta Medica* 30(4): 297–302.

Hilarion. 1982. *Wildflowers, Their Occult Gifts.* Queensville, Canada:Marcus.

Hill, N., C. Stam, and R. A. van Haselen. 1996. "The Efficacy of Prrrikweg Gel in the Treatment of Insect Bites: A Double-Blind, Placebo-Controlled Clinical Trial." *Pharmacy World and Science* 18(1): 35–41.

Hinds, T. E., and R. W. Davidson. 1967. "A New Species of *Ceratocystis* on Aspen." *Mycologia* 59(6): 1102–6.

Holanda Pinto, S. A., L. M. Pinto, M. A. Guedes, et al. 2008. "Antinoceptive Effect of Triterpenoid alpha, beta-Amyrin in Rats on Orofacial Pain Induced by Formalin and Capsaicin." *Phytomedicine* 15(8): 630–34.

Holmes, Peter. 1997. *The Energetics of Western Herbs.* Volume 1. 3rd Edition. Boulder, CO: Snow Lotus.

Hu, Y., and H. Xie. 2016. ["Progress in Study on Effect of Harmine on Bone and Cartilage Metabolism"] *Zhong Nan Da Xue Xue Bao Yi Xue Ban* 41(3): 328–32.

Huang, F., X. Y. Tong, H. M. Deng, H. Nie, R. H. Zhang, and Y. Cai. 2009. "Primary Study on Mechanism of Baicalin on the Th1/Th2 Response in Murine Model of Asthma." *Journal of Chinese Medicinal Materials* 32(9): 1407–10.

Huang, S. T., C. Y. Wang, R. C. Yang, C. J. Chu, H. T. Wu, and J. H. Pang. 2010. "Wogonin, an Active Compound in *Scutellaria baicalensis*, Induces Apoptosis and Reduces Telomerase Activity in the HL-60 Leukemia Cells." *Phytomedicine* 17(1): 47–54.

Huang, Wen-Chung, and Chian-Jiun Liou. 2012. "Dietary Acacetin Reduces Airway Hyperresponsiveness and Eosinophil Infiltration by Modulating Eotaxin-1 and Th2 Cytokines in a Mouse Model of Asthma." *Evidence Based Complementary and Alternative Medicine* 2012. doi:10.1155/2012/910520.

Huang, Y., C. M. Wong, C. W. Lau, et al. 2004. "Inhibition of Nitric Oxide/Cyclic GMP–Mediated Relaxation by Purified Flavnoids, Baicalin, and Baicalein, in Rat Aortic Rings." *Biochemical Pharmacology* 67(4): 787–94.

Hui, K. M., X. H. Wang, and H. Xue. 2000. "Interaction of Flavones from the Roots of *Scutellaria baicalensis* with the Benzodiazepine Site." *Planta Medica* 66(1): 91–93. doi:10.1055/s-0029-1243121.

Huttunen, S., K. Riihinen, J. Kauhanen, and C. Tikkanen-Kaukanen. 2013. "Antimicrobial Activity of Different Finnish Monofloral Honeys against Human Pathogenic Bacteria." *APMIS* 121(9): 827–34.

Huyke, C., M. Laszczyk, A. Scheffler, R. Ernst, and C. M. Schempp. 2006. "Treatment of Actinic Keratoses with Birch Bark Extract: A Pilot Study." *Journal der Deutschen Dermatologischen Gesellschaft* 4(2): 132–36.

Ibrahim, A., M. A. Eldaim, and M. M. Abdel-Daim. 2016. "Nephroprotective Effect of Bee Honey and Royal Jelly against Subchronic Cisplatin Toxicity in Rats." *Cytotechnology* 68(4): 1039–48. doi:10.1007/s10616-015-9860-2.

Im, N. K., D. S. Lee, S. R. Lee, and G. S. Jeong. 2016. "Lupeol Isolated from *Sorbus commixta* Suppresses 1-alpha,25-(OH)2D3-Mediated Osteoclast Differentiation and Bone Loss In Vitro and In Vivo." *Journal of Natural Products* 79(2): 412–20.

Ingraham, Caroline. 2006. *The Animal Aromatics Workbook: Giving Animals the Choice to Select Their Own Natural Medicines.* Hay-on-Wye, UK: Caroline Ingraham.

Ishikawa, T., K. Nishigaya, K. Takami, H. Uchikoshi, I. S. Chen, and I. L. Tsai. 2004. "Isolation of Salicin Derivatives from *Homalium cochinchinensis* and Their Antiviral Activities." *Journal of Natural Products* 67(4): 659–63.

Jaenson, T. G., K. Palsson, and A. K. Borg-Karlson. 2005. "Evaluation of Extracts and Oils of Tick-Repellent Plants from Sweden." *Medical Veterinarian Entomology* 19: 345–52.

Jarboe, C. H., K. A. Zirvi, J. A. Nicholson, and C. M. Schmidt. 1967. "Scopoletin, an Antispasmodic Component of *Viburnum opulus* and *V. prunifolium.*" *Journal of Medicinal Chemistry* 10(3): 488–89.

Jarvis, D. C. 1960. *Arthritis and Folk Medicine.* New York: Holt, Rinehart & Winston.

Ji, S., R. Li, Q. Wang, et al. 2015. "Anti-H1N1 Virus, Cytotoxic and Nrf2 Activation Activities of Chemical Constituents from *Scutellaria baicalensis.*" *Journal of Ethnopharmacology* 176: 475–84.

Jiang, B., R. F. Shen, J. Bi, X. S. Tian, T. Hinchliffe, and Y. Xia. 2015. "Catalpol: A Potential Therapeutic for Neurodegenerative Diseases." *Current Medicinal Chemistry* 22(10): 1278–91.

Jiang, W. L., S. P. Zhang, H. B. Zhu, Jian-Hou, and J. W. Tian. 2010. "Cornin Ameliorates Cerebral Infarction in Rats by Antioxidant Action and Stabilization of Mitochondrial Function." *Phytotherapy Research* 24(4): 547–52. doi:10.1002/ptr.2978.

Jin, Changdong, Wendy Strembiski, Yuliya Kulchytska, Ronald G. Micetich, and Mohsen Daneshtalab. 1999. "Flavonoid Glycosides from *Ledum palustre* L. ssp. *decumbens* (Ait) Hulton." *DARU Journal of Pharmaceutical Sciences* 7(4): 5–8.

Johnson, Leslie Main. 1997. "Health, Wholeness and the Land: Gitksan Traditional Plant Use and Healing." PhD dissertation. Edmonton, Canada: University of Alberta.

Jones, N. P., J. T. Arnason, M. Abou-Zaid, K. Akpagana, P. Sanchez-Vindas, and M. L. Smith. 2000. "Antifungal Activity of Extracts from Medicinal Plants Used by First Nations Peoples of Eastern Canada." *Journal of Ethnopharmacology* 73: 191–98.

Kane, Charles W. 2009. *Herbal Medicine: Trends and Traditions.* Oracle, AZ: Lincoln Town.

Kang, Z., W. Jiang, H. Luan, F. Zhao, and S. Zhang. 2013. "Cornin Induces Angiogenesis through P13K-Akt-eNOS-VEGF Signaling Pathway." *Food and Chemical Toxicology* 58: 340–46.

Kangas, L., N. Saarinen, M. Mutanen, et al. 2002. "Antioxidant and Antitumor Effects of Hydroxymatairesinol (HM-3000, HMR), a Lignan Isolated from the Knots of Spruce." *European Journal of Cancer Prevention* 11 (suppl. 2): S48–57.

Kashan, Z. F., M. Arbabi, M. Delavari, H. Hooshyar, M. Taghizadeh, and Z. Joneydy. 2015. "Effect of *Verbascum thapsus* Ethanol Extract on Induction of Apoptosis in Trichomonas Vaginalis In Vitro." *Infectious Disorders—Drug Targets* 15(2): 125–30.

Keane, Kahlee. 2012. *The Standing People: Field Guide of Medicinal Plants for the Prairie Provinces.* Self-published.

Keinänen, M., and R. Julkunen-Titto. 1996. "Effects of Sample Preparation Method of Birch (*Betula pendula* Roth) Leaf Phenolics." *Journal of Agricultural and Food Chemistry* 44(9): 2724–27.

Keller, K., K. P. Odenthal, and E. Leng-Peschlow. 1985. "Spasmolytische Wirkung des isoasaronfreien Kalmus" [Spasmolytic Effect of Iso-asarone-Free *Calmus*] *Planta Medica* 51(1): 6–9.

Keller, K., and E. Stahl. 1983. "Composition of the Essential Oil from B-asarone Free *Calamus*." *Planta Medica* 47(2): 71–74.

Khaleghi, F., I. Jantan, L. B. Din, W. A. Yaacob, M. A. Khalilzadeh, and S. N. Bukhari. 2014. "Immunomodulatory Effects of 1-(6-Hydroxy-2-Isopropenyl-1-Benzofuran-5-yl)-1-Etha-none from *Petasites hybridus* and Its Synthesized Benzoxazepine." *Journal of Natural Medicine* 68(2): 351–57.

Kharkwal, G. C., C. Pande, G. Tewari, A. Panwar, and V. Pande. 2014. "Composition and Antimicrobial Activity of the Essential Oil of *Heracleum lanatum* Michx. from Uttarakhand Himalaya." *International Journal of Scientific & Technology Research* 3(12): 60–64.

Khoshpey, B., S. Djazayeri, F. Amiri, et al. 2016 "Effect of Royal Jelly Intake on Serum Glucose, Apolipoprotein A-I (ApoA-I), Apolipoprotein B (ApoB), and ApoB/ApoA-I Ratios in Patients with Type 2 Diabetes: A Randomized, Double-Blind Clinical Trial Study." *Canadian Journal of Diabetes* 40(4): 324–28. doi:10.1016/j.jcjd.2016.01.003.

Kim, C. D., J. D. Cha, S. Li, and I. H. Cha. 2015. "The Mechanism of Acacetin-Induced Apoptosis on Oral Squamous Cell Carcinoma." *Archives of Oral Biology* 60(9): 1283–98.

Kim, H., T. H. Han, and S. G. Lee. 2009. "Anti-Inflammatory Activity of a Water Extract of *Acorus calamus* L. Leaves on Keratinocyte HaCaT Cells." *Journal of Ethnopharmacology* 122(1): 149–56.

Kim, H. S., J. M. Lim, J. Y. Kim, Y. Kim, S. Park, and J. Sohn. 2016. "Panaxydol, a Component of Panax Ginseng, Induces Apoptosis in Cancer Cells through EGFR Activation and ER Stress and Inhibits Tumor Growth in Mouse Models." *International Journal of Cancer* 138(6): 1432–41.

Kim, L. S., R. F. Waters, and P. M. Burkholder. 2002. "Immunological Activity of Larch Arabinogalactan and *Echinacea*: A Preliminary, Randomized, Double-Bind, Placebo-Controlled Trial." *Alternative Medicine Review* 7(2): 138–49.

Kim, M. B., C. Kim, W. S. Chung, et al. 2015. "The Hydrolysed Products of Iridoid Glycosides Can Enhance Imatinib Mesylate-Induced Apoptosis in Human Myeloid Leukemia Cells." *Phytotherapy Research* 29(3): 434–43.doi:10.1002/ptr.5272.

Kim, M. H., S. Y. Ryu, M. A. Bae, J. S. Choi, Y. K. Min, and S. H. Kim. 2008. "Baicalein Inhibits Osteoclast Differentiation and Induces Mature Osteoclast Apoptosis." *Food and Chemistry Toxicology* 46(11): 3375–82.

Kim M. J, S. D. Park, A. R. Lee, K. H. Kim, J. H. Jang, and K. S. Kim. 2002. "The Effect of Bee Venom Acupuncture on Protease Activity and Free Radical Damage in Synovial Fluid from Collagen-Induced Arthritis in Rats. *Journal of Korean Society for Acupuncture and Moxibustion* 19:161–75.

Kim, J. Y., S. J. Yu, H. J. Oh, J. Y. Lee, Y. Kim, and J. Sohn. 2011. "Panaxydol Induces Apoptosis through an Increased Intracellular Calcium Level, Activation of JNK and P38 MAPK and NADPH Oxidase-Dependent Generation of Reactive Oxygen Species." *Apoptosis* 16(4): 347–58.

Kirouac, Marie-Victorin. 1935. *Flore laurentienne*. Montreal: Les Frères des Écoles Chrétiennes.

Kiss, A., J. Kowalski, and M. F. Melzig. 2006. "Effect of *Epilobium angustifolium* L. Extracts and Polyphenols on Cell Proliferation and Neutral Endopeptidase Activity in Selected Cell Lines." *Pharmazie* 61: 66–69.

Kiss, T., D. Cadar, and M. Spinu. 2012. "Tick Prevention at a Crossroad: New and Renewed Solutions." *Veterinary Parasitology* 187: 357–66.

Klippel, K. F., D. M. Hiltl, and B. Schipp. 1997. "A Multicentric, Placebo-Controlled, Double-Blind Clinical Trial of beta-Sitosterol (Phytosterol) for the Treatment of Benign Prostatic Hyperplasia. German BPH-Phyto Study Group." *British Journal of Urology* 80(3): 427–32.

Knudtson, Peter, and David T. Suzuki. 2006. *Wisdom of the Elders*. Vancouver: Greystone.

Kochanski, Mors L. 1987. *Northern Bushcraft*. Edmonton, Canada:Lone Pine.

Korkina, L. G., E. Mikhal'chik, M. V. Suprun, S. Pastore, and R. Dal Toso. 2007. "Molecular Mechanisms Underlying Wound Healing and Anti-Inflammatory Properties of Naturally Occurring Biotechnologically Produced Phenylpropanoid Glycosides." *Cellular and Molecular Biology* (France) 53(5): 84–91.

Kostyuk, V., A. Potapovich, T. Suhan, et al. 2008. "Plant Polyphenols against UV-C-Induced Cellular Death." *Planta Medica* 74(5): 509–14.

Krakauer, J., Y. Long, A. Kolbert, S. Thanedar, and J. Southard. 2015. "Presence of L-Canavanine in *Hedysarum alpinum* Seeds and Its Potential Role in the Death of Chris Mccandless." *Wilderness Environmental Medicine* 26(1): 36–42.

Krakauer, Jon. 1997. *Into the Wild*. New York: Anchor.

Kranich, Ernst Michael. 1984. *Planetary Influences upon Plants*. Wyoming, RI: Bio-Dynamic Literature.

Kucinskaite, A., L. Pobłocka-Olech, M. Krauze-Baranowska, M. Sznitowska, A. Savickas, and V. Briedis. 2007. "Evaluation of Biologically Active Compounds in Roots and Rhizomes of *Rhodiola rosea* L. Cultivated in Lithuania." *Medicina* (Lithuania) 43(6): 487–94.

Kuhnlein, H. V., and N. J. Turner. 1987. "Cow-Parsnip (*Heracleum lanatum*), an Indigenous Vegetable of Native People of Northwestern North America." *Journal of Ethnobotany* 6(2): 309–24.

Kuroda, M., K. Iwabuchi, and Y. Mimaki. 2012. "Chemical Constituents of the Aerial Parts of *Scutellaria lateriflora* and Their alpha-Glucosidase Inhibitory Activities." *Natural Products Communication* 7(4): 417–14.

Laidlaw, M., C. A. Cockerline, and D. W. Sepkovic. 2010. "Effects of a Breast-Health Formula Supplement on Estrogen Metabolism in Pre- and Post-Menopausal Women Not Taking Hormonal Contraceptives or Supplements: A Randomized Controlled Trial." *Breast Cancer: Basic and Clinical Research* 4: 85–89.

Lake, Tela Star Hawk. 1988. *Hawk Woman Dancing with the Moon: Sacred Medicine for Today's Woman*. New York: M. Evans.

Lal Shyaula, S., G. Abbas, H. Siddiqui, S. A. Sattar, M. I. Choudhary, and F. Z. Basha. 2012. "Synthesis and Antiglycation Activity of Kaempferol-3-O-Rutinoside (Nicotiflorin)." *Medicinal Chemistry* 8(3): 415–20.

LeClaire, Nancy, and George Cardinal. 1998. *Alberta Elders' Cree Dictionary*. Edited by Earle Waugh. Edmonton, Canada: University of Alberta Press.

Lee, B., J. B. Weon, M. R. Eom, Y. S. Jung, and C. J. Ma. 2015. "Neuroprotective Compounds of *Tilia amurensis*." *Pharmacognosy Magazine* 11(suppl. 2): S303–7.

Lee, C. J., J. H. Seok, G. M. Hur, et al. 2004. "Effects of Ursolic Acid, Betulin, and Sulfur-Containing Compounds on Mucin Release from Airway Goblet Cells." *Planta Medica* 70(12): 1119–22.

Lee, D. K., K. Haggart, F. M. Robb, and B. J. Lipworth. 2004. "Butterbur, a Herbal Remedy, Confers Complementary Anti-Inflammatory Activity in Asthmatic Patients Receiving Inhaled Corticosteroids." *Clinical and Experimental Allergy* 34: 110–14.

Lee, E., R. Emonoto, C. Koshiba, and H. Hirano. 2009. "Inhibition of P-Glycoprotein by Wogonin Is Involved with the Potentiation of Etoposide-Induced Apoptosis in Cancer Cells." *Annals of the New York Academy of Sciences* 1171: 132–36.

Lee, M., J. H. Park, D. S. Min, et al. 2012. "Antifibrotic Activity of Diarylheptanoids from *Betula platyphylla* towards HSC-T6 Cells." *Bioscience Biotechnology Biochemistry* 76(9): 1616–20.

Legault, J., K. Girard-Lalancette, D. Dufour, and A. Pichette. 2013. "Antioxidant Potential of Bark Extracts from Boreal Forest Conifers." *Antioxidants* (Switzerland) 2(3): 77–89.

Lesuisse, Dominique, J. Berjonneau, C. Clot, et al. 1996. "Determination of Oenothein B as the Active-5-alpha-Reductase–Inhibiting Principle of the Folk Medicine *Epilobium parviflorum.*" *Journal of Natural Products* 59: 490–92.

Levin, E. D., S. T. Alaudinov, and V. E. Cherepanova. 1983. "Identification of Prostaglandins E (series 1 and 2) Isolated from the Living Tissues of *Larixsibirica* and *Populus balsamifera.*" *Khimiya Prirodnykh Soedinenii* 5: 567–71.

Li, H., B. Doucet, A. J. Flewelling, et al. 2015. "Antimycobacterial Natural Products from Endophytes of the Medicinal Plant *Aralia nudicaulis.*" *Natural Product Communication* 10(10): 1641–42.

Li, H., T. O'Neill, K. Ellsworth, D. Webster, J. A. Johnson, and C. A. Gray. 2012. "Anti-Mycobacterial Natural Products from *Aralia nudicaulis.*" *Planta Medica* 78(PF37 Abstract).

Li, J., and S. X. Wang. 2016. "Synergistic Enhancement of the Antitumor Activity of 5-Fluorouracil by Bornyl Acetate in SGC-7901 Human Gastric Cancer Cells and the Determination of the Underlying Mechanism of Action." *Journal of the Balkan Union of Oncology* 21(1): 108–17.

Li, J. M., X. Zhang, X. Wang, Y. C. Xie, and L. D. Kong. 2011. "Protective Effects of *Cortex fraxini* Coumarines against Oxonate-Induced Hyperuricemia and Renal Dysfunction in Mice." *European Journal of Pharmacology* 666(1–3): 196–204.

Li, Ji, Yun Zheng, Hong Zhou, Bao-Ning Su, and Rong-Dang Zheng. 1997. "Differentiation of Human Gastric Adenocarcinoma Cell Line Mgc80-3 Induced by Verbascoside." *Planta Medica* 63(6): 499–502.

Li, Peng, Wei-Xi Tian, Xiao-Yan Wang, and Xiao-Feng Ma. 2014. "Inhibitory Effect of Desoxyrhaponticin and Rhaponticin, Two Natural Stilbene Glycosides from the Tibetan Nutritional Food *Rheum tanguticum* Maxim. ex Balf. on Fatty Acid Synthase and Human Breast Cancer Cells." *Food and Function* 5(2): 251–56.

Li, Shilin, Antoine Brault, Mayra Sanchez Villavicencio, and Pierre S. Haddad. 2016. "*Rhododendron groenlandicum* (Labrador Tea), an Antidiabetic Plant from the Traditional Pharmacopoeia of the Canadian Eastern James Bay Cree, Improves Renal Integrity in the Diet-Induced Obese Mouse Model." *Pharmaceutical Biology* 54(10):1998–2006. doi:10.3109/13880209.2015.1137953.

Li, X., K. Cui, X. Sun, X. Li, Q. Zhu, and W. Li. 2010. "Mangiferin Prevents Diabetic Nephropathy in Streptozotocin-Induced Diabetic Rats." *Phytotherapy Research* 24(6): 893–99.

Li, Xia, Zhi-Meng Xu, Zhen-Zhou Jiang, et al. 2014. "Hypoglycemic Effect of Catalpol on High-Fat/Streptozotocin-Induced Diabetic Mice by Increasing Skeletal Muscle Mitochondrial Biogenesis." *Acta Biochimica et Biophysica Sinica* (Shanghai) 46(9): 738–48.

Liang, J. Q., L. Wang, J. C. He, and X. D. Hua. 2016. "Verbascoside Promotes the Regeneration of Tyrosine Hydroxylase–Immunoreactive Neurons in the Substantia Nigra." *Neural Regeneration Research* 11(1): 101–6.

Liao, F., R. L. Zheng, J. J. Gao, and Z. J. Jia. 1999. "Retardation of Skeletal Muscle Fatigue by the Two Phenylpropanoid Glycosides: Verbascoside and Martynoside from *Pedicularis plicata* Maxim." *Phytotherapy Research* 13(7): 621–23.

Lim, S. M., J. J. Jeong, H. S. Choi, H. B. Chang, and D. H. Kim. 2016. "Mangiferin Corrects the Imbalance of Th17/Treg Cells in Mice with TNBS Colitis." *International Immunopharmacology* 34: 220–28.

Lim, Sung Min, Junghee Yoo, Euiju Lee, et al. 2015. "Acupuncture for Spasticity after Stroke: A Systematic Review and Meta-Analysis of Randomized Controlled Trials." *Evidence-Based Complementary and Alternative Medicine* 2015: 870398. doi:10.1155/2015/870398.

Lin, Y.-M., M. T. Flavin, R. Schure, et al. 1999. "Antiviral Activities of Bioflavonoids." *Planta Medica* 65(2): 120–25.

Lindberg, T., O. Anderson, M. Palm, and C. Fagerström. 2015. "A Systematic Review and Meta-Analysis of Dressings Used for Wound Healing: The Efficiency of Honey Compared to Silver on Burns." *Contemporary Nurse* 51(2–3): 121–34.doi:10.1080/10376178.2016.11 71727.

Lipton, R. B., H. Göbel, K. M. Einhäupi, K.Wilks, and A. Mauskop. 2004. "*Petasites hybridus* Root (Butterbur) Is an Effective Preventive Treatment for Migraine." *Neurology* 63(12): 2240–44.

Lirdprapamongkol, Kriengsak, Jan-Peter Kramb, Tuangporn Suthiphongchai, et al. 2009. "Vanillin Suppresses Metastatic Potential of Human Cancer Cells through P13K Inhibition and Decreases Angiogenesis In Vivo." *Journal of Agricultural and Food Chemistry* 57(8): 3055–63. doi:10.1021/jf803366f.

Liu, Iain X., David G. Durham, and R. Michael Richards. 2000. "Baicalin Synergy with beta-Lactam Antibiotics against Methicillin-Resistant *Staphylococcus aureus* and Other beta-Lactam-Resistant Strains of *S. aureus.*" *Journal of Pharmacy and Pharmacology* 52: 361–66. doi:10.1211/0022357001773922.

Liu, J., Y. Cheng, X. Zhang, et al. 2015. "Astragalin Attenuates Allergic Inflammation in a Murine Asthma Model." *Inflammation* 38(5): 2007–16.

Liu, Je-Ruei, Yuan-Chang Yang, Li-Shian Shi, and Chi-Chung Peng. 2008. "Antioxidant Properties of Royal Jelly Associated with Larval Age and Time of Harvest." *Journal of Agricultural and Food Chemistry* 56(23): 11447–52. doi:10.1021/jf802494e.

Liu, K., F. Mei, Y. Wang, et al. 2016. "Quercetin Oppositely Regulates Insulin-Mediated Glucose Disposal in Skeletal Muscle under Normal and Inflammatory Conditions: The Dual Roles of AMPK Activation." *Molecular Nutrition and Food Research* 60(3): 551–65.

Liu, Ko-Yu, Yang-Chang Wu, I. Min Liu, Wen-Chen Yu, and Juei-Tang Cheng. 2008. "Release of Acetylcholine by Syringin, an Active Principle of *Eleutherococcus senticosis*, to Raise Insulin Secretion in Wistar Rats." *Neuroscience Letters* 434(2): 195–99. doi:10.1016/j. neulet.2008.01.054.

Liu, X., and J. Wang. 2011. "Anti-Inflammatory Effects of Irdoid Glycosides Fraction of *Folium syringae* Leaves on TNBS-Induced Colitis in Rats." *Journal of Ethnopharmacology* 133(2): 780–87.

Loers, G., D. V. Yashunsky, N. E. Nifantiev, and M. Schachner. 2014. "Neural Cell Activation by Phenolic Compounds from the Siberian Larch *(Larix sibirica)."Journal of Natural Products* 77(7): 1554–61.

Lubke, L. L., and C. F. Garon. 1997. "Bee Stings as Lyme Inhibitor." *Journal of Clinical Infectious Diseases* 25(suppl. 1): 48–51.

Maggi, F., L. Quassinti, M. Bramucci, et al. 2014. "Composition and Biological Activities of Hogweed (*Heracleum sphondylium* L. ssp. *ternatum* [Velen.] Brummitt) Essential Oil and Its Main Components Octyl Acetate and Octyl Butyrate." *Natural Products Research* 28(17): 1354–63.

Majewska, A., G. Hoser, M. Furmanowa, and N. Ubran'ska. 2005. "Antiproliferative and Antimiotic Effect, S Phase Accumulation, and Induction of Apoptosis and Necrosis after Treatment of Extract from *Rhodiola rosea* Rhizomes on HL-60 Cells." *Journal of Ethnopharmacology* 103: 43–52.

Makino, T., A. Hishida, Y. Goda, and H. Mizukami. 2008. "Comparison of the Major Flavonoid Content of *S. baicalensis, S. lateriflora*, and Their Commercial Products." *Journal of Natural Medicine* 62(3): 294–99.

Manayi, Azadeh, Soodabeh Saeidnia, Seyed Nasser Ostad, et al. 2013. "Chemical Constituents and Cytotoxic Effect of the Main Compounds in *Lythrum salicaria* L." *Zeitschrift für Naturforschung* C 68(9–10): 367–75.

Mannila, E., and A. Talvitie. 1992. "Stilbenes from *Picea abies* Bark." *Phytochemistry* 31(9): 3288–89.

Mao, Jun J., Sharon X. Xie, Jarcy Zee, et al. 2015. "*Rhodiola rosea* versus Sertraline for Major Depressive Disorder: A Randomized Placebo-Controlled Trial." *Phytomedicine* 22(3): 394–99.

Martin, R., M. Hernandez, C. Cordova, and M. L. Nieto. 2012. "Natural Triterpenes Modulate Immune-Inflammatory Markets of Experimental Autoimmune Encephalomyelitis: Therapeutic Implications for Multiple Sclerosis." *British Journal of Pharmacology* 166(5): 1708–23.

Martineau, L. C., D. C. A. Adeyiwola-Spoor, D. Vallerand, A. Afshar, J. T. Arnason, and P. S. Haddad. 2010. "Enhancement of Muscle Cell Glucose Uptake by Medicinal Plant Species of Canada's Native Populations Is Mediated by a Common, Metformin-Like Mechanism." *Journal of Ethnopharmacology* 127(2): 396–406.

Marumoto, S., and M. Miyazawa. 2010. "Beta-Secretase Inhibitory Effects of Furanocoumarins from the Root of *Angelica dahurica*." *Phytotherapy Research* 24(4): 510–13.

Matkowski, A., P. Kus, E. Góralska, and D. Wozniak. 2013. "Mangiferin—A Bioactive Xanthonoid, Not Only from Mango and Not Just Antioxidant." *Mini Reviews in Medicinal Chemistry* 13(3): 439–55.

Matsuda, H., N. Hirata, Y. Kawaguchi, et al. 2005. "Melanogenesis Stimulation in Murine b16 Melanoma Cells by Umberiferae (sic) Plant Extracts and Their Coumarin Constituents." *Biological and Pharmacology Bulletin* 28(7): 1229–33.

Mattioli, L., and M. Perfumi. 2011. "Effects of a *Rhodiola rosea* L. Extract on Acquisition and Expression of Morphine Tolerance and Dependence in Mice." *Journal of Psychopharmacology* 25(3): 411–20.

Mazzio, E. A., and K. F. Soliman. 2009. "In Vitro Screening for the Tumoricidal Properties of International Medicinal Herbs." *Phytotherapy Research* 23(3): 385–98.

McCabe, Vinton. 2007. *The Healing Bouquet: Exploring Bach Flower Remedies.* Laguna Beach, CA: Basic Health.

McCann, M. J., C. I. Gill, T. Linton, D. Berrar, H. McGlynn, and I. R. Rowland. 2008. "Enterolactone Restricts the Proliferation of the LNCaP Human Prostate Cancer Cell Line In Vitro." *Molecular Nutrition Food Research* 52(5): 567–80.

McCune, L. M., and T. Johns. 2002. "Antioxidant Activity in Medicinal Plants Associated with the Symptoms of Diabetes Mellitus Used by the Indigenous Peoples of the North American Boreal Forest." *Journal of Ethnopharmacology* 82(2–3): 197–205.

McCutcheon, Allison R., S. M. Ellis, R. E. W. Hancock, and G. H. N. Towers. 1992. "Antibiotic Screening of Medicinal Plants of the British Columbia Native Peoples." *Journal of Ethnopharmacology* 37(3): 213–23.

———. 1994. "Antifungal Screening of Medicinal Plants of British Columbian Native Peoples." *Journal of Ethnopharmacology* 44(3): 157–69.

McCutcheon, Allison R., T. E. Roberts, E. Gibbons, et al. 1995. "Antiviral Screening of British Columbia Medicinal Plants." *Journal of Ethnopharmacology* 49: 101–10.

McDonald, Jim. 2016. "Sweet Flag/Bitterroot." Jim McDonald, Herbalist. Accessed November 2016. www.herbcraft.org/calamus.html.

McFarland, Phoenix. 2003. *The New Book of Magical Names.* Woodbury, MN: Llewellyn Worldwide.

McGaa, Ed. 2004. *Nature's Way: Native Wisdom for Living in Balance with the Earth.* New York: Harper Collins.

McIlwraith, Thomas F. 1948. *The Bella Coola Indians.* Volume 1. Toronto: University of Toronto Press.

Meili, Dianne. 1991. *Those Who Know: Profiles of Alberta's Native Elders.* Edmonton, Canada: NeWest Press.

Mesaik, M. A., M. K. Azim, and S. Mohiuddin. 2008. "Honey Modulates Oxidative Burst of Professional Phagocytes." *Phytotherapy Research* 22(10): 404–10.

Meyer-Rochow, V. B., and O. Vakkuri. 2002. "Honeybee Heads Weight Less in Winter than in Summer: A Possible Explanation." *Ethology, Ecology and Evolution* 14: 69–71.

Miao, M., L. Guo, X. Yan, T. Wang, and Z. Li. 2016. "Effects of Verbenalin on Prostatitis Mouse Model." *Saudi Journal of Biological Science* 23(1): 148–57.

Miladinovic, D. L., B. S. Ilic, T. M. Mihajilov-Krstev, et al. 2013. "Antibacterial Activity of the Essential Oil of *Heracleum sibiricum.*" *Natural Products Communication* 8(9): 1309–11.

Millspaugh, Charles Frederick. 1887. *American Medicinal Plants: An Illustrated and Descriptive Guide to the American Plants Used as Homeopathic Remedies: Their History, Preparation, Chemistry, and Physiological Effects.* New York: Boericke and Tafel.

Milne, Courtney. 1998. *Visions of the Goddess.* Toronto: Penguin Studio.

Min, B. S., K. H. Bae, Y. H. Kim, H. Myashiro, M. Hattori, and K. Shimotohno. 1999. "Screening of Korean Plants against Human Immunodeficiency Virus Type 1 Protease." *Phytotherapy Research* 13(8): 680–82.

Ming, D. S., B. J. Hillhouse, E. S. Guns, et al. 2005. "Bioactive Compounds from *Rhodiola rosea* (Crassulaceae)." *Phytotherapy Research* 19(9): 740–43.

Mishima, S., K. M. Suzuki, Y. Isohama, et al. 2005. "Royal Jelly Has Estrogenic Effects In Vitro and In Vivo." *Journal of Ethnopharmacology* 101(1–3): 215–20. doi:10.1016/j.jep.2005.04.012.

Mitsunaga, Tohru, Isao Abe, Masanori Kontani, Hiroyuki Ono, and Takaharu Tanaka. 1997. "Inhibitory Effects of Bark Proanthocyanidins on the Activities of Glucosyltransferases of *Streptococcus sobrinus*." *Journal of Wood Chemistry and Technology* 17(3): 327–40.

Miura, T., H. Ichiki, I. Hashimoto, et al. 2001. "Antidiabetic Activity of a Xanthone Compound, Mangiferin." *Phytomedicine* 8(2): 85–87.

Mohammed, G. 2002. *Catnip & Kerosene Grass*. Sault Ste. Marie, Canada: Candlenut.

Molan, P. C. 2006. "The Evidence Supporting the Use of Honey as a Wound Dressing." *International Journal of Lower Extremity Wounds* 5(2): 122.

Molina, V., R. Mas, and D. Carbajal. 2015. "D-002 (Beeswax Alcohols): Concurrent Joint Health Benefits and Gastroprotection." *Indian Journal of Pharmaceutical Sciences* 77(2): 127–34.

Montgomery, Pam. 2008. *Plant Spirit Healing*. Rochester VT: Bear & Co.

Montó, F., C. Arce, M. A. Noguera, et al. 2014. "Action of an Extract from the Seeds of *Fraxinus excelsior* L. on Metabolic Disorders in Hypertensive and Obese Animal Models." *Food and Function* 5(4): 786–96.

Moore, Michael. 1993. *Medicinal Plants of the Pacific West*. Santa Fe, NM: Red Crane.

———. 2003. *Medicinal Plants of the Mountain West*. Revised and Expanded Edition. Santa Fe, NM: Museum of New Mexico Press.

Morrissey, Jenifer. 2000. "Awed by Cottonwoods." Excerpts from *Cottonwoods: Pondering Our Dominant Riparian Trees* 11(1). www.coloradoriparian.org/awed-by-cottonwoods.

Morteza-Semnani, K., M. Saeedi, and M. Akbarzadeh. 2012. "Chemical Composition and Antimicrobial Activity of the Essential Oil of *Verbascum thapsus* L." *Journal of Essential Oil Bearing Plants* 15(3): 373–79.

Moskalenko, S. A. 1987. "Slavic Ethnomedicine in the Soviet Far East. Part 1: Herbal Remedies among Russians/Ukrainians in the Sukhodol Valley, Primorye." *Journal of Ethnopharmacology* 21(3): 231–51.

Mshvidadze, V., J. Legault, S. Lavoie, C. Gauthier, and A. Pichette. 2007. "Anticancer Diarylheptanoid Glycosides from the Inner Bark of *Betula papyrifera*." *Phytochemistry* 68(20): 2531–36.

Mu, X., G. He, Y. Cheng, X. Li, B. Xu, and G. Du. 2009. "Baicalein Exerts Neuroprotective Effects in 6-Hydroxydopamine-Induced Experimental Parkinsonism In Vivo and In Vitro." *Pharmacology Biochemistry and Behavior* 92(4): 642–48.

Muceniece, R., K. Saleniece, J. Rumaks, et al. 2008. "Betulin Binds to gamma-Aminobutyric Acid Receptors and Exerts Anticonvulsant Action in Mice." *Pharmacology, Biochemistry, and Behavior* 90(4): 712–16.

Mucz, M. 2012. *Baba's Kitchen Medicines*. Edmonton, Canada: University of Alberta Press.

Mueller, D., S. Tribel, O. Rudakovski, and E. Richling. 2013. "Influence of Triterpenoids Present in Apple Peel on Inflammatory Gene Expression Associated with Inflammatory Bowel Disease (IBD)." *Food Chemistry* 139(1–4): 339–46.

Münstedt, Karsten, Benjamin Voss, Uwe Kullmer, Ursula Schneider, and Jutta Hübner. 2015. "Bee Pollen and Honey for the Alleviation of Hot Flushes and Other Menopausal Symptoms in Breast Cancer Patients." *Molecular and Clinical Oncology* 3(4): 869–74. doi:10.3892/mco.2015.559.

Muruganandan, S., K. Srinivasan, S. Gupta, P. K. Gupta, and J. Lai. 2005. "Effect of Mangiferin on Hyperglycemia and Atherogenicity in Streptozotocin Diabetic Rats." *Journal of Ethnopharmacology* 97(3): 497–501.

Muthu, R., N. Selvaraj, and M. Vaiyapuri. 2015. "Anti-Inflammatory and Proapoptotic Effects of Umbelliferone in Colon Carcinogenesis." *Human and Experimental Toxicology* 35(10):1041–54. doi:10.1177/0960327115618245.

Na, Li Xin, Qiao Zhang, Shuo Jiang, et al. 2015. "Mangiferin Supplementation Improves Serum Lipid Profiles in Overweight Patients with Hyperlipidemia: A Double-Blind Randomized Controlled Trial." *Scientific Reports* 5:10344. doi:10.1038/srep10344.

Nagai, T., T. Nagashima, N. Suzuki, and R. Inoue. 2005. "Antioxidant Activity and Angiotensin I-Converting Enzyme Inhibition by Enzymatic Hydrolysates from Bee Bread." *Zeitschrift für Naturforschung* C 60: 133–38.

Nagai, T., H. Yamanda, and Y. Otsuka. 1989. "Inhibition of Mouse Liver Sialidase by the Root of *Scutellaria baicalensis*." *Planta Medica* 55(1): 27–29.

Nagyvary, Joseph, Renald N. Guillemette, and Clifford H. Spiegelman. 1984. "Mineral Preservatives in the Wood of Stradivari and Guarneri." *Journals of the Violin Society of America* 7(2): 89–110.

Narimanov, A. A., S. N. Myakisheva, and Kuznetsova. 1991. "Radioprotective Effect of *Archangelica officinalis* Hoffm. and *Ledum palustre* L. Extracts on Mice." *Radiobiologiya* 31(3): 391–93.

Nasir, N. F., T. P. Kannan, S. A. Sulaiman, S. Shamsuddin, A. Azlina, and S. Stangaciu. 2015. "The Relationship between Telomere Length and Beekeeping among Malaysians." *Journal of the American Aging Association* 37(3): 9797. doi:10.1007/s11357-015-9797-6.

Neacsu, M., V. Micol, L. Perez-Fons, S. Wilfor, R. Holmbom, and R. Mallavia. 2007. "A Novel Antioxidant Phenyl Disaccharide from *Populus tremula* Knot Wood." *Molecules* 12(2): 205–17.

Newcombe, C. F. 1897. Unpublished Notes on Haida Plants. New York: Department of Anthropology, American Museum of Natural History.

Niaz, A., W. A. S. Syed, I. Shah, et al. 2012. "Anthelmintic and Relaxant Activities of *Verbascum thapsus* Mullein." *BMC Complementary and Alternative Medicine* 12(29).

Nicholson, J. A., T. D. Darby, and C. H. Jarboe. 1972. "Viopudial, a Hypotensive and Smooth Muscle Antispasmodic from *Viburnum opulus*." *Proceedings for the Society for Experimental Biology and Medicine* 140(2): 457–61.

Nie, B. M., X. Y. Jiang, J. X. Cai, et al. 2008. "Panaxydol and Panaxynol Protect Cultured Cortical Neurons against A-beta$_{(25-35)}$-Induced Toxicity." *Neuropharmacology* 54(5): 845–53.

Niu, H. S., F. L. Hsu, and I. M. Liu. 2008. "Role of Sympathetic Tone in the Loss of Syringin-Induced Plasma Glucose Lowering Action in Conscious Wistar Rats." *Neuroscience Letters* 445(1): 113–16.

Norman, Howard. 1990. *Northern Tales*. New York: Pantheon.

Nowak, R., and T. Krzaczek. 1998. "Pharmacological Research Involving Herbs of *Epilobium angustifolium* L. and *Epilobium parvifolium* Schreb." *Herba Polonica* 1: 5–10.

Oelkers-Ax, R., A. Leins, P. Parzer, et al. 2008. "Butterbur Root Extract and Music Therapy in the Prevention of Childhood Migraine: An Explorative Study." *European Journal of Pain* 12(3): 301–13.

Oh, S. B., C. J. Hwang, S. Y. Song, et al. 2014. "Anticancer Effect of Tectochrysin N NSCLC Cells through Overexpression of Death Receptor and Inactivation of STAT3." *Cancer Letters* 353(1): 95–103.

Ohtsuka, Y., N. Yabunaka, and S. Takayama. 1998. "*Shinrin-Yoku* (Forest-Air Bathing and Walking) Effectively Decreases Blood Glucose Levels in Diabetic Patients." *International Journal of Biometeorology* 41(3): 125–27.

Olsson, E. M., B. Von Scheele, and A. G. Panossian. 2009. "A Randomized, Double-Blind, Placebo-Controlled, Parallel-Group Study of the Standardized Extract Shr-5 of the Roots of *Rhodiola rosea* in the Treatment of Subjects with Stress-Related Fatigue." *Planta Medica* 75(2): 105–12.

O'Neill, T., J. A. Johnson, D. Webster, and C. A. Gray. 2013. "The Canadian Medicinal Plant *Heracleum maximum* Contains Antimycobacterial Diynes and Furanocoumarins." *Journal of Ethnopharmacology* 147(1): 232–37.

Orhan, I., F. Tosun, and B. Sener. 2008. "Coumarin, Anthroquinone and Stilbene Derivatives with Anticholinesterae Activity." *Verlage der Zeitschrift für Naturforschung* C63: 366–70.

Ovodova, R. G., V. V. Goiovchenko, S. V. Popov, A. S. Shashkov, and I. S. Ovodov. 2000. "The Isolation, Preliminary Study of Structure and Physiological Activity of Water-Soluble Polysaccharides from Squeezed Berries of Snowball Tree *Viburnum opulus*." *The Russian Journal of Bioorganic Chemistry* 26(1): 61–7.

Owen, P., and T. Johns. 1999. "Xanthine Oxidase Inhibitory Activity of Northeastern North American Plant Remedies Used for Gout." *Journal of Ethnopharmacology* 64(2): 149–60.

Pajovic, B., N. Radojevic, A. Dimitrovski, S. Tomovic, and M. Vukovic. 2016. "The Therapeutic Potential of Royal Jelly in Benign Prostatic Hyperplasia. Comparison with Contemporary Literature." *Aging Male* (April 5): 1–5. doi:10.3109/13685538.2016.1169400.

Paladini, A. C., M. Marder, H. Viola, C. Wolfman, C. Wasowski, and J. H. Medina. 1999. "Flavonoids and the Central Nervous System: From Forgotten Factors to Potent Anxiolytic Compounds." *Journal of Pharmacy and Pharmacology* 51(5): 519–26.

Pallasdowney, Rhonda. 2002. *The Complete Book of Flower Essences*. Novato, CA: New World Library.

Paola, R. D., G. Oteri, E. Mazzon, et al. 2011. "Effects of Verbascoside, Biotechnically Purified by *Syringa vulgaris* Plant Cell Cultures, in a Rodent Model of Periodontitis." *Journal of Pharmacy and Pharmacology* 63(5): 707–17.

Paper, Jordan D. 2007. *Native North American Religious Traditions: Dancing for Life*. Westport, CT: Praeger.

Parajuli, P., N. Joshee, A. M. Rimando, S. Mittal, and A. K. Yadav. 2009. "In Vitro Antitumor Mechanisms of Various *Scutellaria* Extracts and Constituent Flavonoids." *Planta Medica* 75(1): 41–48.

Parasi, A., E. Tranchita, G. Duranti, et al. 2010. "Effects of Chronic *Rhodiola rosea* Supplementation on Sport Performance and Antioxidant Capacity in Trained Male: Preliminary Results." *Journal of Sports Medicine and Physical Fitness* 50(1): 57–63.

Park, M. H., J. E. Hong, E. S. Park, et al. 2015. "Anticancer Effect of Tectochrysin in Colon Cancer Cell via Suppression of NF-kappa-B Activity and Enhancement of Death Receptor Expression." *Molecular Cancer* 14(124).

Park, S. Y., C. W. Nho, D. Y. Kwon, Y. H. Kang, K. W. Lee, and J. H. Park. 2013. "Maslinic Acid Inhibits the Metastatic Capacity of DU145 Human Prostate Cancer Cells: Possible Mediation via Hypoxia-Inducible Factor-1-alpha Signaling." *British Journal of Nutrition* 109(2): 210–22.

Patel, S. 2016. "Emerging Adjuvant Therapy for Cancer: Propolis and Its Constituents." *Journal of Dietary Supplements* 13(3): 245–68. doi:10.3109/19390211.2015.1008614.

Patil, K. K., R. J. Meshram, N. A. Dhole, and R. N. Gacche. 2016. Role of Dietary Flavonoids in Amelioration of Sugar Induced Cataractogenesis. *Archives of Biochemistry and Biophysics* 593: 1–11.

Patov, S. A., V. V. Punegov, and A. V. Kuchin. 2006. "Synthesis of the *Rhodiola rosea* Glycoside Rosavin." *Chemistry of Natural Compounds* 42(4): 397–99.

Pennacchio, A. M. E., Y. M. Syah, and E. Ghisalberti. 1996. "The Effect of Verbascoside on Cyclic 3′,5′-Adenosine Monophosphate Levels in Isolated Rat Heart." *European Journal of Pharmacology* 305: 169–71.

Peredery, O., and M. A. Persinger. 2004. "Herbal Treatment Following Post-Seizure Induction in Rat by Lithium Pilocarpie: *Scutellaria lateriflora* (Scullcap), *Gelsemium sempervirens* (Gelsemium), and *Datura stramonium* (Jimson Weed) May Prevent Development of Spontaneous Seizures." *Phytotherapy Research* 18(9): 700–5.

Peters, Josephine Grant, and Beverly Ortiz. 2010. *After the First Full Moon in April: A Sourcebook of Herbal Medicine from a California Indian Elder.* New York: Routledge.

Pichette, A., S. Lavoie, P. Morin, V. Mshvildadze, M. Lebrun, and J. Legault. 2006. "New Labdane Diterpenes from the Stem Bark of *Larix laricina*." *Chemical and Pharmaceutical Bulletin* (Tokyo) 54(10): 1429–32.

Pietinen, P., K. Stumpf, S. Männistö, V. Kataja, M. Uusitupa, and H. Adiercreutz. 2001. "Serum Enterolactone and Risk of Breast Cancer: A Case-Control Study in Eastern Finland." *Cancer Epidemiology Biomarkers and Prevention* 10(4): 339–44.

Pisha, E., H. Chai, I. S. Lee, et al. 1995. "Discovery of Betulinic Acid as a Selective Inhibitor of Human Melanoma that Functions by Induction of Apoptosis." *Natural Medicine* 1(10): 1046–51.

Plescia, J., W. Salz, F. Xia, et al. 2005. "Rational Design of Shepherdin, a Novel Anticancer Agent." *Cancer Cell* 7(5): 457–68.

Poaty, B., J. Lahlah, F. Porqueres, and H. Bouafif. 2015. "Composition, Antimicrobial and Antioxidant Activities of Seven Essential Oils from the North American Boreal Forest." *World Journal of Microbiology and Biotechnology* 31(6): 907–19.

Prabhu, S., S. Narayan, and C. S. Devi. 2009. "Mechanism of Protective Action on Mangiferin on Suppression of Inflammatory Response and Lysosomal Instability in Rat Model of Myocardial Infarction." *Phytotherapy Research* 23(6): 56–60.

Prat, H., O. Román, and E. Pino. 1999. ["Comparative Effects of Policosanol and Two HMG-CoA Reductase Inhibitors on Type II Hypercholesterolemia"]. *Revista médica de Chile* 127(3): 286–94.

Prescott, J. H., P. Enriquez, C. Jung, E. Menz, and E. V. Groman. 1995. "Larch Arabinogalactan for Hepatic Drug Delivery: Isolation and Characterization of a 9 kDa Arabinogalactan Fragment." *Carbohydrate Research* 278(1): 113–28.

Punja, S., L. Shamseer, K. Olson, and S. Vohra. 2014. "*Rhodiola rosea* for Mental and Physical Fatigue in Nursing Students: A Randomized Controlled Trial." *PLOS One* (9): e108416. doi:10.1371/journal.pone.0108416.

Qu, D., J. Han, H. Ren, et al. 2016. "Cardioprotective Effects of Astragalin against Myocardial Ischemia/Reperfusion Injury in Isolated Rat Heart." *Oxidative Medicine andCellular Longevity* 2016:8194690. doi:10.1155/2016/8194690.

Radusiene, J., A. Judzentiene, D. Peciulyte, and V. Janulis. 2007. "Essential Oil Composition and Antimicrobial Assay of *Acorus calamus* Leaves from Different Wild Populations." *Plant Genetic Resources: Characterization and Utilization* 5(1): 37–44.

Rafat, Navid, Ali Shabestani Monfared, Maryam Shahidi, and Tayyeb Allahverdi Pourfallah. 2016. "The Modulating Effect of Royal Jelly Consumption against Radiation-Induced Apoptosis in Human Peripheral Blood Leukocytes." *Journal of Medical Physics* 41(1): 52–57. doi:10.4103/0971-6203.177281.

Rahimi, A. R., M. Emad, and G. R. Rezaian. 2008. "Smoke from Leaves of *Populus eurphratica* Olivier vs. Conventional Cryotherapy for the Treatment of Cutaneous Warts: A Pilot, Randomized, Single-Blind, Prospective Study." *International Journal of Dermatology* 47(4): 393–97.

Rahman, M. A., N. H. Kim, H. Yang, and S. O. Huh. 2012. "Angelicin Induces Apoptosis through Intrinsic Caspase-Dependent Pathway in Human SH-SY5Y Neuroblastoma Cells." *Molecular and Cellular Biochemistry* 369(1–2): 95–104.

Rajbhandari, M., R. Mentel, P. K. Jha, et al. 2009. "Antiviral Activity of Some Plants Used in Nepalese Traditional Medicine." *Evidence Based Complementary and Alternative Medicine* 6(4): 517–22.

Ramesh, B., and K. V. Pugalendi. 2006. "Antihyperglemic Effect of Umbelliferone in Streptozotocin-Diabetic Rats." *Journal of Medicinal Food* 9(4): 562–66.

Ramírez, Juan Antonio. 1998. *The Beehive Metaphor: From Gaudí to Le Corbusier*. London: Reaktion.

Ranco, F. 2007. *Muskrat Stew and Other Tales of a Penobscot Life: The Life Story of Fred Ranco*. Orono, ME: Occasional Publications of the Maine Folklife Center.

Ransome, Hilda M. 2004. *The Sacred Bee in Ancient Times and Folklore*. Mineola, NY: Dover.

Rao, Y. T., M. J. Lee, K. Chen, Y. C. Lee, W. S. Wu, and Y. M. Tzeng. 2011. "Insulin-Mimetic Action of Rhoifolin and Cosmosiin Isolated from *Citrusgrandis* (L.) Osbeck Leaves: Enhanced Adiponectin Secretion and Insulin Receptor Phosphorylation in 3T3-L1 Cells." *Evidence-Based Complementary and Alternative Medicine* 2011:624375. doi:10.1093/ecam/nep204.

Rapinski, M., L. Mussallam, J. T. Arnason, P. Haddad, and A. Cuerrier. 2015. "Adipogenic Activity of Wild Populations of *Rhododendron groenlandicum*, a Medicinal Shrub from the James Bay Cree Traditional Pharmacopeia." *Evidence-Based Complementary and Alternative Medicine* 2015: 4924–58.

Rastogi, S., M. M. Pandey, and A. Kumar Singh Rawat. 2015. "Medicinal Plants of the Genus *Betula*—Traditional Uses and a Phytochemical-Pharmacological Review." *Journal of Ethnopharmacology* 159: 62–83. doi:10.1016/j.jep.2014.11.010.

Rattanapitigorn, R., M. Arakawa, and M. Tsuro. 2006. "Vanillin Enhances the Antifungal Effect of Plant Essential Oils against *Botrytis cinerea*." *International Journal of Aromatherapy* 16(3–4): 193–98.

Rau, Henrietta A. Diers. 1968. *Nature's Aid*. New York: Pageant.

Rau, O., M. Wurglics, T. Dingerman, M. Abdel-Tawab, and M. Schubert-Zsilavecz. 2006. "Screening of Herbal Extracts for Activation of the Human Peroxisome Proliferator-Activated Receptor." *Pharmazie* 61(11): 952–56.

Razina, T. G., S. N. Udintsev, T. P. Prishchep, and K. V. Iaremenko. 1987. "Enhancement of the Selectivity of the Action of the Cytostacis Cyclophospane and 5-Fluorouracil by Using an Extract of the Baikal Scullcap in an Experiment." *Voprosy Onkologii* 33(2): 80–84.

Richardson-Boedler, C. 1998. *The Psychological/Constitutional Essences of the Bach Flower Remedies*. San Rafael CA: Kent Homeopathic Associates.

Riede, L., B. Grube, and J. Gruenwald. 2013. "Larch Arabinogalactan Effects on Reducing Incidence of Upper Respiratory Infections." *Current Medical Research Opinion* 29(3): 251–58.

Ritch-Krc, Em, N. J. Turner, and G. H. Towers. 1996. "Carrier Herbal Medicine: An Evaluation of the Antimicrobial and Anticancer Activity in Some Frequently Used Remedies." *Journal of Ethnopharmacology* 52(3): 151–56.

Róbertsdóttir, Anna Rósa. 2016. *Icelandic Herbs and Their Medicinal Uses*. Berkeley, CA: North Atlantic Books.

Rogers, Robert D. 2011. *The Fungal Pharmacy: The Complete Guide to Medicinal Mushrooms and Lichens of North America*. Berkeley, CA: North Atlantic Books.

———. 2014. *Rogers' School of Herbal Medicine: Endocrine*. Volume 7. Edmonton, Canada: Prairie Deva Press.

Rood, Stewart, and Mary Louise Polzin. 2003. "Big Old Cottonwoods." *Canadian Journal of Botany* 81(7): 764–67. doi:10.1139/b03-065.

Rose, Kiva. 2009. "A Golden Torch: Mullein's Healing Light." The Medicine Woman's Roots. November 10. http://bearmedicineherbals.com/a-golden-torch-mullein%E2%80%99s-healing-light.html.

Ryttig, K., P. V. Schlamowitz, O. Warnøe, and F. Wilstrup. 1991. "Gitadyl versus Ibuprofen in Patients with Osteoarthrosis. The Result of a Double-Blind, Randomized Cross-Over Study." *Ugeskrift for Laeger* 153(33): 2298–99.

Saltan, Gülçin, Ipek Süntar, Serkan Ozbilgin, et al. 2016. "*Viburnum opulus* L.: A Remedy for the Treatment of Endometriosis Demonstrated by Rat Model of Surgically-Induced Endometriosis." *Journal of Ethnopharmacology* 193: 450–55.

Samarghandian, S., J. T. Afhari, and S. Davoodi. 2011. "Honey Induces Apoptosis in Renal Cell Carcinoma." *Pharmacognosy Magazine* 25(7): 46–52.

Sanchez-Quesada, C., A. Lopez-Biedma, and J. J. Gaforio. 2015. "The Differential Localization of a Methyl Group Confers a Different Anti-Breast Cancer Activity to Two Triterpenes Present in Olives." *Food and Function Journal* 6(1): 249–56.

Sancho, A. I., R. Foxall, T. Browne, et al. 2006. "Effect of Postharvest Storage on the Expression of the Apple Allergin Mal d1." *Journal of Agricultural and Food Chemistry* 54(16): 5917–23.

Santana Pérez, E., M. Lugones Botell, O. Pérez Stuart, and B. Castillo Brito. 1995. ["Vaginal Parasites and Acute Cervicitis: Local Treatment with Propolis. Preliminary Report"]. *Revista Cubana de Enfermería* 11(1): 51–56.

Saracoglu, I., M. Inoue, I. Callis, and Y. Ogihara. 1995. "Studies on Constituents and Cytostatic Activity of Two Turkish Medicinal Plants, *Phlomis armeniaca* and *Scutellaria salvifolia*." *Biological and Pharmaceutical Bulletin* 18(10): 1396–400.

Sarrell, E. M., A. Mandelberg, and H. A. Cohen. 2001. "Efficacy of Naturopathic Extracts in the Management of Ear Pain Associated with Acute Otitis Media." *Archives of Pediatrics and Adolescent Medicine* 155(7): 796–99.

Sawardekar, S. B., T. C. Patel, and D. Uchil. 2016. "Comparative Evaluation of Antiplatelet Effect of Lycopene with Aspirin and the Effect of Their Combination on Platelet Aggregation: An In Vitro Study." *Indian Journal of Pharmacology* 48(1): 26–31.

Sawicka, T., J. Drozd, J. Prosinska, G. Glinkowska, J. Tautt, and H. Strzelecka. 1995. "Activities of Immunotropic Plant Extracts. III. Effect of Poplar Bud and Leaf Extract on the Maturation of Mouse Thymocytes In Vitro." *Herba Polonica* 41(4): 185–89.

Schapowal, A. 2002. "Randomized Controlled Trial of Butterbur and Cetirizine for Treating Seasonal Allergic Rhinitis." *British Medical Journal* 324(7330): 144–46.

———. 2005. "Study Group. Treating Intermittent Allergic Rhinitis: A Prospective, Randomized, Placebos and Antihistamine-Controlled Study of Butterbur Extract Ze 339." *Phytotherapy Research* 19(6): 530–37.

Schepetkin, I. A., L. N. Kirpotina, L. Jakiw, et al. 2009. "Immunomodulatory Activity of Oenothein B Isolated from *Epilobium angustifolium*." *Journal of Immunology* 183: 6754–66.

Schepetkin, I. A., A. G. Ramstead, L. N. Kirpotina, J. M. Voyich, M. A. Jutila, and M. T. Quinn. 2016. "Therapeutic Potential of Polyphenols from *Epilobium angustifolium* (Fireweed)." *Phytotherapy Research* 30(8):1287–97. doi:10.1002/ptr.5648.

Searls, Damion, ed. 2009. *The Journal of Henry David Thoreau 1837–1861*. New York: New York Review of Books.

Secme, M., C. Erogiu, Y. Dodurga, and G. Bagci. 2016. "Investigation of Anticancer Mechanism of Oleuropein via Cell Cycle and Apoptocic Pathways in SH-SY5Y Neuroblastoma Cells." *Genes* 585(1): 93–99. doi:10.1016/j.gene.2016.03.038.

Sénéchal, H., S. Geny, F. X. Desvaux, et al. 1999. "Genetics and Specific Immune Response in Allergy to Birch Pollen and Food: Evidence of a Strong, Positive Association between Atopy and the HLA Class II Allele HLA-DR7." *Journal of Allergy and Clinical Immunology* 104(2): 395–401.

Senejoux, F., C. Demougeot, M. Cuciureanu, et al. 2013. "Vasorelaxant Effects and Mechanisms of Action of *Heracleum sphondylium* L. (Apiaceae) in Rat Thoracic Aorta." *Journal of Ethnopharmacology* 147(2): 536–39.

Serkedjieva, Julia. 2000. "Combined Anti-Influenza Virus Activity of *Flos verbasci* Infusion and Amantadine Derivatives." *Phytotherapy Research* 14(7): 571–74.

Shah, A. J., and A. H. Gilani. 2010. "Bronchodilatory Effect of *Acorus calamus* (L.) Is Mediated through Multiple Pathways." *Journal of Ethnopharmacology* 131(2): 417–77.

Shang, N., J. A. Guerrero-Analco, L. Musallam, et al. 2012. "Adipogenic Constituents from the Bark of *Larix laricina* (Du Roi, K. Koch; Pinaceae), an Important Medicinal Plant Used Traditionally by the Cree of Eeyou Istchee (Quebec, Canada) for the Treatment of Type 2 Diabetes Symptoms." *Journal of Ethnopharmacology* 141(3): 1051–57. doi:10.1016/j.jep.2012.04.002.

Sheng, G. Q., J. R. Zhang, X. P. Pu, J. Ma, and C. L. Li. 2002. "Protective Effect of Verbascoside on 1-Methyl-4-Phenylpyridinium Ion-Induced Neurotoxicity in PC12 Cells." *European Journal of Pharmacology* 451(2): 119–24.

Shi, Wei, Jiagang Deng, Rongsheng Tong, et al. 2016. "Molecular Mechanisms Underlying Mangiferin-Induced Apoptosis and Cell Cycle Arrest in A549 Human Lung Carcinoma Cells." *Molecular Medicine Reports* 13(4): 3423–32.

Shi, X., G. Chen, X. Liu, et al. 2015. "Scutellarein Inhibits Cancer Cell Metastasis In Vitro and Attenuates the Development of Fibrosarcoma In Vivo." *International Journal of Molecular Medicine* 35(1): 31–38.

Shikov, A. N., G. I. Djachuk, D. V. Sergeev, et al. 2011. "Birch Bark Extract as Therapy for Chronic Hepatitis C: A Pilot Study." *Phytomedicine* 18(10): 807–10. doi:10.1016/j.phymed.2011.01.021.

Shin, K. H., S. S. Lim, and D. K. Kim. 1998. "Effect of Byakangelicin, an Aldose Reductase Inhibitor, on Galactosemic Cataracts, the Polyol Contents and Na$^{(+)}$, K$^{(+)}$ATPase Activity in Sciatic Nerves of Streptozotocin-Induced Diabetic Rats." *Phytomedicine* 5(2): 121–27.

Shin, S. C., C. Li, and J. S. Choi. 2009. "Effects of Baicalein, an Antioxidant, on the Bioavailability of Doxorubicin in Rats: Possible Role of P-glycoprotein Inhibition by Baicalein." *Pharmazie* 64(9): 579–83.

Shook, Edward E. 1978. *Advanced Treatise on Herbology*. Reprinted Mokelume Hill, CA: Health Research, 1999.

Shulgin, Alexander, and Ann Shulgin. 1991. *PiHKAL: A Chemical Love Story*. Berkeley, CA: Transform.

Silvertown, J. 2009. "A New Dawn for Citizen Science." *Trends in Ecology and Evolution* 24: 467–71.

Sipponen, A., O. Kuokkanen, R. Tihonen, H. Kauppinen, and J. J. Jokinen. 2012. "Natural Coniferous Resin Salve Used to Treat Complicated Surgical Wounds: A Pilot Clinical Trial." *International Journal of Dermatology* 51(6): 726–32.

Sipponen, A., M. Rautio, J. J. Jokinen, T. Laakso, P. Saranpaa, and J. Lohi. 2007. "Resin Salve from Norway Spruce—A Potential Method to Treat Infected Chronic Skin Ulcers?" *Drug Metabolism Letters* 1(2): 143–45.

Slanc, P., B. Doljak, S. Kreft, M. Lunder, B. Janes, and B. Strukeji. 2009. "Screening of Selected Food and Medicinal Plant Extracts for Pancreatic Lipase Inhibition." *Phytotherapy Research* 23(6): 874–77.

Smiley, S., D. Alkhani, R. Liu, et al. 2012. "In Vitro Effects of Rhaponticin from the Cree Medicinal Plant, *Larix laricina*, on the Metabolism of the Antidiabetic Drug Gliclazide." Cree Board of Health and Social Services of James Bay. Health Canada. www.creehealth.org/sites/default/files/NHPRSC-2011%20Rhaponticin.pdf.

Smith, Huron H. 1923. *Ethnobotany of the Menomini Indians*. Reprinted Westport, CT: Greenwood, 1970.

Snyder, Gary. 1974. *Turtle Island*. New York: New Directions.

Sokolnicka, I., G. Glinkowska, H. Strzelecka, et al. 1994. "Immunostimulatory Effects of Water-Soluble Extracts of Poplar Buds and Leaves and Their Polyphenolic Compounds." *International Journal of Immunotherapy* 10(2): 83–88.

Sokolov, S., L. F. Belova, A. I. Baginskaia, T. E. Leskova, and T. I. Gorodniuk. 1988. "Pharmacological Properties of the New Antiviral Preparation Alpizarin." *Farmakol Toksikol* 51(4): 93–96.

Soleimani, A., J. Asadi, F. Rostami-Charati, and R. Gharaei. 2015. "High Cytotoxicity and Apoptotic Effects of Natural Bioactive Benzofuran Derivative on the MCF-7 Breast Cancer Cell Line." *Combinatorial Chemistry and High Throughput Screening* 18(5): 505–13.

Song, D. K., J. Y. Kim, G. Li, et al. 2005. "Agents Protecting against Sepsis from the Roots of *Angelica dahurica*." *Biological and Pharmacology Bulletin* 28(2): 380–82.

Song, X., J. He, H. Xu, et al. 2016. "The Antiviral Effects of Acteoside and the Underlying IFN-Y-Inducing Action." *Food and Function* 2016(7): 3017–30. doi:10.1039/C6FO00335D.

Song, Y. S., C. Jin, K. J. Jung, and E. H. Park. 2002. "Estrogenic Effects of Ethanol and Ether Extracts of Propolis." *Journal of Ethnopharmacology* 82(2–3): 89–95.

Song, Y. Y., Y. Li, and H. Q. Zhang. 2010. "Therapeutic Effect of Syringin on Adjuvant Arthritis in Rats and Its Mechanism." *Yao Xue Xue Bao (ActaPharmaceutica Sinica)* 45(8): 1006–11.

Spasov, A. A., G. K. Wikman, V. B. Mandrikov, I. A. Mironova, and V. V. Neumoin. 2000. "A Double-Blind, Placebo-Controlled Pilot Study of the Stimulating and Adaptogenic Effect of *Rhodiola rosea* SHR-5 Extract on the Fatigue of Students Caused by Stress During an Examination Period with a Repeated Low-Dose Regimen." *Phytomedicine* 7(2): 85–89.

Spoor, D. C. A., L. C. Martineau, C. Leduc, et al. 2006. "Selected Plant Species from the Cree Pharmacopoeia of Northern Quebec Possess Anti-Diabetic Potential." *Canadian Journal of Physiology and Pharmacology* 84(8–9): 847–58.

Staneva, J., M. Todorova, N. Neykov, and L. Evstatieva. 2009. "Ultrasonically Assisted Extraction of Total Phenols and Flavonoids from *Rhodiola rosea*." *Natural Product Communications* 4(7): 935–38.

Steiner, Rudolf. 1933. *Nine Lectures on Bees Given in 1923 to the Workmen at the Goetheanum*. Bray, UK: Anthroposophical Agricultural Foundation.

Steinmetz, E. F. 1954. *Materia Medica Vegetabilis*. Amsterdam: Steinmetz.

Stolarczyk, M., M. Naruszewicz, and A. K. Kiss. 2013. "Extracts from *Epilobium* sp. Herbs Induce Apoptosis in Human Hormone-Dependent Prostate Cancer Cells by Activating the Mitochondrial Pathway." *Journal of Pharmacy and Pharmacology* 65: 1044–54.

Storm, Hyemeyohsts. 1972. *Seven Arrows*. New York: Ballantine.

Su, Q., W. Tao, H. Wang, Y. Chen, H. Huang, and G. Chen. 2016. "Umbelliferone Attenuates Unpredictable Chronic Mild Stress-Induced Insulin Resistance in Rats." *International Union of Biochemistry and Molecular Biology LIFE* 68(5): 329–409. doi:10.1002/iub.1496.

Subrahmanyam, M. 1991. "Topical Application of Honey in Treatment of Burns." *British Journal of Surgery* 76(4): 497–98.

Sumiyoshi, M., M. Sakanaka, M. Taniguchi, K. Baba, and Y.Kimura. 2014. "Antitumor Effects of Various Furanocoumarins Isolated from the Roots, Seeds, and Fruits of *Angelica* And *Cnidum* Species under Ultraviolet A Irradiation." *Journal of Natural Medicine* 68(1): 83–94.

Sun, K., X. H. Tang, and Y. K. Xie. 2015. "Paclitaxel Combined with Harmine Inhibits the Migration and Invasion of Gastric Cancer Cells through Down-Regulation of Cyclooxygenase-2 Expression." *Oncology Letters* 10(3): 1649–54.

Suzuki, A., K. Matsunaga, Y Mimaki, Y. Sashida, and Y. Ohizumi. 1999. "Properties of Amentoflavone, a Potent Caffeine-Like Ca^{2+} Releaser in Skeletal Muscle Sarcoplasmic Reticulum." *European Journal of Pharmacology* 372(1): 97–102.

Swanton, J. R. 1905. *Haida Texts and Myths*. Smithsonian Institute Bulletin 29. Washington, DC: Bureau of American Ethnology.

Szczeklik, Andrzej, Adam Zagajewski, John Martin, and Antonia Lloyd-Jones. 2012. *Kore: On Sickness, the Sick, and the Search for the Soul of Medicine*. Berkeley, CA: Counterpoint.

Szott-Rogers, Laurie. 2004. *The Path of the Devas*. Edmonton, Canada: Prairie Deva Press.

Szwajgier, D. 2015. "Anticholinesterase Activity of Selected Phenolic Acids and Flavonoids— Interaction Testing in Model Solutions." *Annals of Agricultural and Environmental Medicine* 22(4): 690–94.

Takaki-Doi, S., K. Hashimoto, M. Yamamura, and C. Kamei. 2009. "Antihypertensive Activities of Royal Jelly Protein Hydrolysate and Its Fractions in Spontaneously Hypertensive Rats." *Acta Medica Okayama* 63(1): 57–64.

Takeda, T., M. Tsubaki, T. Kino, et al. 2016. "Mangiferin Enhances the Sensitivity of Human Multiple Myeloma Cells to Anticancer Drugs through Suppression of the Nuclear Factor kappa-B Pathway." *International Journal of Oncology* 48(6):2704-12. doi:10.3892/ijo.2016.3470.

Tang, J. J., J. G. Li, W. Qi, et al. 2011. "Inhibition of SREBP by a Small Molecule, Betulin, Improves Hyperlipidemia and Insulin Resistance and Reduces Atherosclerotic Plaques." *Cell Metabolism* 13(1): 44–56.

Tao, Y. H., D. Y. Jiang, H. B. Xu, and X. L. Yang. 2008. "Inhibitory Effect of *Erigeron breviscapus* Extract and Its Flavonoid Components on GABA Shunt Enzymes." *Phytomedicine* 15(1–2): 92–97.

Tarragó, T., N. Kichik, B. Classen, R. Prades, M.Teixidó, and E. Girait. 2008. "Baicalin, a Prodrug Able to Reach the CNS, Is a Prolyl Oligopeptidase Inhibitor." *Bioorganic and Medicinal Chemistry* 16(15): 7516–24.

Tavares, D. C., W. M. Lira, C. B. Santini, C. S. Takahashi, and J. K. Bastos. 2007. "Effects of Propolis Crude Hydroalcoholic Extract on Chromosomal Aberrations Induced by Doxorubicin in Rats." *Planta Medica* 73(15): 1531–36.

Tedlock, Barbara. 2005. *The Woman in the Shaman's Body: Reclaiming the Feminine in Religion and Medicine*. New York: Bantam.

Teit, James A. 1912. *Mythology of the Thompson Indians*. Edited by Franz Boas. New York: G. E. Stechert.

Tendland, Y., S. Pellerin, P. Haddad, and A. Cuerrier. 2012. "Impacts of Experimental Leaf Harvesting on a North American Medicinal Shrub, *Rhododendron groenlandicum*." *Botany* 90(3): 347–51.

Thien, F. C., R. Leung, B. A. Baldo, J. A. Weiner, R. Plomley, and D. Czarny. 1996. "Asthma and Anaphylaxis Induced by Royal Jelly." *Clinical and Experimental Allergy* 26(2): 216–22.

Thirupathi, A., P. C. Silveira, R. T. Nesi, and R. A. Pinho. 2016. "Beta-Amyrin, a Pentacyclic Triterpene, Exhibits Anti-Fibrotic, Anti-Inflammatory, and Anti-Apoptotic Effect on Dimethyl Nitrosamine-Induced Hepatic Fibrosis in Male Rats." *Human and Experimental Toxicology* March 2016. doi:10.1177/0960327116638727.

Thoreau, Henry David. 1848. "Ktaadn, and the Maine Woods." *Union Magazine of Literature and Art* 3(1).

Thoreau, Henry David, Bradford Torrey, and Franklin Benjamin Sanborn. 1906. *The Writings of Henry David Thoreau*. Volume 16. Boston: Houghton, Mifflin.

Throop, Priscilla. 1998. *Hildegard von Bingen's Physica: The Complete English Translation of Her Classic Work on Health and Healing*. Rochester, VT: Healing Arts.

Thu, O. K., O. Spigset, O. G. Nilsen, and B. Hellum. 2016. "Effect of Commercial *Rhodiola rosea* on CYP Enzyme Activity in Humans." *European Journal of Clinical Pharmacology* 72(3): 295–300.

Tkachenko, K. G. 2006. "Antiviral Activity of the Essential Oils of Some *Heracleum* L. Species." *Journal of Herbs, Spices and Medicinal Plants* 12(3): 1–12.

———. 2009. "Essential Oils from Roots of Certain *Heracleum* Species." *Chemistry of Natural Compounds* 45(4): 578–81.

Tracz, Orysiz. 2001. "The Things We Do … The *Kalyna* in Ukrainian Folk Medicine and Folklore." *The Ukrainian Weekly*. June 3.

Treadwell, E. M., and T. P. Clausen. 2008. "Is *Hedysarum mackenzii* (Wild Sweet Pea) Actually Toxic?" *Ethnobotany Research and Applications* 6: 319–21.

Treben, M. 1982. *Health through God's Pharmacy*. Steyr, Austria: Wilhelm Ennsthaler.

Treshow, M., and K. Harper. 1974. "Longevity of Perennial Forbs and Grasses." *Oikos* 25(1): 93–96.

Tressider, Jack. 2000. *Symbols and Their Meanings*. New York: Friedman/Fairfax.

Tuglu, D., E. Yilmaz, E. Yuvanc, et al. 2014. "*Viburnum opulus*: Could It Be a New Alternative, Such as Lemon Juice, to Pharmacological Therapy in Hypocitraturic Stone Patients?" *Archivio Italiano di Urologia e Andrologia* 86(4): 297–99.

Turker, A. U., and N. D. Camper. 2002. "Biological Activity of Common Mullein, a Medicinal Plant." *Journal of Ethnopharmacology* 82(2-3): 117–25.

Turner, Nancy J. 2014. *Ancient Pathways, Ancestral Knowledge*. Volume 2. Montreal: McGill-Queen's University Press.

Turner, Nancy J., and Barbara S. Efrat. 1982. *Ethnobotany of the Hesquiat Indians of Vancouver Island. Culture Recovery Report*. No. 2. Victoria, Canada: British Columbia Provincial Museum.

Udani, J. K., B. B. Singh, M. Barrett, and V. J. Singh. 2010. "Proprietary Arabinogalactan Extract Increases Antibody Response to the Pneumonia Vaccine: A Randomized, Double-Blind, Placebo-Controlled, Pilot Study on Healthy Volunteers." *Nutrition Journal* 9(32).

Uhari, Matti, T. Tapianen, and T. Kontiokari. 2000. "Xylitol in Preventing Acute Otitis Media." *Vaccine* 19(suppl. 1): S144–47.

Ulger, H., T. Ertekin, O. Karaca, et al. 2013. "Influence of *Gilaburu* (*Viburnum opulus*) Juice on 1,2-Dimethylhydrazine (DMH)-Induced Colon Cancer." *Toxicology and Industrial Health* 29(9): 824–29.

Urban, N., L. Wang, S. Kwiek, J. Rademann, W. M. Kuebler, and M. Schaefer. 2016. "Identification and Validation of Larixyl Acetate as a Potent TRPC6 Inhibitor." *Molecular Pharmacology* 89(1): 197–213.

Usow, Nach. 1958. "Normalisiert die Tinktur Schnell den Blutdruck, Dieso Rk. Halt bei den Versuchsstieren (Hunden) Langero Zeit an.—Baicalin und Wogonin Sollen Diuretisch Wirken." *Farmakologija i Toxikologija* 21(2): 31–34.

Utterback, G., R. Zackarias, S. Timraz, and D. Mershman. 2014. "Butterbur Extract: Prophylactic Treatment for Childhood Migraines." *Complementary Therapies in Clinical Practice* 20(1): 61–64.

Vandal, J., M. M. Abou-Zaid, G. Ferroni, and L. G. Leduc. 2015. "Antimicrobial Activity of Natural Products from the Flora of Northern Ontario, Canada." *Pharmaceutical Biology* 53(6): 800–6.

Van Deusen, Kira. 2009. *Kiviuq: An Inuit Hero and His Siberian Cousins.* Montreal: McGill-Queen's University Press.

Van Dierman, Daphne, A. Marston, J. Bravo, M. Reist, P. A. Carrupt, and K. Hostettmann. 2009. "Monoamine Oxidase Inhibition by *Rhodiola rosea* L. Roots." *Journal of Ethnopharmacology* 122(2): 397–401.

Vanharanta, M., S. Voutilainen, T. H. Rissanen, H. Adlercreutz, and J. T. Salonen. 2003. "Risk of Cardiovascular Disease-Related and All-Cause Death According to Serum Concentrations of Enterolactone: Kuopio Ischaemic Heart Disease Risk Factor Study." *Archives of Internal Medicine* 163(9): 1099–1104.

Van Hoof, L., J. Totte, J. Corthout, et al. 1989. "Plant Antiviral Agents VI. Isolation of Antiviral Phenolic Glucosides from Populus Cultivar Beaupre by Droplet Counter-Current Chromatography." *Journal of Natural Products* 52(4): 875–78.

Vareed, S. K., M. K. Reddy, R. E. Schutzki, and M. G. Nair. 2006. "Anthocyanins in *Cornus alternifolia, Cornus controversa, Cornus kousa,* and *Cornus florida* Fruits with Health Benefits." *Life Sciences* 78(7): 777–84.

Vareed, S. K., R. E. Schutzki, and M. G. Nair. 2007. "Lipid Peroxidation, Cyclooxygenase Enzyme and Tumor Cell Proliferatory Inhibitory Compounds in *Cornus kousa* Fruits." *Phytomedicine* 14(10): 706–9.

Vermeulen, Frans, and Linda Johnston. 2011. *Plants: Homeopathic and Medicinal Uses from a Botanical Family Perspective.* Glasgow, Scotland: Saltire.

Villar, I. C., R. Jiménez, M. Galisteo, M. F. Garcia-Suara, A. Zarzuelo, and J. Duarte. 2002. "Effects of Chronic Chrysin Treatment in Spontaneously Hypertensive Rats." *Planta Medica* 68(9): 847–50.

Vlad, L., A. Munta, and I. G. Crisan. 1977. "Digitalis Like Cardiotonic Action of *Viburnum* spp. Extracts." *Planta Medica* 31(3): 228–31.

Vogel, A. 1986. *Nature: Your Guide to Healthy Living.* Teufen, Switzerland: A. Vogel.

Vunduk, Jovana, Anita Klaus, Maja Kozarski, et al. 2015. "Did the Iceman Know Better? Screening of the Medicinal Properties of the Birch Polypore Medicinal Mushroom, *Piptoporus betulinus* (Higher Basidiomycetes)." *International Journal of Medicinal Mushrooms* 17(12): 1113–25.

Vyas, A., K. Syeda, A. Ahmad, S. Padhye, and F. H. Sarkar. 2012. "Perspectives on Medicinal Properties of Mangiferin." *Mini Reviews in Medicinal Chemistry* 12(5): 412–25.

Vynograd, N., I. Vynograd, and Z. Sosnowski. 2000. "A Comparative Multi-Centre Study of the Efficacy of Propolis, Acyclovir and Placebo in the Treatment of Genital Herpes (HSV)." *Phytomedicine* 7(1): 1–6.

Wagner, H., M. Wierer, and R. Bauer. 1986. "In Vitro Inhibition of Prostaglandin Biosynthesis by Essential Oils and Phenolic Compounds." *Planta Medica* 3: 184–87.

Walker, Barbara G. 1988. *The Woman's Dictionary of Symbols and Sacred Objects*. San Francisco: HarperSanFrancisco.

Wang, C. C., J. E. Lai, L. G. Chen, K. Y. Yen, and L. L. Yang. 2000. "Inducible Nitric Oxide Synthase Inhibitors of Chinese Herbs. Part 2: Naturally Occurring Furanocoumarins." *Bioorganic and Medicinal Chemistry* 8(12): 2701–7.

Wang, G. J., Y. L. Lin, C. H. Chen, X. C. Wu, J. F. Liao, and J. Ren. 2010. "Cellular Calcium Regulatory Machinery of Vasorelaxation Elicited by Petasin." *Clinical and Experimental Pharmacology and Physiology* 37(3): 309–15.

Wang, H., Y. Ding, J. Zhou, X. Sun, and S. Wang. 2009. "The In Vitro and In Vivo Antiviral Effects of Salidroside from *Rhodiola rosea* L. against Coxsackievirus B3." *Phytomedicine* 16(2–3): 146–55.

Wang, J., Y. Cui, W. Feng, et al. 2014. "Involvement of the Central Monoaminergic System in the Antidepressant-Like Effect of Catapol in Mice." *Bioscience Trends* 8(5): 248–52.

Wang, J., Q. Li, G. Ivanochko, and Y. Huang. 2006. "Anticancer Effect of Extracts from a North American Medicinal Plant—Wild Sarsaparilla." *Anticancer Research* 26(3A): 2157–64.

Wang, J., S. Li, Q. Wang, B. Xin, and H. Wang. 2007. "Trophic Effect of Bee Pollen on Small Intestine in Broiler Chickens." *Journal of Medicinal Food* 10(2): 276–80.doi:10.1089/jmf.2006.215.

Wang, Junfeng, Rui Lu, Jian Yang, et al. 2015. "TRPC6 Specifically Interacts with APP to Inhibit Its Cleavage by Y-Secretase and Reduce AB Production." *Nature Communications* 6:8876. doi:10.1038/ncomms9876.

Wang, Peng, Juan-Carlos Alvarez-Perez, Dan P. Felsenfeld, et al. 2015. "A High-Throughput Chemical Screen Reveals that Harmine-Mediated Inhibition of DYRK1A Increases Human Pancreatic Beta Cell Replication." *Nature Medicine* 21(4): 383–88.

Wang, Qian, Yu-Tian Wang, Shao-Ping Pu, and Y. T. Zheng. 2004. "Zinc Coupling Potentiates Anti-HIV-1 Activity of Baicalin." *Biochemistry Biophysics Research Communication* 324: 605–10.

Wang, W. W., L. Lu, T. H. Bao, et al. 2016. "Scutellarin Alleviates Behavioral Deficits in a Mouse Model of Multiple Sclerosis, Possibly through Protecting Neural Stem Cells." *Journal of Molecular Neuroscience* 58(2): 210–20.

Wang, Xue, Haribalan Perumalsamy, Hyung-Wook Kwon, Young-Eun Na, and Young-Jun Ahn. 2015. "Effects and Possible Mechanisms of Action of Acacetin on the Behavior and Eye Morphology of *Drosophila* Models of Alzheimer's Disease." *Scientific Reports* 2015(5): 1612–17.

Wardecki, T., P. Werner, M. Thomas, et al. 2016. "Influence of Birch Bark Triterpenes on Keratinocytes and Fibroblasts from Diabetic and Nondiabetic Donors." *Journal of Natural Products* 79(4): 1112–23.

Webster, D., T. D. Lee, J. Moore, et al. 2010. "Antimycobacterial Screening of Traditional Medicinal Plants Using the Microplate Resazurin Assay." *Canadian Journal of Microbiology* 56(6): 487–94.

Webster, D., P. Taschereau, T. D. Lee, and T. Jurgens. 2006. "Immunostimulant Properties of *Heracleum maximum* Bartr." *Journal of Ethnopharmacology* 106(3): 360–63.

Weiss, Rudolf Fritz. 1988. *Herbal Medicine*. Beaconsfield, UK: Beaconsfield.

Wildi, E., T. Langer, W. Schaffner, and K. B. Büter. 1998. "Quantitative Analysis of Petasin and Pyrrolizidine Alkaloids in Leaves and Rhizomes of in Situ-Grown *Petasites hybridus* Plants." *Planta Medica* 64(3): 264–67.

Williamson, Darcy. 2011. *130 Medicinal Plant Monographs of the Northwest*. McCall, ID: From the Forest.

Wolfman, C., H. Viola, A. Paladini, F. Dajas, and J. H. Medina. 1994. "Possible Anxiolytic Effects of Chrysin, a Central Benzodiazepine Receptor Ligand Isolated from *Passiflora coerulea*." *Pharmacology Biochemistry and Behavior* 47(1): 1–4.

Wolfson, P., and D. L. Hoffmann. 2003. "An Investigation into the Efficacy of *Scutellaria lateriflora* in Healthy Volunteers." *Alternative Therapies in Health and Medicine* 9(2): 74–78.

Wood, Matthew. 1997. *The Book of Herbal Wisdom*. Berkeley, CA: North Atlantic Books.

———. 2008. *The Earthwise Herbal: A Complete Guide to Old World Medicinal Plants*. Berkeley, CA: North Atlantic Books.

———. 2009. *The Earthwise Herbal: A Complete Guide to New World Medicinal Plants*. Berkeley, CA: North Atlantic Books.

Wu, H. S., D. F. Zhu, C. X. Zhou, C. R. Feng, Y. J. Lou, and Q. J. He. 2009. "Insulin Sensitizing Activity of Ethyl Acetate Fraction of *Acorus calamus* L. In Vitro and In Vivo." *Journal of Ethnopharmacology* 123(2): 288–92.

Wu, Hao-Shu, Ying-Yin Li, Lin-Jia Weng, Chang-Xin Zhou, Qiao-Jun He, and Yi-Jia Lou. 2007. "A Fraction of *Acorus calamus* L. Extract Devoid of beta-Asarone Enhances Adipocyte Differentiation in 3T3-L1 Cells." *Phytotherapy Research* 21(6): 562–64. doi:10.1002/ptr.2112.

Wu, X., B. Zhao, Y. Cheng, et al. 2015. "Melittin Induces PTCH1 Expression by Down-Regulating MeCP2 in Human Hepatocellular Carcinoma SMMC-7721 Cells." *Toxicology and Applied Pharmacology* 288(1): 74–83. doi:10.1016/j.taap.2015.07.010.

Wu, Y. D., and Y. J. Lou. 2007. "Brassinolide, a Plant Sterol from Pollen of *Brassica napus* L., Induces Apoptosis in Human Prostate Cancer PC-3 Cells." *Pharmazie* 62(5): 392–95.

Wu, Y. X., and X. Fang. 2010. "Apigenin, Chrysin and Luteolin Selectively Inhibit Chymotrypsin-Like and Trypsin-Like Proteasome Catalytic Activities in Tumor Cells." *Planta Medica* 76(2): 128–32.

Wulff, Mary, and Gregory L. Tilford. 2009. *Herbs for Pets: The Natural Way to Enhance Your Pet's Life.* Irvine, CA: i5 Press.

Xiao, Pei-Gen, and Ke-Ji Chen. 1987. "Recent Advances in Clinical Studies of Chinese Medicinal Herbs 1. Drugs Affecting the Cardiovascular System." *Phytotherapy Research* 1(2): 53–57.

Xu, Y., Y. Xu, H. Luan, Y. Jiang, X. Tian, and S. Zhang. 2016. "Cardioprotection against Experimental Myocardial Ischemic Injury Using Cornin." *Brazilian Journal of Medical and Biological Research* 49(2): e5039.

Yamamoto, M. 2006. ["Yamamoto and Dung Vanilla."] [*Japan Probe Aroma Research*] 7: 258–80.

Yan, Q. 2010. "Chinese Medicine for Drug Addiction Treatment and the Preparation Method." *Faming ZhuanliShenqing* CN 101703647 A 20100512.

Yang, E. J., S. I. Kim, H. Y. Ku, et al. 2010. "Syringin from Stem Bark of *Fraxinus rhynchophylla* Protects A-beta$_{(25-35)}$–Induced Toxicity in Neuronal Cells." *Archives of Pharmaceutical Research* 33(4): 531–38.

Yang, L. L., Y. C. Lang, C. W. Chang, et al. 2002. "Effects of Sphondin, Isolated from Heracleum Laciniatum On IL-1-beta–Induced Cyclooxygenase-2 Expression in Human Pulmonary Epithelial Cells." *Life Sciences* 72(2): 199–213.

Yang, X. W., B. Xu, F. X. Ran, R. Q. Wang, J. Wu, and J. R. Cui. 2007. Inhibitory Effects of 11 Coumarin Compounds against Growth of Human Bladder Carcinoma Cell Line E-J In Vitro. *Zhong Xi Yi Jie He Xue Bao* 5(1): 56–60.

Yano, S., H. Tachibana, and K. Yamada. 2005. "Flavones Suppress the Expression of the High-Affinity IgE Receptor Fc-epsilon-R1 in Human Basophilic KU812 Cells." *Journal of Agriculture Food Chemistry* 53(5): 1812–17.

Yin, D., W. Yao, S. Chen, R. Hu, and X. Gao. 2009. "Salidroside, the Main Active Compound of *Rhodiola* Plants, Inhibits High Glucose-Induced Mesangial Cell Proliferation." *Planta Medica* 75(11): 1191–95.

Yoshida, T., H. Ito, T. Hatano, et al. 1996. "New Hydrolysable Tannins, Shephagenins A and B, from *Shepherdia argentea* as HIV-1 Reverse Transcriptase Inhibitors." *Chemical & Pharmaceutical Bulletin* 44: 1436–39.

Yoshimi, N., K. Matsunaga, M. Katayama, et al.. 2001. "The Inhibitory Effects of Mangiferin, a Naturally Occurring Glucosylxanthone, in Bowel Carcinogenesis of Male F344 Rats." *Cancer Letters* 163(2): 163–70.

You, S. P., L. Ma, J. Zhao, S. L. Zhang, and T. Liu. 2016. "Phenylethanol Glycosides from *Cistanche tubulosa* Suppress Hepatic Stellate Cell Activation and Block the Conduction of Signaling Pathways in TGF-beta/smad as Potential Anti-Hepatic Fibrosis Agents." *Molecules* 21(1).

Young, David, Grant Ingram, and Lise Swartz. 1989. *Cry of the Eagle: Encounters with a Cree Healer.* Toronto: University of Toronto Press.

Young, David, Robert Rogers, and Russell Willier. 2015. *A Cree Healer and His Medicine Bundle: Revelations of Indigenous Wisdom.* Berkeley, CA: North Atlantic Books.

Young, Jane, and Alex Hawley. 2004. *Plants and Medicines of Sophie Thomas: Based on the Traditional Knowledge of Sophie Thomas, Saik'uzElder and Healer.* Second Edition. Prince George, Canada: University of Northern British Columbia.

Zakharov, N. A., N. M. Pridantseva, A. A. Khokhlova and V. G.Nikolaeva. 1980. "Use of a Tincture of Birch Buds for Treating Suppurative Wounds." *Vestnik Khirurgii Imemi I. I. Grekova* 124(1): 82–85.

Zaklos-Szyda, M., I. Majewska, M. Redzynia, and M. Koziolkiewicz. 2015. "Antidiabetic Effect of Polyphenol Extracts from Selected Edible Plants as alpha-Amylase, alpha-Glucosidase, and PTP1B Inhibitors, and Beta Pancreatic Cells Cytoprotective Agents—a Comparative Study." *Current Topics in Medicinal Chemistry* 15(23): 2431–44.

Zanoli, P., R. Avallone, and M. Baraldi. 2000. "Behavioral Characterization of the Flavonoids Apigenin and Chrysin." *Fitoterapia* 71(suppl. 1): 117–23.

Zaugg, J., E. Eickmeier, S. N. Ebrahimi, I. Baburin, S. Hering, and M. Hamburger. 2011. "Positive GABA(A) Receptor Modulators from *Acorus calamus* and Structural Analysis of (+)-Dioxosarcoguaiacol by 1D and 2D NMR and Molecular Modeling." *Journal of Natural Products* 74(6): 1437–43.

Zeldin, Theodore. 2012. *An Intimate History of Humanity*. New York: Random House.

Zeng, H., P. Huang, X. Wang, J. Wu, M. Wu, and J. Huang. 2015. "Galangin-Induced Down-Regulation of BACE1 by Epigenetic Mechanisms in SH-SY5Y Cells." *Neuroscience* 294: 172–81.

Zgórniak-Nowosielska, I., J. Grzybek, N. Manolova, J. Serkedjieva, and B. Zawilińska.1991. "Antiviral Activity of Flos Verbasci Infusion against Influenza and Herpes Simplex Viruses." *Archivum immunologiae et therapiae experimentalis* (Warsaw) 39(1–2): 103–8.

Zgrajka, W., M. Turska, G. Rajtar, M. Majdan, and J. Parada-Turska. 2013. "Kynurenic Acid Content in Antirheumatic Herbs." *Annals of Agricultural and Environmental Medicine* 20(4): 800–2.

Zhang, F., Z. Jia, Z. Y. Deng, Y. Wei, R. Zheng, and L. J. Yu. 2002. "In Vitro Modulation of Telomerase Activity, Telomere Length, and Cell Cycle in MKN45 Cells by Verbascoside." *Planta Medica* 68(2): 115–18.

Zhang, Q., X. H. Zhao, and Z. J. Wang. 2008. "Flavones and Flavonols Exert Cytotoxic Effects on a Human Esophageal Adenocarcinoma Cell Line (OE33) by Causing G2/M Arrest and Inducing Apoptosis." *Food and Chemical Toxicology* 46(6): 2042–53.

Zhang, Z., X. Y. Lian, S.Li, and J. L. Stringer. 2009."Characterization of Chemical Ingredients and Anticonvulsant Activity of American Scullcap (*Scutellaria lateriflora*)." *Phytomedicine* 16(5): 485–93.

Zhao, G., A. Shi, Z. Fan, and Y. Du. 2015. "Salidroside Inhibits the Growth of Human Breast Cancer In Vitro and In Vivo." *Oncology Report* 33(5): 2553–60.

Zhao, J., A. K. Dasmahapatra, S. I. Khan, and I. A. Khan. 2008. "Anti-Aromatase Activity of the Constituents from Damiana (*Turnera diffusa*)." *Journal of Ethnopharmacology* 120(3): 387–93.

Zhao, X.,H. Li, J. Wang, Y. Guo, B. Liu, X. Deng, and X. Niu. 2016. "Verbascoside Alleviates Pneumococcal Pneumonia by Reducing Pneumolysin Oligomers." *Molecular Pharmacology* 89(3): 376–87.

Zhao, Y. L., S. F. Wang, Y. Li, Q. X. He, K. C. Liu, Y. P. Yang, and X. L. Li. 2011. "Isolation of Chemical Constituents from the Aerial Parts of *Verbascum thapsus* and Their Antiangiogenic and Antiproliferative Activities." *Archives of Pharmacological Research* 34(5): 703–7.

Zheng, M. S., and Z. Y. Lu. 1989. ["Antiviral Effect of Mangiferin and Isomangiferin on Herpes Simplex Virus"]. *Zhongguo Yao Li Xue Bao (Acta Pharmacologica Sinica)* 10(1): 85–90.

Zheng, R. L., P. F. Wang, J. Li, Z. M. Liu, and Z. J. Jia. 1993. "Inhibition of the Autoxidation of Linoleic Acid by Phenylpropanoid Glycosides from *Pedicularis* in Micelles." *Chemistry and Physics in Lipids* 65(2): 151–54.

Zheng, Y. M., A. X. Lu, J. Z. Shen, A. H. Kwok, and W. S. Ho. 2016. "Imperatorin Exhibits Anticancer Activities in Human Colon Cancer Cells via the Caspase Cascade." *Oncology Reports* 35(4):1995–2002. doi:10.3892/or.2016.4586.

Zhou, Z., N. Han, Z. Liu, Z. Song, P. Wu, J. Shao, J. M. Zhang, and J. Yin. 2016. "The Antibacterial Activity of Syringopicroside, Its Metabolites, and Natural Analogues from Syringae Folium." *Fitoterapia* 110: 20–25.

Zhu, Judy T. T., Roy C. Y. Choi, Jun Li, Heidi Q. H. Xie, Cathy W. C. Bi, et al. 2009. "Estrogenic and Neuroprotective Properties of Scutellarin from Erigeron Breviscapus: A Drug against Postmenopausal Symptoms and Alzheimer's Disease." *Planta Medica* 75(4): 1489–93.

Zubeldia, J. M., H. A. Nabi, M. Jiménez del Rio, and J. Genovese. 2010. "Exploring New Applications for *Rhodiola rosea*: Can We Improve the Quality of Life of Patients with Short-Term Hypothyroidism Induced by Hormone Withdrawal?" *Journal of Medicinal Food* 13(6): 287–92. doi:10.1089/jmf.2009.028.

Index

About the Author

ROBERT DALE ROGERS has been an herbalist for over forty-five years, specializing in the plants and mushrooms of the boreal forest. He has a bachelor of science in botany and spent eighteen years in clinical practice. Robert is the author of over forty books and teaches earth spirit medicine at the Northern Star College in Edmonton, Alberta, Canada. Robert is a long-standing professional member of the American Herbalist Guild and an assistant clinical professor in family medicine at the University of Alberta, his alma mater.

Robert conducts plant and mushroom walks throughout North America and writes occasionally for the magazine *Fungi* and the *Journal of the American Herbalists Guild*. Some of his peer-reviewed papers can be read or downloaded at www.academia.edu/robertdalerogers. He lives in Edmonton with his beautiful and talented wife, Laurie, and out-of-control cat, Ceres. In 2015 he was honored an Herbal Elder of Canada by the Canadian Council of Herbal Associations. You may contact the author by emailing scents@telusplanet.net.

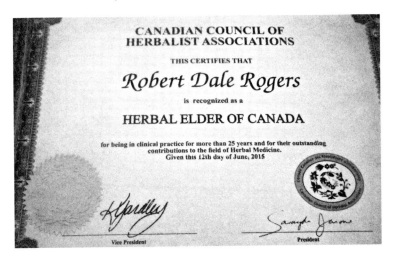

About North Atlantic Books

North Atlantic Books (NAB) is an independent, nonprofit publisher committed to a bold exploration of the relationships between mind, body, spirit, and nature. Founded in 1974, NAB aims to nurture a holistic view of the arts, sciences, humanities, and healing. To make a donation or to learn more about our books, authors, events, and newsletter, please visit www.northatlanticbooks.com.

For more information on books, authors, events, and to sign up for our newsletter, please visit www.northatlanticbooks.com.

North Atlantic Books is the publishing arm of the Society for the Study of Native Arts and Sciences, a 501(c)(3) nonprofit educational organization that promotes cross-cultural perspectives linking scientific, social, and artistic fields. To learn how you can support us, please visit our website.